Continuous Glucose Monitoring

Weiping Jia
Editor

Continuous Glucose Monitoring

SSTP

Springer

Editor
Weiping Jia
Department of Endocrinology and Metabolism
Shanghai Clinical Center for Diabetes
Shanghai Diabetes Institute
Shanghai Jiao Tong University Affiliated Sixth People's Hospital
Shanghai
China

ISBN 978-981-10-7073-0 ISBN 978-981-10-7074-7 (eBook)
https://doi.org/10.1007/978-981-10-7074-7

Library of Congress Control Number: 2018945466

Printed on acid-free paper

This Springer imprint is published by the registered company Springer Nature Singapore Pte Ltd.
The registered company address is: 152 Beach Road, #21-01/04 Gateway East, Singapore 189721, Singapore

Foreword 1

Since Banting and Best won the Nobel Prize for their discovery of insulin, there have been many small, iterative advances in diabetes management. However, there have been only a few major breakthroughs that have revolutionized our ability to better control glucose over that same period of time. One of those is continuous glucose monitoring (CGM). Whether used in masked (professional) or real-time (personal) mode, CGM permits the healthcare professional and patient to understand the relationship among the three key elements of metabolic control, i.e., behavior (meals, exercise, stress, etc.), medication (injectable or oral), and glucose levels, in ways not possible with meter-based blood glucose monitoring. CGM is both an educational tool for the patient and healthcare provider (HCP) and a management tool for the HCP regardless of whether the patient has type 1 or type 2 diabetes.

Numerous studies have shown that masked (professional) CGM—essentially a Holter monitor for glucose—adds significant value in the management in both type 1 and type 2 diabetes regardless of whether or not the patient is taking insulin. In addition, it is critical in evaluating the efficacy and safety of not only new pharmaceuticals but also psycho-educational interventions. By the data being masked from the patient the true, real-world effect of the intervention can be determined. Real-time (personal) CGM provides significant information to the patient whether they are receiving insulin by injection or pump. It also has been shown to benefit those with type 2 diabetes not on insulin where it acts as a behavior modification tool.

The future of CGM is discussed in the last chapter. I foresee four major directions in CGM use:

1. CGM will be a bridge to an era when we will use actual glucose metrics (mean, standard deviation, severity of hypo- and hyperglycemia, and times-in-ranges) rather than a surrogate marker (A1C) to evaluate diabetes control. It is well known that there are many problems with using A1C, not the least of which is that there is a wide range of mean blood glucose for a given A1C, e.g., for an A1C of 8% the mean can be from 120 to 200 mg/dL (6.7-11.1 mmol/L) because of different glycation rates, red cell turnover, and other as yet undefined genetic factors. While A1C will remain a touchstone for our understanding of how it correlates with diabetes complications, CGM-derived metrics will permit healthcare providers to make changes between the typical quarterly A1C determination.

2. There will continue to be iterative improvements in CGM accuracy, longevity, and footprint with the use of optical, fluorescence, and hydrogel technologies that permit miniaturization and prolongation of sensor life by months to years.
3. CGM drives artificial pancreas systems. Indeed, we have just entered that era with the US FDA's approval of the MiniMed Medtronic Hybrid Closed Loop system (670G), which automates basal insulin delivery and suspends insulin delivery based on CGM data. Many groups around the world are actively investigating novel algorithms as well as ways to incorporate other relevant hormones like glucagon, pramlintide, and exenatide into artificial pancreas systems.
4. CGM will be used to assess dysglycemia in patients without diabetes including those with prediabetes and obesity, and it is possible that CGM-derived criteria for the diagnosis of these metabolic disorders will be created to supplement the traditional criteria. CGM is likely to be used to educate nondiabetic yet dysglycemic patients about how to modify their lifestyle behaviors. It is also reasonable to think that CGM will be used in wellness efforts by a wide spectrum of individuals without metabolic abnormalities.

Professor Jia and her colleagues have been international leaders in the use of CGM. Their multiple publications in leading scientific journals have provided important insights about diabetes both in China and internationally. Importantly, they have used CGM to establish norms for the population and published one of the first guidelines in how CGM can be used to benefit patients with diabetes and related conditions. This book provides a comprehensive description of the science and clinical use of CGM by one of the world's experts in CGM and is essential reading for anyone treating patients with diabetes.

Robert A. Vigersky
Washington D.C.
United States of America

Foreword 2

Various types of diabetes with different etiologies or pathogenesis share a common pathophysiological feature, that is, the elevation of blood glucose levels. For more than half a century, measurement of venous or capillary glucose levels or glycated hemoglobin has been the major methods to monitor impaired glucose metabolism. Recent years have witnessed the rapid development of continuous glucose monitoring (CGM) technology, which detects glucose in subcutaneous interstitial fluid through a specialized sensor. As is known to all, blood flows from the capillaries to the veins, and interstitial fluid acts as a bridge in the diffusion of glucose between capillaries and cells of the tissue. Elevation of glucose levels in interstitial fluid, due to impaired glucose uptake or excessive glucose release into the interstitial fluid, represents the basic pathogenesis of the increased plasma glucose concentration in diabetes mellitus. Therefore, understanding intraday and interday trends of interstitial fluid glucose is the stepping stone to in-depth comprehension of normal or impaired glucose metabolism and the metabolism of glucose-related substances. From a hundred years ago when urine glucose testing was initially performed to now, the feasible means for daily routine monitoring of abnormal glucose metabolism remain imperfect and are still in progress.

The evaluation of the accuracy of CGM shows that the technology can reflect the trend in blood glucose fluctuations. Thus, in China, CGM was once referred to as dynamic glucose monitoring technology. CGM helps to understand the trend in glucose fluctuations, as well as to detect occult hyperglycemia and hypoglycemia, which are usually not detected by traditional glucose monitoring methods. Therefore, CGM allows more precise management of diabetes by controlling hyperglycemia, reducing hypoglycemia events, decreasing glucose fluctuations, and finally preventing the occurrence and development of diabetes complications that jeopardize the health and life span of patients.

The technology of CGM is among the great achievements of glucose monitoring technologies for diabetes. Since 1999 when the retrospective CGM system was first launched, CGM technology has played a positive role in promoting progress in diabetes management. In order to expand the knowledge of CGM technology and to facilitate the scientific, standardized, and reasonable use of CGM technology, the authors compiled this book based on their long-term original researches and clinical experience, as well as the scientific findings from domestic and international counterparts.

The authors of this book introduced their initial work on the establishment of the normal reference ranges for CGM parameters in Chinese population. Indeed, the definition of the "normal" value is the key to judging "abnormalities." In the early years of clinical application of CGM technology, there was a lack of normal reference values for CGM parameters and the reference range of finger-stick glucose value was apparently not suitable to CGM measurements. These limitations significantly hindered the interpretation of CGM results and the clinical application of this technology. Previously, the authors carried out a multicenter study and obtained large amounts of normal CGM data and established the CGM normal reference range for the first time worldwide. In the book, the authors introduce their innovative work and compare and analyze similar findings from domestic and international counterparts in different ethnic groups. These studies lay the foundation for scientific application of CGM and rational explanation for CGM results, and solve the key problems in making the best use of CGM technology in clinical practice.

Moreover, the authors introduce their CGM reporting and management system in details, which was developed independently with intellectual property rights. Scientific interpretation of CGM data and its graphical display are important to the clinical use of the technology as are the presentation of a comprehensive display of glucose metrics and standardized reports. By illustrating clinical cases, the authors introduce their CGM reporting system and explain how to interpret or analyze CGM profiles. Their reporting system includes an analysis software, which can calculate CGM-derived metrics and generate a standardized CGM report automatically. All these efforts enable clinicians to understand the trend of blood glucose fluctuations in patients.

Furthermore, the clinical significance and application of CGM metrics proposed by domestic and international scholars are reviewed in the book. The authors also summarize the advantages and concerns of several parameters based on the clinical trials conducted by themselves.

In the book, the current clinical application of CGM technology is discussed in detail. The book also demonstrates the use of CGM measurements in various situations of abnormal glucose metabolism, as well as the role of CGM in evaluating the efficacy of different hypoglycemic therapies.

I would like to thank my colleagues in Shanghai Clinical Center for Diabetes who have engaged in glucose monitoring studies and related clinical work for their persistent devotion and efforts to promote the development of CGM in China. It is expected that this book will help all the readers gain a comprehensive understanding of the CGM system and promote the standardized and wide application of CGM in clinical practice, thereby contributing to the improvement of diabetes management in China.

Shanghai, China Kunsan Xiang

Preface

Blood glucose monitoring is an important part of diabetes management. It plays an essential role in the assessment of glucose metabolism disorders, thereby guiding the optimization of the magagement of diabetes. As blood glucose level changes continuously, neither the glucose values at certain time points nor glycated hemoglobin reflects the dynamic fluctuations in blood glucose throughout the day. Indeed, the capture of continuous glucose monitoring has always been a dream pursued by both patients and clinicians for a long time. As in the early 1960s, Clark and Lyons first put forward the concept of a glucose sensor. The designed sensor consisted of a thin layer of glucose oxidase (GOD), an oxygen electrode, an inner oxygen semipermeable membrane, and an outer dialysis membrane. The glucose concentration could be calculated by measuring the change in the local oxygen concentrations. In 1967, Updike and Hicks further improved the detection assay and measured glucose concentrations in biological fluids of an animal model for the first time. Subsequently, continuous glucose monitoring (CGM) technology has become increasingly sophisticated and accurate and has been gradually promoted from the experimental monitoring to clinical application.

In 1999, a CGM system was approved by the US Food and Drug Administration (FDA) for clinical use, allowing a convenient, panoramic view of all-day changes in blood glucose for the first time. Since 2005, the real-time CGM system has been applied in clinical practice. In addition to real-time display of monitoring results, it integrates alarm and predictive alert features, providing a guarantee for the safety of treatment. At the same time, the development of CGM technology promotes the creation of algorithms that can modify the rate of continuous insulin infusion. Moreover, with the application of CGM technology, investigators have been able to study the normal patterns of glucose variation and how they differ under different clinical circumstances.

In 2001, we started to apply CGM in clinical practice in China for the first time. We found some challenges that need to be addressed. For example, the lack of normal reference range for CGM parameters, the absence of standardized interpretation methods for CGM graphs, and the complex and time-consuming process of CGM data analysis. In addition, little experience exists regarding the clinical indications for this new technique, the methods for assessing the accuracy of CGM data, and how the data should be used to guide decisions in clinical practice. To address these challenges, we established the normal reference values of CGM parameters by a national multicenter study, which was the first reported evidence domestically and internationally. We also analyzed the patterns of blood glucose fluctuations in different metabolic disorders, carried out standardized protocols for CGM graphs interpretation, and designed a series of supporting software and management systems independently to simplify the time-consuming data analysis process. We have published more than 50 papers related to CGM in domestic and international journals, established a CGM database containing more than 15,000 cases, and accumulated a wealth of clinical experience. In order to further enhance the knowledge of CGM technology among professional medical staff in the fields of endocrinology and metabolism, we have compiled this book to facilitate the scientific, standardized, and proper utilization of CGM technology.

The book firstly focuses on the basic knowledge of CGM technology, and then introduces the advantages and applications of the CGM system with clinical cases. In the book, we introduce the principles, the operation methods, the management procedures, and indications of CGM. Also, the alarms settings and responses to the alarms, interpretation of CGM results, the analysis of clinical cases, the relative researches and prospects are also discussed. This book is edited mainly based on our original research results and specifically focuses on the clinical application. It illustrates CGM knowledge in the form of clinical cases and graphs, with the aim of becoming a reference book guiding the application of CGM technology in clinical practice and scientific research.

All the clinical trials carried out by the authors in this book have been reported to the Ethics Committee of Shanghai Jiao Tong University Affiliated Sixth People's Hospital already and were in accordance with the Good Clinical Practice and Standards of China Association for Ethical Studies (approval number: 2007-45).

I would like to thank my colleagues in the Department of Endocrinology and Metabolism and Shanghai Diabetes Institute who have engaged in the glucose monitoring and clinical work for years for their continuous dedication. In addition, my colleague Jie Li and graduate students Xingxing He, Hang Su, Lingwen Ying, Jiahui Peng, Lingli Cai, Yiming Si, Dongjun Dai, Yun Shen, and others who have contributed in the careful editing and chart proofing. Specifically, my mentor, the Chinese Academy of Engineering member, Professor Kunsan Xiang, and the former president of the Endocrine Society, Professor Robert A. Vigersky, wrote the foreword for this book. Also, many thanks to my editors Ling Wan, Jianshe Zeng, Lujing Kong, et al. in the Shanghai Scientific and Technical Publishers for their help and support.

There might be some inevitable shortcomings and omissions exist in the book. We sincerely hope that readers will share their valuable advice and suggestions for future improvements.

Shanghai, China Weiping Jia

Contents

About the Editor and Associate Editors

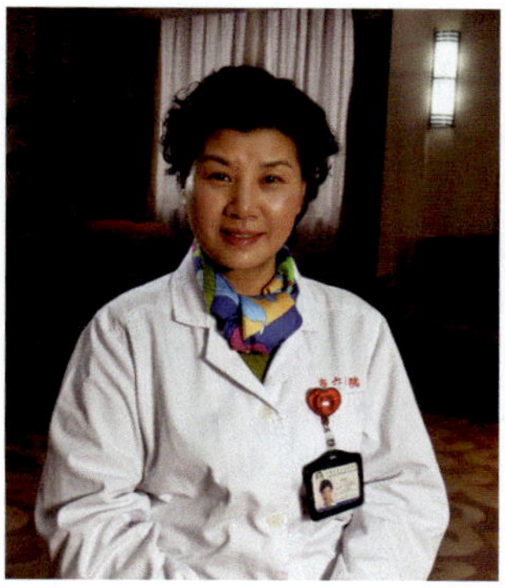

Weiping Jia is a Chinese endocrinologist, professor of medicine at Shanghai Jiao Tong University, president of the Shanghai Sixth People's Hospital, director of the Shanghai Clinical Center for Diabetes, and director of Shanghai Diabetes Institute. Professor Jia also serves as the president of Chinese Diabetes Society, chief editor of the *Chinese Journal of Internal Medicine*, associate editor of *Diabetes Research and Clinical Practice*, as well as an editorial board member of *Lancet Diabetes Endocrinology*. She is the chief editor of the *Chinese National Guideline for Prevention and Treatment of Type 2 Diabetes Mellitus (2017 Edition)* and the *Chinese National Guideline for Primary Healthcare of Diabetes (2018 Edition)*. Her research interests include the diagnosis and monitoring of diabetes as well as identification of genetic risk factors for diabetes. She established new diagnostic standards for diabetes and abdominal obesity, discovered novel T2DM genetic susceptibility loci, and established normal reference values for continuous glucose monitoring in Chinese population. She has published over 100 research articles in international journals, including *Diabetes*, *Diabetes Care*, *Diabetologia*, *JCEM*, *BMJ*, *Lancet Diabetes Endocrinol*, and *JACC*. Her research has been funded by the Natural Science Foundation of China (NSFC), the National Basic Research Program of China, and the European Association for the Study of Diabetes (EASD). She is the Co-PI of research projects funded by the US National Institute of Health (NIH). Since 2015, she has been the PI of the Construction of Prevention and Treatment of Diabetes Healthcare System in Shanghai, the largest community-based screening program for complications of diabetes in China which covers over 200,000 patients.

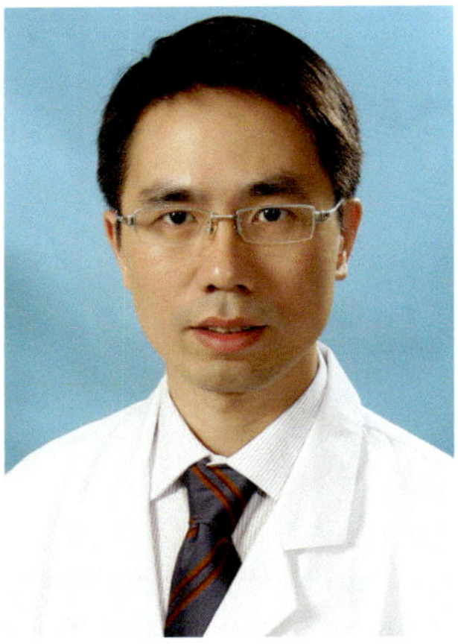

Jian Zhou is the associated professor of medicine at Shanghai Jiao Tong University and the deputy director of the Department of Endocrinology and Metabolism, Shanghai Jiao Tong University Affiliated Sixth People's Hospital. He also serves as the member of the Youth Committee of Chinese Society of Endocrinology, the secretary and committee member of Shanghai Diabetes Society, an editorial board member of *Cardiovascular Diabetology*, and the corresponding editor of *Chinese Medical Journal, Chinese Journal of Endocrinology and Metabolism*, and *Chinese Journal of Diabetes*. His career has focused on diabetes and obesity, and he has taken the leading role in promoting the new technology of Continuous Glucose Monitoring in China. He was the first researcher who proposed to establish the normal reference values of Continuous Glucose Monitoring parameters and published the relevant results in Chinese population on *Diabetes Care*. He has published more than 90 research articles (as first or corresponding author), among which 30 were cited by international peer-reviewed journals.

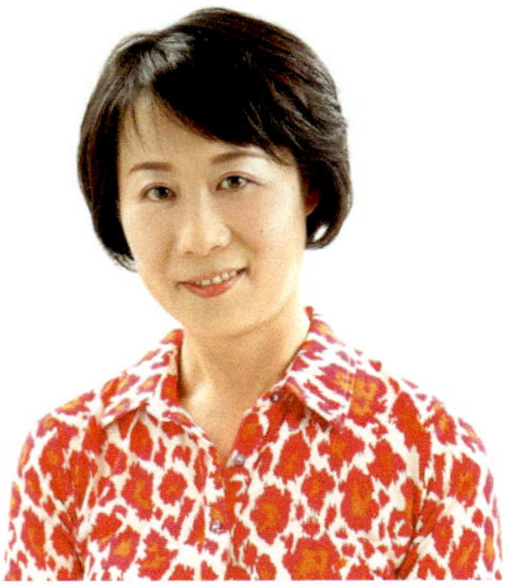

Yuqian Bao is a Chinese endocrinologist, professor of medicine at Shanghai Jiao Tong University, the director of the Department of Endocrinology and Metabolism, Shanghai Jiao Tong University Affiliated Sixth People's Hospital, and the executive deputy director of Shanghai Clinical Center for Diabetes. She also serves as the vice chairman of Specialty Subcommittee of Diabetes Prevention and Control of Chinese Preventive Medicine Association, member of Chinese Society of Endocrinology, and the president of Shanghai Diabetes Society. Her career has focused on obesity, and she was professionally trained in key research areas.

Her team established the accurate diagnostic criteria of central obesity (abdominal obesity) for the first time in Chinese population and defined the corresponding waist circumference cutoffs, which were adopted by the "Criteria of weight for adults" (WS/T 428-2013) issued by National Health and Family Planning Commission of the People's Republic of China in 2013. She was also the first researcher who proposed to use glycated hemoglobin A1c as a supplemental index for the diagnosis of diabetes in Chinese population and published the relevant results in the *British Medical Journal*. Moreover, she has established the hyperglycemic clamp technique as the precise method to evaluate pancreatic β-cell function in Chinese population. In recent years, her team has founded a model of comprehensive management of metabolic surgery, also called the "Shanghai Model" by local and international researchers.

Contributors

W. Jia Department of Endocrinology and Metabolism, Shanghai Clinical Center for Diabetes, Shanghai Diabetes Institute, Shanghai Jiao Tong University Affiliated Sixth People's Hospital, Shanghai, China

J. Zhou Department of Endocrinology and Metabolism, Shanghai Clinical Center for Diabetes, Shanghai Diabetes Institute, Shanghai Jiao Tong University Affiliated Sixth People's Hospital, Shanghai, China

Y. Bao Department of Endocrinology and Metabolism, Shanghai Clinical Center for Diabetes, Shanghai Diabetes Institute, Shanghai Jiao Tong University Affiliated Sixth People's Hospital, Shanghai, China

X. J. Ma Department of Endocrinology and Metabolism, Shanghai Clinical Center for Diabetes, Shanghai Diabetes Institute, Shanghai Jiao Tong University Affiliated Sixth People's Hospital, Shanghai, China

Y. F. Mo Department of Endocrinology and Metabolism, Shanghai Clinical Center for Diabetes, Shanghai Diabetes Institute, Shanghai Jiao Tong University Affiliated Sixth People's Hospital, Shanghai, China

J. Y. Lu Department of Endocrinology and Metabolism, Shanghai Clinical Center for Diabetes, Shanghai Diabetes Institute, Shanghai Jiao Tong University Affiliated Sixth People's Hospital, Shanghai, China

Y. F. Wang Department of Endocrinology and Metabolism, Shanghai Clinical Center for Diabetes, Shanghai Diabetes Institute, Shanghai Jiao Tong University Affiliated Sixth People's Hospital, Shanghai, China

H. Y. Yu Department of Endocrinology and Metabolism, Shanghai Clinical Center for Diabetes, Shanghai Diabetes Institute, Shanghai Jiao Tong University Affiliated Sixth People's Hospital, Shanghai, China

L. Zhang Department of Endocrinology and Metabolism, Shanghai Clinical Center for Diabetes, Shanghai Diabetes Institute, Shanghai Jiao Tong University Affiliated Sixth People's Hospital, Shanghai, China

M. Li Department of Endocrinology and Metabolism, Shanghai Clinical Center for Diabetes, Shanghai Diabetes Institute, Shanghai Jiao Tong University Affiliated Sixth People's Hospital, Shanghai, China

J. F. Han Department of Endocrinology and Metabolism, Shanghai Clinical Center for Diabetes, Shanghai Diabetes Institute, Shanghai Jiao Tong University Affiliated Sixth People's Hospital, Shanghai, China

F. Gao Department of Endocrinology and Metabolism, Shanghai Clinical Center for Diabetes, Shanghai Diabetes Institute, Shanghai Jiao Tong University Affiliated Sixth People's Hospital, Shanghai, China

W. Lu Department of Endocrinology and Metabolism, Shanghai Clinical Center for Diabetes, Shanghai Diabetes Institute, Shanghai Jiao Tong University Affiliated Sixth People's Hospital, Shanghai, China

Determination of Glucose and Continuous Glucose Monitoring

1

Y. F. Wang and W. Jia

Glucose is the main source of energy for human activities. Under normal circumstances, the blood glucose level in the body is relatively constant, generally maintained at 3.9–6.1 mmol/L before meals and 7.8–8.3 mmol/L after meals. Diabetes is a group of disorders characterized by chronic elevation of blood glucose. Thus, determination of blood glucose is a basic method for the diagnosis, treatment, and follow-up of diabetes. Due to the limitations of detection technologies, until recent years, it was not possible to observe a panoramic view of subtle changes in blood glucose and, thus, not possible to gain an in-depth understanding of the changes in blood glucose among diabetic patients. At present, a widely used technology is continuous glucose monitoring (CGM) technology, which monitors the glucose concentrations in subcutaneous tissue interstitial fluid (referred to as interstitial fluid) through a glucose sensor. This technology is able to provide continuous, comprehensive, and reliable all-day glucose profiles, thereby allowing for an understanding of trends in blood glucose fluctuations, and to detect occult hyperglycemia and hypoglycemia that cannot be detected by traditional blood glucose monitoring methods [1]. This chapter introduces the metabolism and regulation of glucose in the body, explains the detection of interstitial fluid glucose concentration, and analyzes the principle of CGM technology and its differences from traditional blood glucose monitoring methods, in order to help readers understand the CGM technology more comprehensively.

1.1 Metabolism and Regulation of Glucose

1.1.1 Glucose Metabolism

Glucose is a carbohydrate molecule composed of six carbon atoms. The chemical formula is $C_6H_{12}O_6$; the molecular weight is 180.16; the density is 1.54 g/cm^3; the melting point is 146 °C; and it is easy to dissolve in water. Glucose is the most extensively utilized and stored carbohydrate molecule and also the basic carrier for energy supply and transportation in the body. Carbohydrates are important sources of energy for the body, and more than 70% of the energy needed is derived from carbohydrates in food. Glucose is a digestive product of carbohydrates, and as smallest unit of carbohydrate, it is absorbed into blood circula-

Y. F. Wang (✉) · W. Jia (✉)
Department of Endocrinology and Metabolism, Shanghai Clinical Center for Diabetes, Shanghai Diabetes Institute, Shanghai Jiao Tong University Affiliated Sixth People's Hospital, Shanghai, China
e-mail: wpjia@sjtu.edu.cn

W. Jia (ed.), *Continuous Glucose Monitoring*, https://doi.org/10.1007/978-981-10-7074-7_1

tion and then oxidized and utilized by organs, tissues, and cells. Excessive glucose is stored in the muscles and liver in the form of glycogen. Muscle glycogen is an energy reservior that is readily available for utilization at any time in the skeletal muscle; it accommodates the need for energy in emergency situations. On the other hand, the glucose is absorbed by the small intestinal mucosa, transported to the liver via the portal vein, and finally synthesized into liver glycogen for storage. The liver glycogen level keeps a dynamic balance with glucose homeostasis under the tight control of numerous neurohumoral factors. Generally, in a healthy adult, the liver glycogen store is about 100 g, and it becomes depleted within 24 h in the fasting state. Liver glycogen decomposition accounts for 50% of hepatic glucose output during overnight fasting. With prolonged fasting time, liver glycogen is gradually consumed and is almost depleted after fasting up to 40 h. In the case of gradually decreasing glycogen, hepatic gluconeogenesis is enhanced, leading to the synthesis of glucose from materials such as fatty acid degradation products and three-carbon gluconeogenic intermediates (such as lactic acid, pyruvic acid, and glycerol) converted from glycogenic amino acids.

There are various pathways for glucose metabolism based on different oxidation status. The common pathways of glucose metabolism include anaerobic glycolysis, aerobic oxidation, pentose phosphate pathway, uronic acid pathway, polyol pathway, glycogen synthesis and decomposition, gluconeogenesis, hexose metabolic pathway, and others. When tissue oxygenation is inadequate, the glucose is only decomposed into lactic acid, and the release of free energy is 1/18 that of aerobic oxidation. This energy supply pathway is known as anaerobic glycolysis of glucose. Although anaerobic glycolysis produces a small, limited amount of energy, it is extremely important for the human body under hypoxic conditions, since it is the only effective means of energy production without the use of oxygen. When the oxygen supply is sufficient, the glucose can be completely oxidized into the final products of carbon dioxide and water, releasing substantial energy. This process is called aerobic oxidation of glucose. Usually, most cells or tissues obtain energy through aerobic glucose metabolism. Blood glucose mainly comes from (1) foods. Dietary carbohydrates provide 60–70% of the whole body energy, (2) glycogen decomposition, and (3) gluconeogenesis during a long period of starvation.

Blood glucose is mainly (1) oxidatively decomposed for energy supply; (2) used for glycogen synthesis in the liver, muscle, and other tissues; (3) converted to other types of carbohydrates and derivatives, such as ribose, amino sugar, and uronic acid; (4) converted to nonsugar substances, such as fat, nonessential amino acids, etc.; and (5) discharged in the urine when the blood glucose concentration is too high and exceeds the renal glucose threshold (usually >8.9–10.0 mmol/L; Fig. 1.1).

1.1.2 Glucose Regulation

In the human body, blood glucose is maintained at a relatively constant level, which is essential for the utilization of glucose in various organs and tissues, especially brain tissue, bone marrow, nerve cells, and red blood cells. There is a dynamic equilibrium mechanism in the body that finely regulates the balance of blood glucose production and release, which is also known as glucose homeostasis (Fig. 1.2). Since many tissues store very little glycogen, they need to uptake glucose from the blood to meet the needs of metabolism and various functional activities whenever necessary. Glucose in the blood is transported to various cells and tissues mainly through facilitated diffusion. If the blood glucose concentration is too low, conditions are not conducive for glucose transport across the cell membrane into various tissues; if the blood glucose concentration is too high, glucose is discharged in the urine through the kidneys. The human brain consumes a considerable amount of energy but stores very little glycogen. It normally derives almost all of its energy from the aerobic oxidation of glucose in the blood. Therefore, low blood

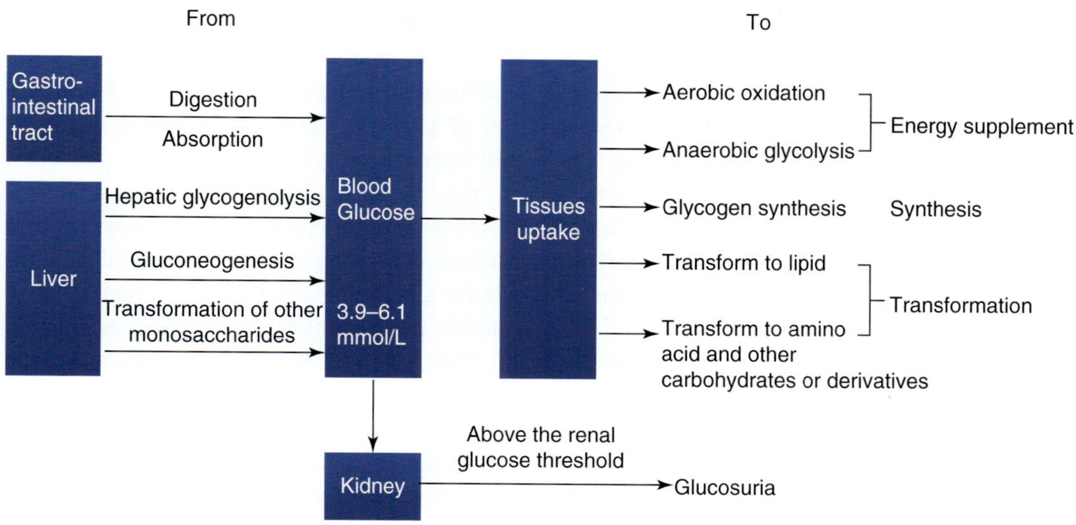

Fig. 1.1 Pathways of glucose metabolism

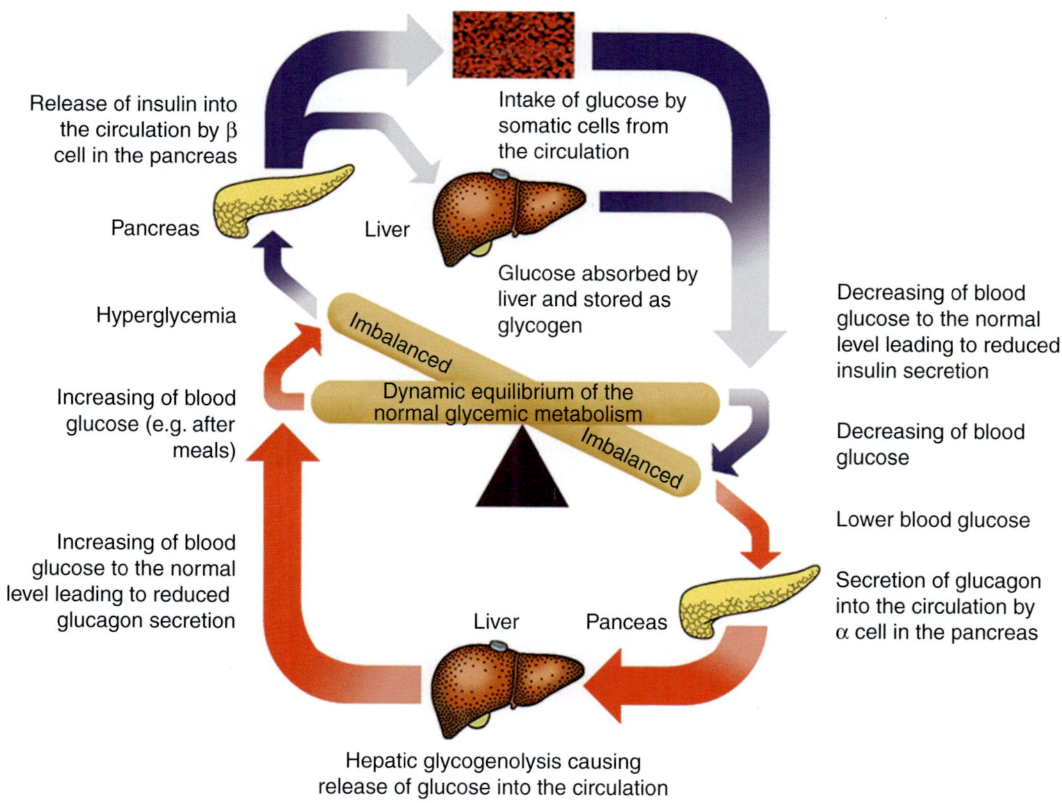

Fig. 1.2 Schematic diagram of blood glucose regulation

glucose can cause coma, convulsions, and irreversible damage to brain tissue. In addition, specific cell types, such as mature red blood cells, have no functional aerobic oxidase system due to the lack of mitochondria. They metabolize glucose mainly via glycolysis under normal circumstances. That mainly explains why the blood glucose concentration typically decreases if the blood cells are not separated in a timely manner from in vitro blood samples.

The body maintains blood glucose homeostasis under tight regulation by nerves, hormones, and the liver. During this process, the hypothalamus and nerves serve as a command center, hormones as main factors, and the liver as an important organ for precisely regulating glucose levels. The hypothalamus directly acts on the adrenal medulla, islet cells, and liver via the splanchnic nerves and vagus nerve and regulates blood glucose through modulating the secretion of related hormones (Fig. 1.3). The main hormones involved in the regulation of glucose metabolism include insulin, glucagon, adrenaline, cortisol, growth hormone, and others. Insulin is the hormone that has the hypoglycemic effect in the body. It decreases the blood glucose level by reducing glucose production via inhibition of glycogenolysis and gluconeogenesis as well as enhancing glucose uptake and utilization by the muscles, liver, and adipose tissue. Moreover, insulin can promote the formation of transmembrane glucose gradient through intracellular glucose phosphorylation, which leads to glucose transportation from blood circulation into liver cells. This process facilitates hepatic glycogen production and inhibits gluconeogenesis, thereby reducing hepatic glucose output. Glucagon, adrenaline, cortisol, and growth hormone all have effects on blood glucose that are opposite to insulin and thus are known as hyperglycemic hormones. In healthy individuals, insulin secretion increases when the blood glucose level is elevated and decreases when the blood glucose level is decreased. Hyperglycemic hormones act in an opposite fashion to insulin. These hormones work closely together to maintain homeostatic glucose levels, i.e., are increased when hypoglycemia develops. For this reason,

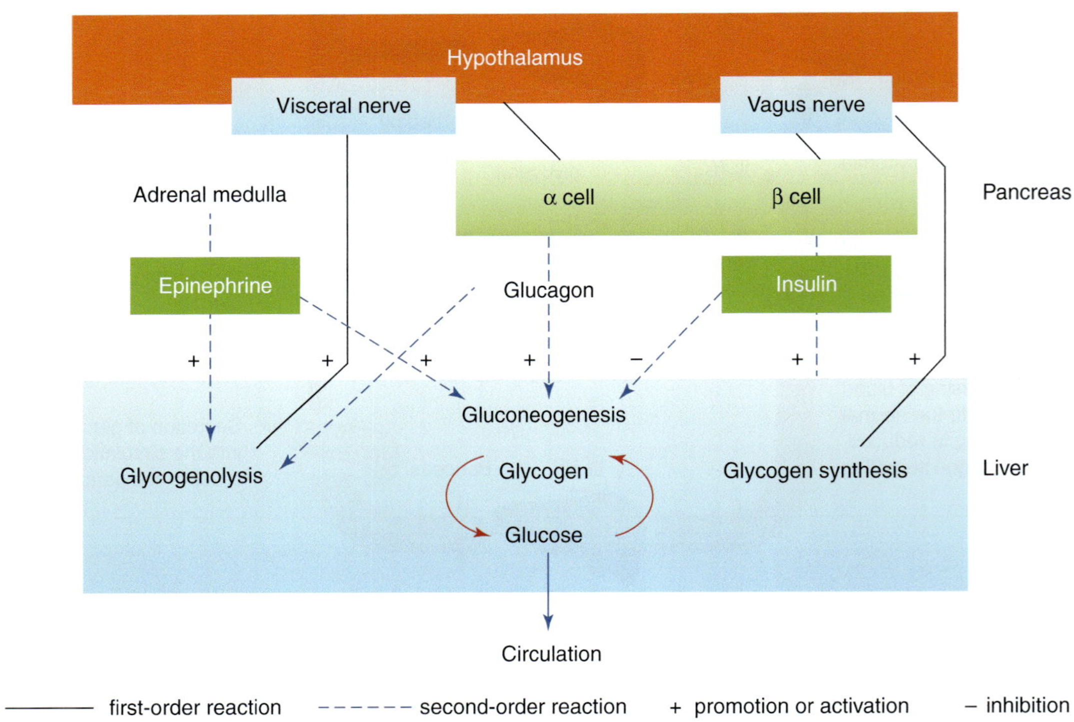

Fig. 1.3 Main mechanism underlying blood glucose regulation

they are also called counter-regulatory hormones. When the blood glucose concentration exceeds the normal value, synthesis of glycogen from glucose is increased for storage; when the blood glucose concentration is below the normal level, the stored hepatic glycogen is immediately broken down to release glucose into the blood, increasing the blood glucose level. Hepatic glycogen will soon be depleted when the endogenous glucose consumption sharply increases (such as during strenuous exercise), while glucose intake or absorption is seriously inadequate, for example, during starvation. At this time, the liver can synthesize glycogen utilizing nonsugar substances such as lactic acid, pyruvate, glycerol, and a part of glycogenic amino acids, through a process known as gluconeogenesis, which contributes to keeping adequate levels of glycogen in the liver. If the body takes in or absorbs a large amount of sugar, far exceeding the consumption capacity of the body, the glucose may be transformed into fat for storage.

1.2 Detection of Interstitial Fluid Glucose Concentration and Its Clinical Significance

The interstitial fluid refers to the total volume of extracellular fluid outside of the blood vessels but excludes the plasma volume, and it accounts for 15% of the bodyweight in adults. The interstitial fluid contains basically similar ingredients as plasma, allowing the exchange of metabolites and nutrients between them, but it does not contain red blood cells and contains only a small amount of protein. Under normal circumstances, the vast majority of interstitial fluid can rapidly exchange with blood or intracellular fluid, known as functional extracellular fluid (Fig. 1.4). Thus, it plays an important role in maintaining fluid and electrolyte balances in the body. A part of interstitial fluid becomes lymph fluid and is absorbed back into systemic circulation via lymph vessels. There is also a small part of the interstitial fluid, accounting for only approximately 10% of the interstitial fluid, which plays only a small role in maintaining the balance of fluid and electrolytes.

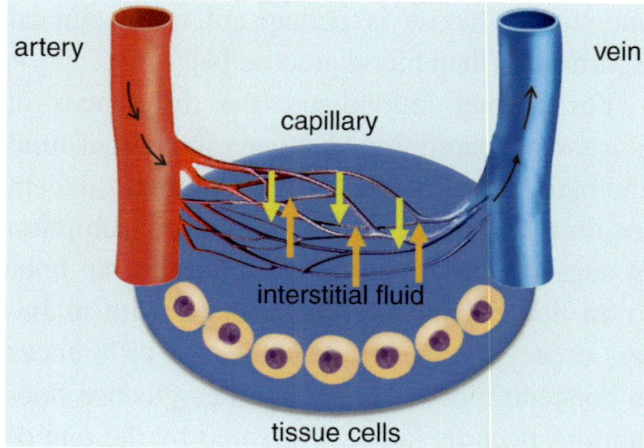

Fig. 1.4 Illustration of exchange between capillaries and the interstitial fluid

This type of interstitial fluid is known as "nonfunctional extracellular fluid."

Glucose in the blood transfuses into the interstitial fluid by facilitated diffusion, and interstitial glucose is consumed or returned back to plasma. The glucose concentrations in blood and subcutaneous interstitial fluid are highly correlated. Thus, it is possible to continuously monitor subcutaneous interstitial fluid glucose to reflect the changes of blood glucose concentrations [2, 3]. The interstitial fluid glucose physiologically lags 4–10 min behind plasma glucose [3–5]. When the blood glucose changes rapidly, the balance between plasma and interstitial fluid glucose will be broken, and rebalance takes a relatively long time, which will exacerbate the lagging time between them.

However, there are some situations, such as during hypoglycemia, when changes in blood glucose concentrations lag behind interstitial fluid glucose concentrations. That is, when blood glucose becomes extremely low, the concentrations of glucose in other parts of the body may be even lower. On one hand, glucose consumption occurs in tissues and cells with insufficient glucose supply, resulting in low transport velocity in relation to glucose consumption in cells, which has been proven by experimental research and in some patients with type 1 diabetes [4, 6]. On the other hand, insulin stimulates the utilization of glucose by cells, causing a decrease in interstitial glucose prior to blood glucose. Since interstitial fluid is the "first site" of cells and tissues that utilizes glucose, from this perspective, monitoring interstitial glucose is perhaps of more clinical significance than blood glucose [4].

For normal individuals, the differences in glucose concentrations between interstitial fluid and blood are very small, even negligible, except for on a few occasions, e.g., after consumption of sugary beverages (within about half an hour to an hour). However, for patients with diabetes, especially type 1 diabetes, the differences in concentrations are increased as glucose fluctuations become larger. Measured by the rate of change in blood glucose, the faster the blood glucose changes, the longer the lagging time is, leading to increased differences and worse correlations between blood glucose and interstitial fluid glucose [3, 4, 7, 8]. Therefore, when the interstitial fluid glucose concentration is inconsistent with the blood glucose concentration, for instance, during hypoglycemic events, will there be any clinical value in measuring glucose concentration in the interstitial fluid by sensors? In fact, the interstitial fluid is the main place where the body utilizes glucose and suffers damage by glucose abnormalities (e.g., hyperglycemia or hypoglycemia). Therefore, it is able to truly reflect the degree of glucose changes pathophysiologically. In clinical practice, measuring blood glucose instead of interstitial glucose is not because the former is superior than the later, but because there has been no reliable and convenient method to measure interstitial glucose level in the past [3, 4].

1.3 Principle and Classification of CGM Technology

The detection methods for measuring interstitial fluid glucose concentration are mainly divided into two categories. One is minimally invasive technology, which involves continuously monitoring interstitial glucose concentrations with a subcutaneous glucose sensor, also known as a CGM system. CGM systems can be classified as retrospective CGM systems, real-time CGM systems, and flash glucose monitoring system [1, 9, 10]. The other is noninvasive technology, which involves extracting glucose across the skin to monitor glycemia using weak current electrodes close against the skin, also known as reverse iontophoresis or the microdialysis technique [11].

In 1999, the first retrospective CGM system was approved by the US Food and Drug Administration (FDA), and it was later approved by China Food and Drug Administration (CFDA) in 2001 for clinical application and research. The retrospective CGM system consists of a glucose sensor, a cable, a blood glucose recorder, an information extractor, and analysis software. The sensor is composed of a semipermeable membrane, glucose oxidase (GOD), and a microelectrode, on which chemical reactions are initiated with interstitial fluid glucose to generate electrical signals upon subcutaneous implantation at the umbilical level. Moreover, with the help of analysis software, CGM can be used to view and analyze multiday glucose trends and daily glucose profiles and also to detect imperceptible hyperglycemia, hypoglycemia, and glucose variability, truly reflecting the glucose changes in patients. Therefore, CGM has been widely used in clinical practice [12].

In 2002, the first GlucoWatch G2 Biographer (GW2B) was approved by the US FDA. It is slightly larger in appearance than the average watch. When worn on the wrist, the watch contacts with the human skin through a layer of gel pad, where two electrodes are set. Micro-current extracts interstitial glucose molecules from the skin when they pass through the electrodes, and glucose interacts with the GOD to generate an electrical current. The device automatically detects the glucose level every 10 min for up to 13 h continuously. When the glucose concentration is too high or too low, the device will give an alarm. Although the glucose watch has been approved by the FDA for children over 7 years of age, one-fourth of measurements still have a deviation >30%. Thus, it is improper to adjust the insulin dose based solely on a single glucose reading. Because of the relative inaccuracy and uncomfortableness of this device, it is no longer being manufactured [4, 11, 13].

1.4 Different Glucose Concentration Displayed in Human Body

The samples for glucose concentration determination are not limited to arterial or venous blood but also include peripheral capillary blood, urine, interstitial fluid, saliva, and tears [14, 15]. Blood samples can be further subdivided into whole blood, plasma, and serum. Different blood samples can display different glucose concentrations due to various reasons.

1.4.1 Glucose Concentrations in Three Major Types of Blood Vessels

1.4.1.1 Venous Blood Glucose

The venous blood is the blood flowing in the veins of the systemic circulation and the blood flowing through the pulmonary artery into the right ventricle during pulmonary circulation. The venous blood is dark red, and it contains substantial metabolic wastes, such as carbon dioxide, urea, and others. The venous blood glucose level is the estimated glucose level after utilization of glucose by tissues, and it is an important indicator for the screening and diagnosis of diabetes and evaluation of glycemic control.

1.4.1.2 Arterial Blood Glucose

Arterial blood is the blood flowing in the arteries of the systemic circulation and the blood flowing through the pulmonary vein into the left atrium during pulmonary circulation. Arterial blood is bright red with high oxygen and low carbon dioxide concentrations. Arterial blood glucose is easily affected by various factors such as food intake and emotional changes.

1.4.1.3 Capillary Blood Glucose

Usually, the sample collection sites for detecting capillary blood glucose include fingers, earlobes, palm (including the thenar and hypothenar), toes, forearms, thighs, and other parts. Among them, capillaries are more abundant in fingers, earlobes, palms, and toes. The tip of the finger is the most common site for puncture due to convenience (Fig. 1.5). In addition, the forearm, upper arm, and thigh contain a less dense distribution of nerve endings and are potentially less sensitive to pain. These sites can be used as alternatives site sampling. However, no clear evidence has shown that alternative site sampling can enhance adherence [16–19] or improve glycemic control [18]. A drawback of alternative site testing is that it may be inaccurate in times of fluctuating blood glucose levels. Thus, alternate sites are not recommended in the following situations: right after insulin administration, 1-2h after food intake, exercising and the presence of hypoglycemic symptoms [20, 21]. Furthermore, these alternate sites should never be used to calibrate a CGM.

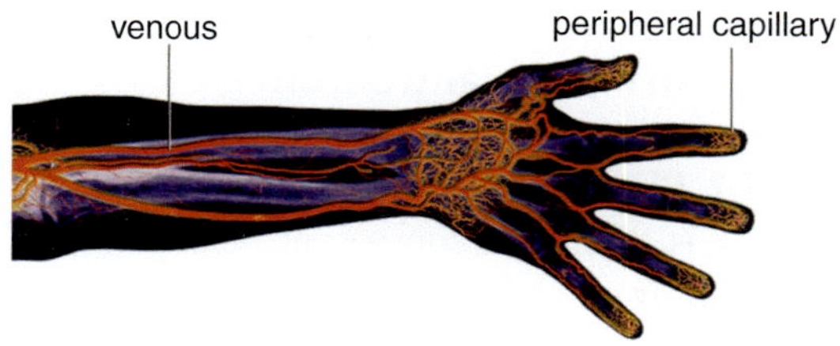

Fig. 1.5 Schematic diagram of different blood sampling sites

Capillaries are at the intersections of arteries and veins, and the blood composition is closer to arterial blood. Capillary, arterial, and venous blood glucose values are almost equal after fasting for 8–10 h. After food intake or consumption of sugar, the glucose absorbed in the intestine is transported through the vena cava back to the heart, then flows through the arteries into peripheral capillaries where glucose is consumed by tissues, and finally flows out into the vein. Accordingly, arterial blood glucose is about 8% higher than venous blood glucose, and the difference peaks at 0.5–1.0 h after food intake or sugar consumption. The arterial and venous blood glucose concentrations become equal at 3 h after food intake or sugar consumption.

1.4.2 Glucose Concentrations in Plasma and Serum

1.4.2.1 Plasma Glucose

Plasma is the liquid component of blood. It is separated from anticoagulated fresh blood samples by centrifugation or sedimentation followed by a collection of slight yellow or colorless fluid in supernatants. Water is the main constituent of blood plasma; it makes up 90–92% of its volume. The dissolved substrates in plasma include plasma protein, glucose, inorganic salts, hormones, carbon dioxide, and others. Detection of plasma glucose concentration is an important means for diabetes diagnosis. The World Health Organization (WHO) guidelines on diabetes recommend the use of venous plasma glucose for the diagnosis of diabetes.

1.4.2.2 Serum Glucose

The serum is the clear, light yellow liquid, separated out of blood after coagulation. The blood sample in a test tube will rapidly solidify in the absence of anticoagulants due to the activation of the coagulation reaction. After clot contraction, the light yellow, transparent liquid surrounding the clot is serum. It can also be obtained by centrifugation after the addition of coagulants.

1.4.2.3 Comparison of Plasma Versus Serum Glucose

The serum does not contain fibrinogen that can be converted into fibrin. That is the most significant difference between plasma and serum. Theoretically, plasma and serum glucose concentrations are the same. In reality though, the serum glucose concentration is often slightly lower, because the blood cells in plasma are separated and removed immediately after sample collection, thus avoiding glucose glycolysis in blood, whereas for serum samples, 1–3 h are usually required for blood coagulation and clot contraction before centrifugation, during which glucose glycolysis may occur. The plasma components should be separated as soon as possible after sample collection. Due to ongoing glycolysis, the red blood cells continuously consume glucose in plasma, leading to a 5–7% reduction in plasma glucose per hour, if the in vitro whole blood sample is not separated in a timely manner.

1.4.2.4 Comparison of Plasma Versus Whole Blood Glucose

Plasma and serum differ from whole blood in that the cellular components have been removed. The whole blood and plasma have the same molar concentration of glucose. Glucose is soluble only in water, and cells contain less water content than plasma does, so the concentration of glucose per unit volume of plasma is greater than that of blood cells. Glucose can easily diffuse through the membrane of red blood cells. The plasma glucose concentration is about 11% higher than that in the whole blood, and in return, the whole blood glucose value is 10–15% lower than that in plasma or serum. For samples with the same plasma glucose concentration, the whole blood glucose value is reversely correlated with hematocrit; that is, high hematocrit leads to a low blood glucose value and vice versa (Table 1.1) [22, 23]. Whole blood thus has a lower glucose concentration by approximately 12% compared to plasma at a normal hematocrit of 35–45%. In the past, glucose meters usually displayed whole blood glucose readings, and now the readings on glucose meters mostly have been converted into plasma glucose values [24] (Fig. 1.6).

1.4.2.5 Urine Glucose

Urine glucose refers to the glucose level in the urine. In some parts of the world, urine glucose has been the most commonly used method for diabetes monitoring. When the blood flows through the kidneys, the plasma glucose filters through the glomeruli into tubules, and the majority of glucose in the renal tubules is reabsorbed

Table 1.1 Differences between whole blood glucose and plasma glucose at different hematocrit levels

Hematocrit (%)	Whole blood glucose values (mmol/L)	Plasma glucose values (mmol/L)
25	9.40	10.0
35	9.16	10.0
45	8.92	10.0
55	8.68	10.0
65	8.44	10.0

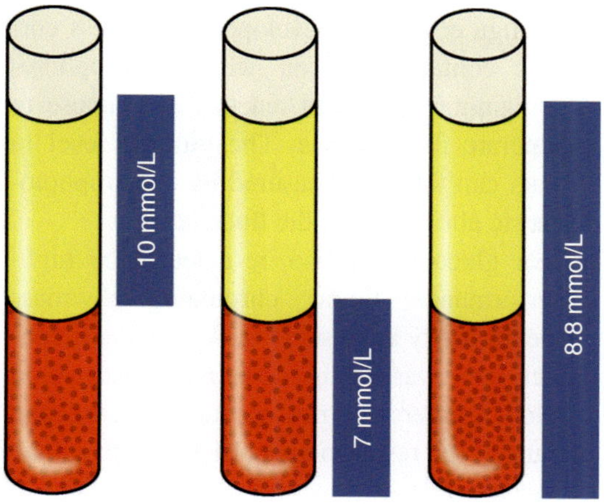

Fig. 1.6 Whole blood glucose and plasma glucose

into the blood. In normal individuals, the daily excretion of glucose was between 32 and 93 mg, which is undetectable and mostly tests as negative in the qualitative test. Glucose excretion greater than 0.83 mmol per 24 h is defined as glucosuria and usually tests as positive in the qualitative test.

Renal threshold for glucose excretion refers to the lowest blood glucose level that correlates with the first detectable appearance of urine glucose. Glycosuria appears when the blood glucose rises above this level and vice versa. The renal threshold for glucose excretion in normal individuals is 8.9–10.0 mmol/L. However, patients with kidney diseases and the elderly may have an increased renal glucose threshold due to a deceased glomerular filtration rate. For some elderly patients with diabetes, even if the blood glucose is more than 13.9 mmol/L, their urine glucose can be negative. On the contrary, renal glycosuria may occur because of the lowering of the renal threshold for glucose excretion, manifested by the presence of urine glucose without hyperglycemia. For instance, some pregnant women, especially primiparas, experience glycosuria because the renal threshold normally decreases during pregnancy. Finally, the urine glucose represents an average of the glucose excretion over the time since the last voiding rather than accurately reflecting the blood glucose at the time of urination. Previously, "double voiding" was used to overcome this problem.

1.4.2.6 Cerebrospinal Fluid (CSF) Glucose

Normal CSF glucose levels vary between 2.5 and 4.4 mmol/L, which is about 50–80% of levels in the blood. Decreased glucose concentrations in CSF are seen in patients with bacterial or cryptococcal meningitis and malignant brain tumors and are related to accelerated glycolysis. Increased glucose concentrations in CSF are seen in hyperglycemia, viral infections of the central nervous system, brain trauma, posterior fossa tumors or tumors at the bottom of the third ventricle, hyperpyrexia, and other conditions, which are related to increased blood-brain barrier permeability.

The CSF/blood glucose ratio is normally maintained relatively constant, which used to be explained by the theory that the free transport of glucose across the blood-brain barrier. However, currently it is recognized that this transport is not based on simple dispersion, but membrane transportation, known as carrier-mediated transport or carrier-mediated dispersion. The glucose level in CSF depends on the following factors: (1) blood glucose concentration, (2) blood-brain barrier permeability, (3) the degree of glucose glycolysis in CSF, and (4) the capacity of the transport system.

1.4.2.7 Salivary Glucose

Saliva is secreted from the salivary glands (parotid gland, submandibular gland, sublingual gland, and minor salivary glands). It moisturizes food, protects the membranes of the mouth, and facilitates digestion. The saliva has a relatively complex chemical composition, which is partially similar to plasma, including urea, creatinine, uric acid, calcium, inorganic phosphorus, and some steroids or therapeutic drugs. Due to the capacity for noninvasive collection and easy accessibility, saliva has been used for monitoring certain plasma components or concentrations of therapeutic drugs [14].

Studies have shown an increased permeability in the parotid basement membrane in type 1 diabetes [25]. When the blood glucose rises, large amounts of glucose flow into saliva with saliva secretion. In ten cases of newly diagnosed type 1 diabetes aged 4–15 years old, the saliva glucose level was found to be significantly higher than that in normal individuals, which might be helpful for the early diagnosis of type 1 diabetes mellitus. After insulin treatment, plasma glucose concentration decreases, accompanied by a decrease in the saliva glucose concentration, indicating that good glycemic control is associated with a decreased salivary glucose concentration. Moreover, the duration of diabetes may also have an impact on the saliva glucose concentration. In some patients with a longer duration of diabetes, similar to the renal threshold for glucose, saliva secretion also has a threshold of 8–15 mmol/L, at which level the glands promote glucose secretion. Saliva, as a specimen that is easy to access and can be collected noninvasively, can be a substitute for plasma in the determination of certain plasma ingredients. If a correlation between salivary and plasma glucose levels can be established, it is expected that the saliva glucose concentration can be used for glucose monitoring in diabetes patients, in an attempt to reduce frequent blood sampling and alleviate pain.

1.4.2.8 Tear Glucose

The determination of glucose in tear fluids has many advantages, including high sensitivity, noninvasiveness, easy accessibility, simple operation, stable glucose level, and fewer influential factors, under the premise of a unified collection method. In normal subjects, the glucose levels in the tears averaged 0.14 ± 0.07 mmol/L, and diabetes patients have an increased tear glucose level of 0.32 ± 0.18 mmol/L.

At present, there are a variety of methods for detecting tear glucose, and three methods are mainly used:

1. March et al. [26] first developed glucose-sensing corneal contact lenses based on the intensity of fluorescence. When the tear glucose rises, the fluorescence signal on the corneal contact lens is enhanced, but it does not represent a specific value of tear glucose.
2. Badugu et al. [27] developed a colorless corneal contact lens, on which fluorophore-containing boric acid reacts with glucose to generate fluorescence. The glucose level in tears can thus be measured by spectrophotometric absorption of the fluorescence.
3. Tear glucose can also be detected by high-performance liquid chromatography/mass spectrometry analysis [14]. A new smart contact lens was being developed that would allow wearers to measure tear glucose and transfer the result to a recorder or apps on the phone wirelessly.

1.4.3 Glycemic Parameters Reflecting Different Time Periods

In addition to reflecting instant glucose concentrations, urine glucose can reflect the mean blood glucose (MBG) over the previous 2–6 h. CGM can display continuous changes in blood glucose for 3–7 days; 1,5-anhydroglucitol (1,5-AG) can represent the MBG over the previous 1–2 weeks; and glycated albumin (GA) and glycated hemoglobin A_{1c} (HbA_{1c}) can reflect the average blood glucose levels over the previous 2–3 weeks and 2–3 months, respectively (Fig. 1.7). 1,5-AG is a 1-deoxy form of glucopyranose with a structure similar to glucose. Importantly, patients with diabetes mellitus

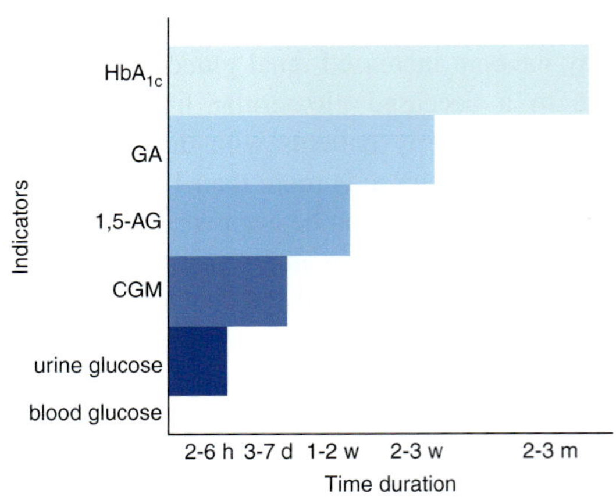

Fig. 1.7 Glycemic parameters reflecting different time periods

exhibit significantly lower levels of 1,5-AG than normoglycemic individuals. 1,5-AG was approved by the US FDA in 2003 as a short-term marker of glycemic control [15, 28].

References

1. Chinese Diabetes Society. Clinical application guide of blood glucose monitoring in China (Edition 2015). Chin J Diabetes. 2015;7:603–13. https://doi.org/10.3760/cma.j.issn.1674-5809.2015.10.004.
2. Jansson PA, Fowelin J, Smith U, Lonnroth P. Characterization by microdialysis of intracellular glucose level in subcutaneous tissue in humans. Am J Phys. 1988;255:E218–20.
3. Dye L, Mansfield M, Lasikiewicz N, Mahawish L, Schnell R, Talbot D, Chauhan H, Croden F, Lawton C. Correspondence of continuous interstitial glucose measurement against arterialised and capillary glucose following an oral glucose tolerance test in healthy volunteers. Br J Nutr. 2010;103:134–40. https://doi.org/10.1017/S0007114509991504.
4. Boyne MS, Silver DM, Kaplan J, Saudek CD. Timing of changes in interstitial and venous blood glucose measured with a continuous subcutaneous glucose sensor. Diabetes. 2003;52:2790–4.
5. Cengiz E, Tamborlane WV. A tale of two compartments: interstitial versus blood glucose monitoring. Diabetes Technol Ther. 2009;11(Suppl 1):11–6. https://doi.org/10.1089/dia.2009.0002.
6. Sternberg F, Meyerhoff C, Mennel FJ, Mayer H, Bischof F, Pfeiffer EF. Does fall in tissue glucose precede fall in blood glucose? Diabetologia. 1996;39:609–12.
7. Zhou J, Jia WP, Yu M, Yu HY, Bao YQ, Ma XJ, Lu W, Hu C, Xiang KS. The reference values of glycemic parameters for continuous glucose monitoring and its clinical application. Zhong hua Nei Ke Za Zhi. 2007;46:189–92.
8. Zhou J, Li H, Ran X, Yang W, Li Q, Peng Y, Li Y, Gao X, Luan X, Wang W, Jia W. Reference values for continuous glucose monitoring in Chinese subjects. Diabetes Care. 2009;32:1188–93. https://doi.org/10.2337/dc09-0076.
9. Kilpatrick ES, Rigby AS, Goode K, Atkin SL. Relating mean blood glucose and glucose variability to the risk of multiple episodes of hypoglycemia in type 1 diabetes. Diabetologia. 2007;50:2553–61. https://doi.org/10.1007/s00125-007-0820-z.
10. Ji L, Guo X, Guo L, Ren Q, Yu N, Zhang J. A multicenter evaluation of the performance and usability of a novel glucose monitoring system in chinese adults with diabetes. J Diabetes Sci Technol. 2017;11:290–5. https://doi.org/10.1177/1932296816662884.
11. Chase HP, Beck R, Tamborlane W, Buckingham B, Mauras N, Tsalikian E, Wysocki T, Weinzimer S, Kollman C, Ruedy K, Xing D. A randomized multicenter trial comparing the GlucoWatch biographer with standard glucose monitoring in children with type 1 diabetes. Diabetes Care. 2005;28:1101–6.
12. Zhou J, Lv X, Mu Y, Wang X, Li J, Zhang X, Wu J, Bao Y, Jia W. The accuracy and efficacy of real-time continuous glucose monitoring sensor in Chinese diabetes patients: a multicenter study. Diabetes Technol Ther. 2012;14:710–8. https://doi.org/10.1089/dia.2012.0014.
13. Diabetes Research in Children Network (DirecNet) Study Group. Accuracy of the GlucoWatch G2 biographer and the continuous glucose monitoring system during hypoglycemia: experience of the diabetes research in children network. Diabetes Care. 2004;27:722–6.
14. Corrie SR, Coffey JW, Islam J, Markey KA, Kendall MA. Blood, sweat, and tears: developing clinically relevant protein biosensors for integrated body fluid analysis. Analyst. 2015;140:4350–64. https://doi.org/10.1039/c5an00464k.
15. Ma X, Hu X, Zhou J, Hao Y, Luo Y, Lu Z, Bao Y, Jia W. Glycated albumin is more closely correlated with coronary artery disease than 1,5-anhydroglucitol and glycated hemoglobin A1c. Cardiovasc Diabetol. 2015;14:16. https://doi.org/10.1186/s12933-014-0166-z.
16. Vigersky RA. Glucose monitoring. In: Umpierrez GE, editor. Therapy for diabetes mellitus and related disorders. 6th ed. Alexandria: American Diabetes Association; 2014. p. 28–50.
17. Bennion N, Christensen NK, McGarraugh G. Alternate site glucose testing: a crossover design. Diabetes Technol Ther. 2002;4:25–33.
18. Knapp PE, Showers KM, Phipps JC, Speckman JL, Sternthal E, Freund KM, Ash AS, Apovian CM. Self-monitoring of blood glucose with finger tip versus alternative site sampling: effect on glycemic control in insulin-using patients with type 2 diabetes. Diabetes Technol Ther. 2009;11:219–25.
19. Suzuki Y, Atsumi Y, Matusoka K. Alternative site testing increases compliance of SMBG (preliminary study of 3 years cohort trials). Diabetes Res Clin Pract. 2003;59:233–4.
20. Bina DM, Anderson RL, Johnson ML, Bergenstal RM, Kendall DM. Clinical impact of prandial state, exercise, and site preparation on the equivalence of alternative-site blood glucose testing. Diabetes Care. 2003;26:981–5.
21. Jungheim K, Koschinsky T. Glucose monitoring at the arm: risky delays of hypoglycemia and hyperglycemia detection. Diabetes Care. 2002;25:956–60.
22. Tonyushkina K, Nichols JH. Glucose meters: a review of technical challenges to obtaining accurate results. J Diabetes Sci Technol. 2009;3:971–80. https://doi.org/10.1177/193229680900300446.

23. Tang Z, Lee JH, Louie RF, Kost GJ. Effects of different hematocrit levels on glucose measurements with handheld meters for point-of-care testing. Arch Pathol Lab Med. 2000;124:1135–40. https://doi.org/10.1043/0003-9985(2000)124<1135:EODHLO>2.0.CO;2.
24. Ginsberg BH. Factors affecting blood glucose monitoring: sources of errors in measurement. J Diabetes Sci Technol. 2009;3:903–13. https://doi.org/10.1177/193229680900300438.
25. Belazi MA, Galli TA, Drakoulakos D, Fleva A, Papanayiotou PH. Salivary alterations in insulin-dependent diabetes mellitus. Int J Paediatr Dent. 1998;8:29–33.
26. March WF, Mueller A, Herbrechtsmeier P. Clinical trial of a noninvasive contact lens glucose sensor. Diabetes Technol Ther. 2004;6:782–9. https://doi.org/10.1089/dia.2004.6.782.
27. Badugu R, Lakowicz JR, Geddes CD. A glucose-sensing contact lens: from bench top to patient. Curr Opin Biotechnol. 2005;16:100–7. https://doi.org/10.1016/j.copbio.2004.12.007.
28. Su H, Ma X, Yin J, Wang Y, He X, Bao Y, Zhou J, Jia W. Serum 1,5-anhydroglucitol levels slightly increase rather than decrease after a glucose load in subjects with different glucose tolerance status. Acta Diabetol. 2017;54:463–70. https://doi.org/10.1007/s00592-017-0968-z.

2 Introduction of Continuous Glucose Monitoring Technology

J. Y. Lu and Y. Bao

Glucose monitoring is an important part of diabetes management, from self-monitoring of fasting and postprandial 2-h blood glucose to continuous glucose monitoring (CGM). Other metrics for monitoring diabetes include glycated hemoglobin A_{1c} (HbA_{1c}) and glycated albumin (GA). Among these, self-monitoring of blood glucose (SMBG) is the basic form of glucose monitoring, whereas HbA_{1c} is a gold standard for assessing glycemic control. However, HbA_{1c} and SMBG have their own limitations. The HbA_{1c} reflects the mean blood glucose (MBG) level over the past 2–3 months. Thus, there is a "delayed effect" for assessing the efficacy of a treatment. Moreover, HbA_{1c} cannot accurately predict the risk of hypoglycemia, nor does it fully reflect the characteristics of blood glucose fluctuations. SMBG is unable to fully exhibit the blood glucose profile of a whole day. Therefore, in recent years, the development of CGM technology has become an important supplement to traditional glucose monitoring methods because of the limit on the amount of SMBG patients are willing to do. CGM is gradually being popularized and applied in clinical practice.

CGM identifies the glucose concentrations in subcutaneous interstitial fluid through a glucose sensor. It is able to provide continuous, comprehensive, and reliable all-day glucose profiles, thereby allowing for an understanding of trends in blood glucose fluctuations and the detection of occult hyperglycemia and hypoglycemia. Therefore, the main feature of CGM technology is that it indirectly reflects blood glucose levels by measuring interstitial fluid glucose concentrations with glucose sensors, in contrast with SMBG. The main characteristics of the two glucose monitoring methods are shown in Table 2.1.

2.1 Development of CGM Technology

The development of CGM has been largely dependent on the evolution of glucose sensors. For the sake of sensitivity, repeatability, and reliability, the vast majority of glucose sensors are designed based on an electrochemical principle that was first proposed by Clark and Lyons in 1962 [2]. Glucose oxidase (GOD) has a very high specificity for glucose. GOD has many advantages, including being easily accessible, inexpensive, and resistant to extreme temperature, pH values, and ionic strength. Moreover, the requirements for industrial production of GOD are minimal [3, 4]. Thus, it is the most widely used catalytic enzyme for the determination of glucose. All GOD-based glucose sensors work via the following chemical reactions: GOD catalyzes the oxidation of β-D-glucose to produce gluconic acid; concomitantly, oxygen is reduced

J. Y. Lu · Y. Bao (✉)
Department of Endocrinology and Metabolism, Shanghai Clinical Center for Diabetes, Shanghai Diabetes Institute, Shanghai Jiao Tong University Affiliated Sixth People's Hospital, Shanghai, China
e-mail: yqbao@sjtu.edu.cn

W. Jia (ed.), *Continuous Glucose Monitoring*, https://doi.org/10.1007/978-981-10-7074-7_2

Table 2.1 Comparison of the characteristics of SMBG and CGM [1]

	SMBG	CGM
Performance	• Glucose detection by disposable test strips	• Continuous 24-h monitoring through glucose senor
	• Some glucose analyzers have data storage function and glycemic data output function through the software	• Data are downloaded into a computer for qualitative and quantitative analysis of glycemic profiles
Features	• Reflects glucose value at a time point, like a "snapshot"	• Reflects continuous glycemic changes, like a "movie"
	• Sporadic glycemic data, partially reflecting the glycemic changes with diet, drugs, exercise, etc.	• Continuous glycemic data, fully reflecting the glycemic changes with diet, drugs, exercise, etc.
	• Retrospective analysis based on the output of glucose values	• Reflects the direction or speed of glucose changes and helps patients to understand the overall trends and individualized features of glucose changes
Measurement methods	• Measures blood glucose	• Measures glucose concentration in subcutaneous interstitial fluid to indirectly reflect blood glucose level
	• Uses test strips and a pricker, mostly at the fingertip or other sites	• Sensors are implanted in the subcutaneous tissue at the abdomen (mostly) or arm

to generate hydrogen peroxide (H_2O_2); the reaction process is accompanied by electron transfer between substances; and the amount of electron transfer is associated with the glucose concentration. Sensor-based methods for glucose detection are based on (1) measuring the consumption of oxygen, (2) measuring the quantity of H_2O_2 generation, and (3) measuring electron transfer between GOD and the electrode with redox mediators.

With the development of technology, the electrochemical glucose sensor has evolved to the third generation.

The first-generation glucose sensor: the concept of the sensor for measuring glucose levels was first proposed by Clark and Lyons in 1962 [2]. This glucose sensor was composed of a thin layer of GOD, an oxygen electrode, an inner oxygen semipermeable membrane, and an outer dialysis membrane. The change in the measured oxygen concentration was proportional to the glucose concentration. In 1967, Updike and Hicks [5] significantly simplified the electrochemical glucose assay by immobilizing and thereby stabilizing GOD in a polyacrylamide gel on the oxygen electrode and for the first time measured glucose concentration in biological fluids. The first commercial glucose sensor was introduced by Yellow Springs Instrument (YSI) for the direct measurement of glucose in 1975 and was based on the amperometric detection of H_2O_2. This analyzer was almost exclusively applied in clinical laboratories because of its high cost due to the expensive platinum electrode.

The second-generation glucose sensors: in the second-generation sensor, the oxidation process of the GOD is mediated by redox mediators. Oxygen is no longer involved in the enzymatic reaction; instead, redox mediators carry electrons from the GOD to the surface of the working electrode, generating an electric current with strength proportional to the glucose concentration. In 1984, Cass et al. [6] successfully used ferrocene as a redox mediator, which was a landmark event in the development of second-generation glucose sensors. The first electrochemical glucose analyzer for SMBG, the ExacTech blood glucose meter, was launched by Medisense Inc. in 1987 [7] and significantly improved the management of diabetes.

The third-generation glucose sensors: the third-generation glucose sensors are based on direct electron transfer between the GOD and the working electrode without redox mediators [8]. The evolution of this technology directly led to the development of an in vivo implantable CGM system.

In 1974, Albisser et al. [9] first put forward the idea of in vitro CGM in their artificial pancreas project. In 1982, Shichiri et al. [10] buried the glucose sensor in the subcutaneous area of a diabetic dog and connected it to an insulin pump, for the first time achieving in vivo CGM. The first subcutaneously implanted glucose sensor was introduced by MiniMed (Northridge, CA, USA, currently a subordinate of Medtronic) in 1999 and approved by the US Food and Drug Administration (FDA), initiating the clinical application of a CGM system. According to the placement of the glucose sensor and the transmitter that connects to the sensor, CGM systems are generally divided into minimally invasive and noninvasive. At present, the minimally invasive CGM systems are most commonly used, with a subcutaneously (mostly at the abdomen) implantable needle-type sensor measuring glucose concentrations in interstitial fluid, which can indirectly reflect the blood glucose level. The life span of implantable glucose sensors is 3–14 days. This device can display updated real-time glucose concentrations every 1–5 min and requires calibration by fingertip glucose levels for one to four times every day.

2.2 Technical Characteristics of CGM System

Several main CGM systems (Fig. 2.1) and their parameters and characteristics are listed as follows [11] (Table 2.2).

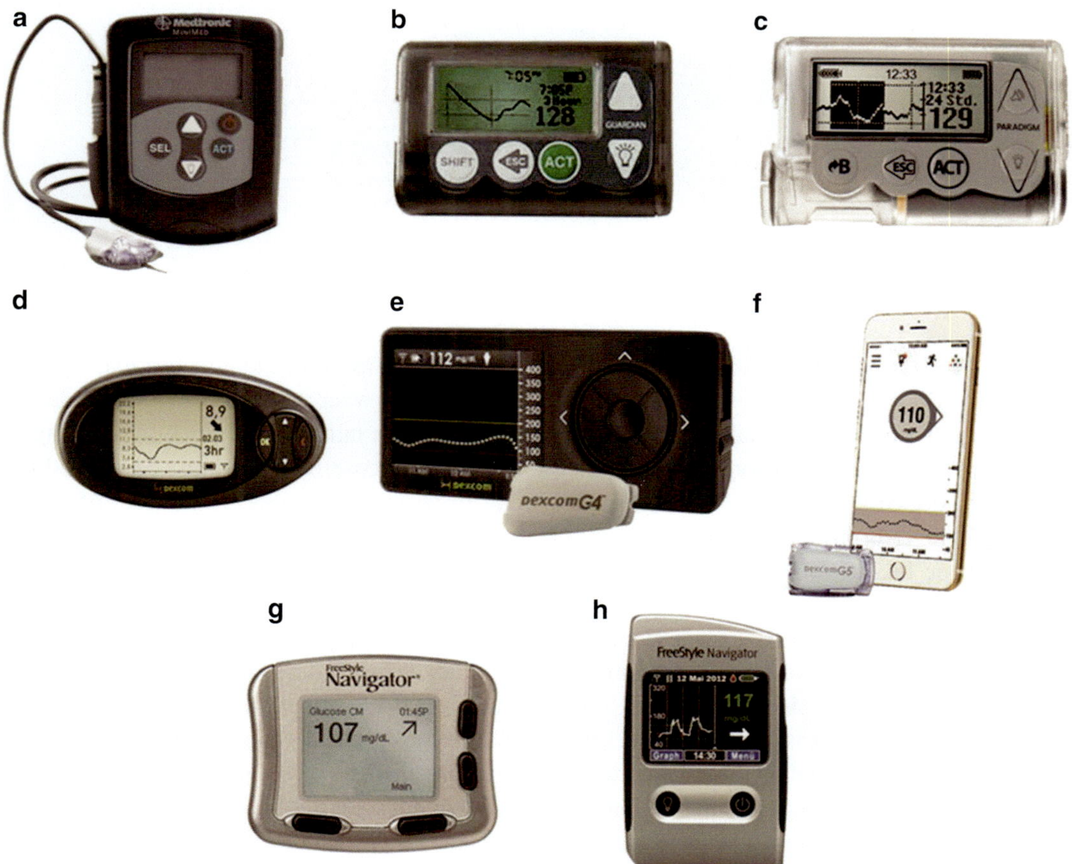

Fig. 2.1 The main CGM systems on the market. Notes: (**a**) Medtronic Inc. CGMS Gold; (**b**) Medtronic Inc. Guardian REAL-Time; (**c**) Medtronic Inc. Paradigm REAL-Time; (**d**) Dexcom SEVEN PLUS; (**e**) Dexcom G4 PLATINUM; (**f**) Dexcom G5 Mobile; (**g**) Abbott FreeStyle Navigator; (**h**) Abbott FreeStyle Navigator II

Table 2.2 Technical characteristics of common CGM systems on the market [11]

Parameters	CGMS Gold	Guardian REAL-Time	SEVEN Plus	G4 Platinum	FreeStyle Navigator	FreeStyle Navigator II
Time to market (year)	2003	2009	2009	2012	2008	2011
Life span of glucose sensor (h)	72	72	128	128	120	120
Initialization time (h)	2	2	2	2	10	10
Detection frequency (min)	5	5	5	5	1	1
Frequency of calibration required (times)	12	12	16	16	4	4
Retrospective or real time	Retrospective	Real time	Real time	Real time	Real time	Real time
High/low glucose alarm	No	Yes	Yes	Yes	Yes	Yes
Predictive alert feature	No	Yes	Yes	Yes	Yes	Yes
Integration with insulin pump	No	Yes	No	Yes	No	No

Reprint with permission from International Journal of Endocrinology and Metabolism

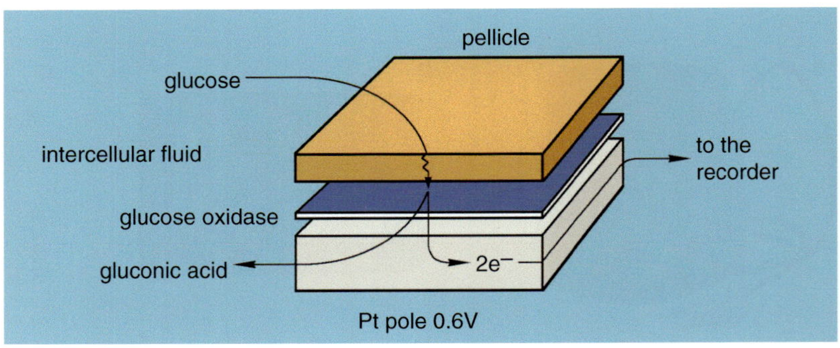

Fig. 2.2 The monitoring principle of CGM technology

2.2.1 Medtronic Inc.

In 1999, the first commercialized subcutaneously implanted glucose sensor, or the so-called retrospective CGM system, was introduced by MiniMed Inc. (Northridge, CA, USA, acquired by Medtronic Inc. in 2001). Its upgraded product, CGMS Gold, was approved in 2003. The CGM system consists of a glucose sensor, a cable, a glucose recorder, an information extractor, and an analysis software and other components. The sensor is composed of a semipermeable membrane, GOD, and a microelectrode, on which a chemical reaction is initiated with interstitial fluid glucose to generate electrical signals upon subcutaneous implantation at the umbilical level (Fig. 2.2). The recorder receives electrical signal every 10 s through the cable and converts it into a glucose value every 5 min for up to 288 glucose readings per day. Subjects wear the recorder for 72 h; during which time, a minimum of three to four fingertip blood glucose readings must be entered per day in order to calibrate the device. Also, the events that may affect the blood glucose fluctuations, such as meal intake, exercise, hypoglycemic agents, and hypoglycemic episodes, are recorded in a logbook for entry into the system's software. After 3 days, the data can be downloaded to a computer by a data extractor and analyzed by special analysis software; thus the dynamic changes of blood glucose over 3 consecutive days are obtained. The accurate glycemic data are presented in the form of graphs, pie charts, and tables, combined with the marked events that affect the changes in blood glucose, quantitatively and qualitatively reflecting the glycemic characteristics of the subjects.

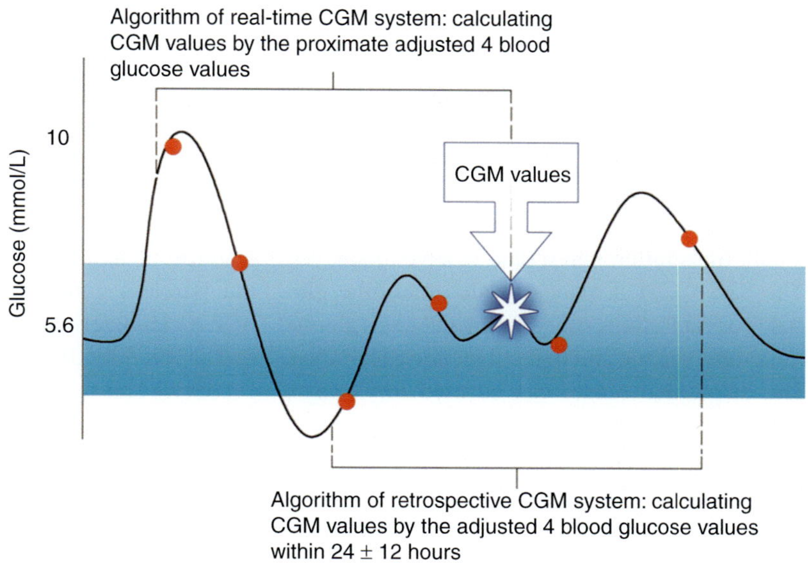

Fig. 2.3 The different CGM glucose values calculated by a retrospective algorithm and a real-time algorithm

In 2011, a new generation of retrospective iPro2 system came onto the market and was approved to enter the Chinese market by the China Food and Drug Administration (CFDA) in 2015. The iPro2 system has advantages of small size, easy to wear, concealed carry, simple operation, higher accuracy, and high-speed data loading via USB, as compared with other retrospective CGM system. However, iPro2 still needs calibration two to four times a day.

In 2004, Medtronic launched the Guardian CGM system, which has been approved by the US FDA. In contrast to CGMS Gold, the biggest advantage of the Guardian CGM system is the integration of the alarm function for hyperglycemia and hypoglycemia. The Guardian REAL-Time CGM System was approved by the US FDA in 2005, and the updated version of Guardian REAL-Time CGM was approved in 2009 and formally entered the Chinese market in 2013. The data transmitter and receiver are connected wirelessly. In addition to the alarm function, the Guardian REAL-Time CGM integrates real-time display function, which can present glucose curves at 3, 6, 12, and 24 h. In addition, another important advantage of this system is its predictive alert feature for hyperglycemia or hypoglycemia (up to 30 min in advance), by the indication of the number of upper and lower arrows, which suggests the trend and speed of blood glucose changes. The start-up initialization is 2 h and requires calibrations with blood glucose values at the second and eighth hours after installation and at every 12 h thereafter. It is worth noting that, due to the real-time display feature, the algorithm for the real-time CGM system is different from that of the retrospective CGM system (Fig. 2.3).

In 2006, Medtronic launched the Paradigm REAL-Time dynamic insulin pump system and, for the first time, achieved integration of real-time CGM and an insulin pump. Since then, Medtronic has introduced the Paradigm Veo system, which automatically suspends insulin infusion while glucose is below the preset value. In September 2016, the FDA approved the MiniMed 670G system, the world's first semiautomatic, closed-loop CGM-insulin pump system certified by the US FDA. This semiautomatic system automatically adjusts insulin basal rates every 5 min based on real-time CGM measurements; however, it still requires a manual bolus of insulin to be administered before meals. This system is applicable to type 1 diabetes patients aged 14 years old and above. Patients using the MiniMed 670G must calibrate the sensor at least every 12 h, change the glucose sensor weekly, and refill the insulin reservoir every 3 days.

2.2.2 Dexcom Inc.

The STS CGM system was developed by Dexcom Inc. (San Diego, CA, USA) and approved by the US FDA in 2006 as the first generation of the commercial Dexcom CGM system. It consists of a glucose sensor, a sensor introducer needle, a data transmitter, and a data receiver/displayer. The STS CGM displays updated real-time glucose concentrations every 5 min and gives alarms for hypoglycemic and hyperglycemic excursions. The disposable sensor can be used for 3 days, with an initialization time of 2 h.

SEVEN is the second-generation Dexcom CGM system to be approved by the US FDA for up to 7 days of continual use. This improvement diminishes the frequency of sensor replacement and resultantly reduces the economic burden on patients as well as the discomfort caused by the replacement of the glucose sensor. SEVEN PLUS is an upgraded version, and it integrates a predictive alert feature.

In 2012, Dexcom Inc. introduced the G4 PLATINUM system whose monitoring accuracy was increased by 20% and weight was reduced by about 30% compared with the SEVEN PLUS system. The glucose sensor, transmitter, and receiver are smaller; the diameter of the glucose sensor is similar to that of a hair. The maximum distance between the transmitter and receiver in wireless communication is up to 6 m. In the initial 30 min after the initialization, it requires two calibrations with a fingertip glucose value and recalibration every 12 h thereafter.

In 2015, Dexcom released its latest product, the G5 Mobile system. The biggest feature of this system is the use of a corresponding application on smartphone as the data receiver, and the monitoring results can be shared with others, thus greatly simplifying the operation of CGM.

2.2.3 Abbott Inc.

The FreeStyle Navigator is the first-generation CGM system produced by Abbott Inc. (Alameda, CA, USA), which was launched in 2008. The system detects glucose once every minute and updates in real time. The life span of the implantable glucose sensors is 5 days, and the measured range is 1.1–19.4 mmol/L (20–350 mg/dL). It requires four calibrations with fingertip glucose values (10, 12, 24, and 72 h after installation). The data transmitter is waterproof and connected to the data receiver via wireless communication. In addition, one of the characteristics of FreeStyle Navigator is that it can directly detect fingertip glucose with FreeStyle Lite test strips, making the calibration of glucose convenient. The system also has predictive alerts within 30 min before reaching a low or high glucose alarm. Unlike the Guardian RT, the FreeStyle Navigator does not display the speed of glucose changes by the number of upper and lower arrows. It displays only one arrow, a horizontal arrow representing the rate of glucose change <1 mg/(dL•min); an upward or downward arrow represents the rate >2 mg/(dL•min), and an inclined arrow indicates that the rate of glucose change is between 1 and 2 mg/(dL•min). It should be noted that after the system is attached, a 10-h start-up initialization period is required (although improvement has been made to reduce to 1 h in some updated version); in contrast, other similar products typically take only 2 h for glucose sensor initialization.

The FreeStyle Navigator II is the second-generation CGM product from Abbott Inc. It is designed to offer improved volume, weight, comfort, and functionality, compared with the first-generation CGM. One of the key features of the FreeStyle Navigator II is that the system is unaffected by daily activities. The user can swim, bathe, or even exercise when wearing it. The maximum distance between the transmitter and receiver in wireless communication is up to 30 m, which is very convenient for use and facilitates adherence.

In September 2016, the US FDA approved the Abbott Libre Pro Professional CGM system. It is a retrospective CGM, with a glucose sensor designed for wear for up to 14 days, during which glucose calibration is not necessary.

References

1. Chinese Diabetes Society. Chinese clinical guideline for continuous glucose monitoring (2012). Chin J Diabetes Mellitus. 2012;4:582–90. https://doi.org/10.3760/cma.j.issn.1674-5809.2012.10.003.
2. Clark LC Jr, Lyons C. Electrode systems for continuous monitoring in cardiovascular surgery. Ann N Y Acad Sci. 1962;102:29–45.
3. Bankar SB, Bule MV, Singhal RS, Ananthanarayan L. Glucose oxidase–an overview. Biotechnol Adv. 2009;27:489–501. https://doi.org/10.1016/j.biotechadv.2009.04.003.
4. Heller A, Feldman B. Electrochemical glucose sensors and their applications in diabetes management. Chem Rev. 2008;108:2482–505. https://doi.org/10.1021/cr068069y.
5. Updike SJ, Hicks GP. The enzyme electrode. Nature. 1967;214:986–8.
6. Cass AE, Davis G, Francis GD, Hill HA, Aston WJ, Higgins IJ, Plotkin EV, Scott LD, Turner AP. Ferrocene-mediated enzyme electrode for amperometric determination of glucose. Anal Chem. 1984;56:667–71.
7. Matthews DR, Holman RR, Bown E, Steemson J, Watson A, Hughes S, Scott D. Pen-sized digital 30-second blood glucose meter. Lancet. 1987;1:778–9.
8. Palmisano F, Zambonin PG, Centonze D, Quinto M. A disposable, reagentless, third-generation glucose biosensor based on overoxidized poly (pyrrole) /tetrathiafulvalene–tetracyanoquinodimethane composite. Anal Chem. 2002;74:5913–8.
9. Albisser AM, Leibel BS, Ewart TG, Davidovac Z, Botz CK, Zingg W, Schipper H, Gander R. Clinical control of diabetes by the artificial pancreas. Diabetes. 1974;23:397–404.
10. Shichiri M, Kawamori R, Yamasaki Y, Hakui N, Abe H. Wearable artificial endocrine pancreas with needle-type glucose sensor. Lancet. 1982;2:1129–31.
11. Liu XF, Liu C. Comparison of several common continuous glucose monitoring systems. Int J Endocrinol Metab. 2009;29:197–200. https://doi.org/10.3760/cma.j.issn.1673-4157.2009.03.015.

3 Accuracy Assessment of Continuous Glucose Monitoring Technology

J. Zhou and W. Jia

Continuous glucose monitoring (CGM) has gradually been applied in clinical practice in recent years. CGM continuously monitors the glucose concentrations in subcutaneous interstitial fluid through a glucose sensor. It can detect occult hyperglycemia, hypoglycemia, and the trends in glycemic changes that cannot be routinely detected by self-monitoring of blood glucose (SMBG), thereby more comprehensively reflecting the characteristics of glycemic fluctuations. Only when CGM measurements truly reflect the glycemic level of a patient can it guide decisions on treatment to achieve better glycemic control. Therefore, the accuracy of CGM is of great importance in diabetes management. This chapter introduces the methods used for assessing the accuracy of CGM technology in clinical practice.

3.1 Accuracy Assessment Methods Commonly Used in Clinical Practice

Accuracy assessment includes both data accuracy and clinical accuracy. Data accuracy refers to the consistency of the measured data with the matching reference data. At present, the accuracy assessment methods for SMBG data commonly include linear regression and correlation coefficient method, International Organization for Standardization (ISO) accuracy standards, and absolute and relative differences. Among these, the linear regression and correlation coefficient methods are widely used as tools for accuracy evaluation. However, this method ignores the systematic error between the two inspection methods. When two methods are used to detect the same sample, even if the correlation is very high, the possibility of detection error between the two methods cannot be ruled out. In other words, two methods with a high correlation cannot be alternately used in clinical practice.

Clinical accuracy refers to the accuracy of medical decisions made based on test results. The high consistency between two test results leads to the right clinical decision and vice versa. The Clarke error grid analysis was originally developed for clinical accuracy of SMBG [1]. The Clarke error grid is divided into five zones (A, B, C, D, and E) with the reference blood glucose value [usually Yellow Springs Instrument (YSI) values] as the abscissa and CGM measurements as the ordinates (Fig. 3.1) [2]. The clinical significance of each zone is as follows: region A includes those values within 20% of the reference sensor [usually against Yellow Springs Instrument (YSI)], indicating that the CGM measurements have no effect on clinical decision and thus meet the analytical accuracy requirements. Region B

J. Zhou · W. Jia (✉)
Department of Endocrinology and Metabolism, Shanghai Clinical Center for Diabetes, Shanghai Diabetes Institute, Shanghai Jiao Tong University Affiliated Sixth People's Hospital, Shanghai, China
e-mail: wpjia@sjtu.edu.cn

W. Jia (ed.), *Continuous Glucose Monitoring*, https://doi.org/10.1007/978-981-10-7074-7_3

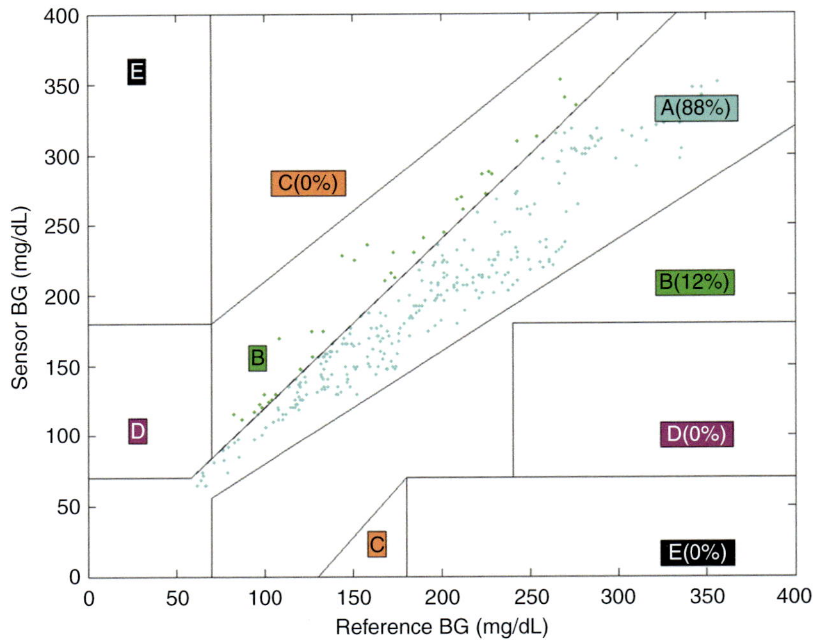

Fig. 3.1 Clarke error grid analysis of paired YSI–retrospective CGM data

contains values that deviate from the reference by >20%, but altered clinical actions have little or no effect on clinical outcome or would not lead to inappropriate treatment. Region C contains those values that deviate from the reference by >20%, and changes in clinical behaviors are likely to affect clinical outcomes; that is to say, the test results are biased and lead to unnecessary or wrong treatment. Region D includes those values indicating a potentially dangerous failure to detect hypoglycemia or hyperglycemia or to achieve target glycemic goal, and changes in clinical decision will be at major risk of medical malpractice. Region E contains those measurements that indicate serious risk of clinical consequences. The higher the percentage of results in regions A and B, the more clinically accurate the test is.

3.2 Accuracy Assessment Methods for CGM Technology

Compared with SMBG, CGM can not only offer immediate glucose values but, more importantly, can reflect the changes in blood glucose along a timeline. To this end, the use of traditional methods alone, such as correlation analysis, cannot fully evaluate the CGM glucose measurements (rate accuracy, the direction of glucose changes, delay effect, etc.). Therefore, researchers have developed new accuracy assessment methods to evaluate CGM results, including consensus error grid analysis and continuous error grid analysis.

The consensus error grid analysis [3], so-called because it represents the consensus opinion about risk from 100 diabetes experts, is similar to the Clarke error grid analysis; however, its distribution of risk zone looks fan-shaped, radiating from the 45° line with increasing risk. Thus, this pattern contains no discontinuities in risk categories. The risk categories, in order of increasing severity, were defined as follows: zone A, no effect on clinical action; zone B, altered clinical action but little or no effect on clinical outcome; zone C, altered clinical action likely to effect clinical outcome; zone D, altered clinical action could have significant medical risk; and zone E, altered clinical action could have dangerous consequences. Previously, we evaluated the point and trend accuracy of a retrospective CGM system against YSI glucose measurements in 11 patients with type 2 diabetes mellitus by frequent venous blood sampling. The results of consensus error grid analysis are shown in Fig. 3.2 [2]. The results showed that 100% of paired YSI–CGM data fell in zones A and B (96.2% in zone A, 3.8% in zone B). Further analysis showed that the accuracy of the CGM system varied with blood glucose range: more than 96% of paired values fell within zone A when glucose >6.6 mmol/L, and 100% and 89.7% of values fell within zone A when glucose concentrations were 2.2–4.4 mmol/L and 4.4–6.6 mmol/L, respectively (Table 3.1).

Continuous glucose-error grid analysis (CG-EGA) is a new method for clinical evaluation of CGM system established by Kovatchev et al. [4] in 2004 based on traditional error grid analysis. It evaluates the accuracy of CGM measurements in terms of both point glucose values and trends in glucose changes (speed and direction). The CG-EGA combines point and rate accuracy separately for each of the three critical blood glucose ranges: hypoglycemia (blood glucose ≤3.9 mmol/L), euglycemia (3.9 mmol/L < blood glucose ≤10 mmol/L), and hyperglycemia (glucose >10 mmol/L) using distinct matrices of point versus rate accuracy. These matrices reflect the relative importance of point versus rate accuracy in different clinical situations. In summary, the metrics of CGM accuracy can be classified into

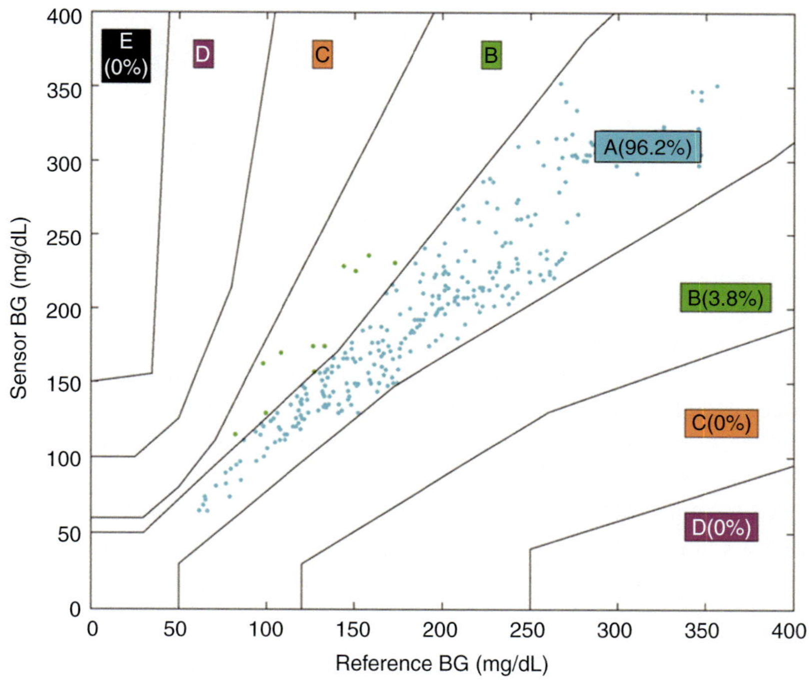

Fig. 3.2 Consensus error grid analysis of paired YSI–retrospective CGM data ($n = 319$) [2] (Reprint with permission from Chinese Journal of Diabetes Mellitus)

Table 3.1 Consensus error grid analysis of paired YSI–retrospective CGM data at different glycemic ranges [number of pairs (%)] [2]

	YSI value				
	Total	2.2–4.4 mmol/L	>4.4–6.6 mmol/L	>6.6–13.3 mmol/L	>13.3–22.2 mmol/L
A + B	319 (100.0)	10 (100.0)	39 (100.0)	199 (100.0)	71 (100.0)
A	307 (96.2)	10 (100.0)	35 (89.7)	191 (96.0)	71 (100.0)
B	12 (3.8)	0 (0.0)	4 (10.3)	8 (4.0)	0 (0.0)
C	0 (0.0)	0 (0.0)	0 (0.0)	0 (0.0)	0 (0.0)
D	0 (0.0)	0 (0.0)	0 (0.0)	0 (0.0)	0 (0.0)
E	0 (0.0)	0 (0.0)	0 (0.0)	0 (0.0)	0 (0.0)
Total	319 (100.0)	10 (3.1)	39 (12.2)	199 (62.4)	71 (22.3)

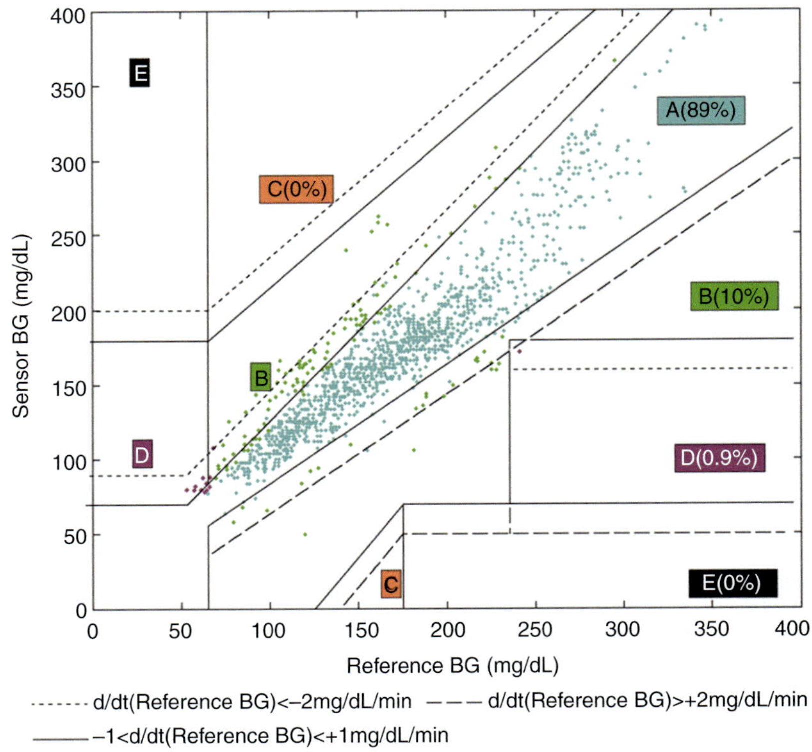

Fig. 3.3 Continuous glucose-error grid analysis of paired YSI–real-time CGM data ($n = 1317$) [5] (Reprint with permission from Diabetes Technology & Therapeutics)

a 2 × 2 (numerical-clinical) × (point-rate) accuracy table. The higher the percentage of results in zones A and B, the more clinically accurate the glucose system is. We conducted a multicenter study to evaluate the accuracy of a real-time CGM system. The CG-EGA showed that 99% of paired YSI–sensor values fell in zones A and B (89% in zone A, 10% in zone B) (Fig. 3.3). In addition, the analysis based on the rate of change in blood glucose showed that 96.9% of paired YSI–sensor values fell in zones A and B (90% in zone A, 6.9% in zone B) (Fig. 3.4) [5].

3.3 Accuracy Assessment of CGM Monitoring Results

The accuracy of CGM results should be assessed prior to data analysis. Only when the sensor glucose values are confirmed to be valid can they be used to guide the treatment of patients. At present, for different CGM instruments, the accuracy assessments of monitoring results are different. For the Medtronic retrospective CGM system, clinicians can use the analysis software to evaluate the accuracy of glucose sensor data. The criteria for "optimal accuracy" are:

1. At least three paired sensor glucose and meter glucose values and a correlation coefficient between the paired sensor glucose and meter glucose values ≥0.79.
2. When the range (maximum to minimum) of meter glucose values is ≥5.6 mmol/L, the mean absolute relative difference (MAD) is ≤28%.
3. When the range of meter glucose values is <5.6 mmol/L, the MAD is ≤18%; at that time, the correlation coefficient (R value) between the paired sensor glucose and meter glucose values is presented in the form of "n/a."

If the CGM glucose measurements fail to meet the above "optimal accuracy" criteria, this will be presented in the final report. Therefore, clinicians need to adjust hypoglycemic regimen according to clinical judgment.

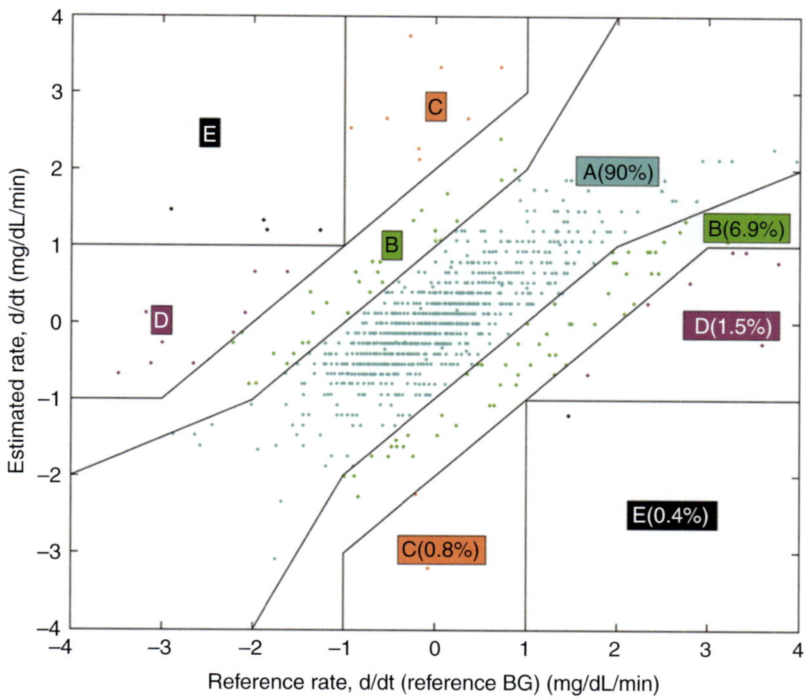

Fig. 3.4 Continuous glucose-error grid analysis of paired YSI–real-time CGM data: rate accuracy ($n = 1317$) [5]

3.4 Factors Affecting the Accuracy of CGM Measurements

Various factors can affect the accuracy of CGM measurements. The accuracy of CGM largely relies on the technical level of the sensor as well as the CGM algorithm. The retrospective CGM system adopts a retrospective algorithm. The biggest difference between the retrospective algorithm and real-time algorithm is that the retrospective algorithm can correct the CGM values for a specific period of time according to the trend of all original data when calculating CGM results. Therefore, the accuracy of a retrospective CGM system is generally higher than that of a real-time CGM system. In addition, the common influencing factors include:

1. The life span of the sensor. The accuracy is significantly decreased if the sensor is not exchanged in a timely manner.
2. CGM sensor glucose values are commonly calibrated using SMBG glucose values. Thus, any factor affecting the detection of SMBG values can also affect the accuracy of CGM.
3. If the user incorrectly enters blood glucose value for calibration, one way to approach this question is to reenter the correct calibration blood glucose value as soon as possible. For the Medtronic retrospective CGM system, if the user enters calibration blood glucose values twice within 10 min, the device automatically ignores the first input and takes the second input value for calibration.
4. During periods of dramatic glycemic fluctuations (such as the use of drugs that affect blood glucose, consumption of a sweet beverage or snack, excessive exercise, hypoglycemia, etc.), calibration with the blood glucose value may affect the accuracy of CGM. It is therefore advisable not to enter a calibration blood glucose value during a time when the blood glucose changes rapidly.
5. Delayed input of calibration blood glucose value should be avoided.
6. The interstitial fluid glucose level physiologically lags behind the plasma glucose level,

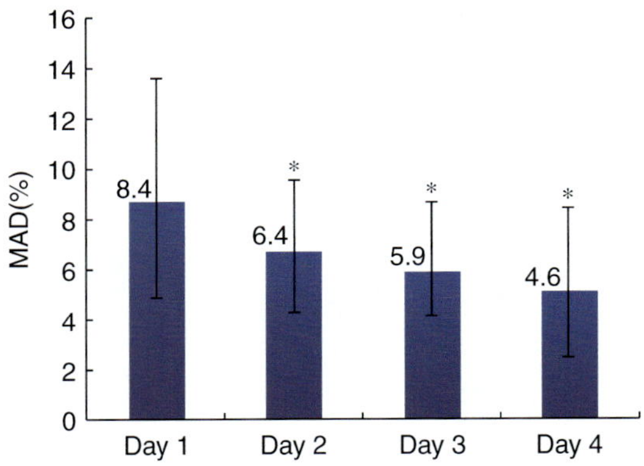

Fig. 3.5 Comparison of MAD values for daily CGM results in 530 patients with type 2 diabetes mellitus. $*P < 0.05$ vs. intragroup MAD value at previous day [6] (Reprint with permission from West China Medical Journal)

especially when the blood glucose changes rapidly. Calibration with a blood glucose value at the time immediately after initialization completion, that is, when the electron signals are unstable and the glycemic readings fluctuate sharply, will result in CGM sensor glucose measurements obviously lagging behind actual glucose levels.

We reviewed the retrospective CGM data of 530 patients with type 2 diabetes and evaluated the accuracy of CGM results using MAD [6]. The results showed that the MAD value decreased gradually with prolonged monitoring, suggesting that the accuracy of CGM gradually increased (Fig. 3.5). In addition, the MAD value in the intensive insulin therapy group was higher than that in the oral medication group, suggesting that the accuracy of CGM might also be associated with the hypoglycemic regimen, probably due to an increased glycemic variability in patients with intensive insulin therapy, which has a certain impact on accuracy.

Statement on Consent for Participation

All the clinical trials carried out by the authors in this book have been reported to the Ethics Committee of Shanghai Jiao Tong University Affiliated Sixth People's Hospital already and were in accordance with the Good Clinical Practice and Standards of China Association for Ethical Studies (approval number: 2007-45).

References

1. Clarke WL, Cox D, Gonder-Frederick LA, Carter W, Pohl SL. Evaluating clinical accuracy of systems for self-monitoring of blood glucose. Diabetes Care. 1987;10:622–8.
2. Zhou J, Bao YQ, Ma XJ, Lu W, Hao YP, Zhou M, Mo YF, Hu C, Xiang KS, Jia WP. Accuracy assessment of continuous glucose monitoring by frequent venous blood collection in patients with type 2 diabetes mellitus. Chin J Diabetes Mellit. 2012;4:523–8. https://doi.org/10.3760/cma.j.issn.1674-5809.2012.09.004.
3. Parkes JL, Slatin SL, Pardo S, Ginsberg BH. A new consensus error grid to evaluate the clinical significance of inaccuracies in the measurement of blood glucose. Diabetes Care. 2000;23:1143–8.
4. Kovatchev BP, Gonder-Frederick LA, Cox DJ, Clarke WL. Evaluating the accuracy of continuous glucose-monitoring sensors: continuous glucose-error grid analysis illustrated by TheraSense Freestyle Navigator data. Diabetes Care. 2004;27:1922–8.
5. Zhou J, Lv X, Mu Y, Wang X, Li J, Zhang X, Wu J, Bao Y, Jia W. The accuracy and efficacy of real-time continuous glucose monitoring sensor in Chinese diabetes patients: a multicenter study. Diabetes Technol Ther. 2012;14:710–8. https://doi.org/10.1089/dia.2012.0014.
6. Lu W, Zhou J, Ma XJ, Pan JM, Zhu W, Lu FD, Bao YQ, Jia WP. Assessment of the accuracy of continuous glucose monitoring and its correlated factor. West China Med J. 2011;26:811–4.

4 Operation Standards for Continuous Glucose Monitoring

W. Lu and Y. Bao

4.1 Operation Specifications for Medtronic CGM Systems

Medtronic CGM Systems are usually classified to retrospective CGMS (for example, CGM Gold, iPro2) and real-time CGMS (for example, Guardian REAL-Time, Medtronic Paradigm 722 insulin pump system) (Fig. 4.1). Take iPro2 system as an example, performing CGM on a patient usually includes these steps: patient selection, arrangement of follow-up visits, sensor insertion, data recording, data upload, and interpretation of the report (Fig. 4.2). Both medical practitioners and patients will work together to make the best use of the CGMS.

4.2 Sensor Implantation Site

The selection of the sensor implantation site is a prerequisite for successful implantation of the continuous glucose monitoring (CGM) sensor. For adults with diabetes, the CGM sensor is usually inserted into the subcutaneous fat tissue in the lower abdomen. The sensor should not be implanted at sites for insulin injection or insulin pump infusion or at areas within 5 cm around the umbilicus. Patients also should avoid tight or restrictive clothing that may cause friction at the implantation site. Sites with scar or atrophy tissues or sites that move violently during exercise or activity are not suitable for sensor implantation. However, for children with type 1 diabetes, considering the need for long-term injection of insulin in the abdomen and to prevent accidental removal of sensor by children, the recommended implantation site for the sensor is the upper outside aspect of the hip, that is, the muscle injection site, where CGM is least affected by sleep and exercise [1, 2] (Fig. 4.3).

4.3 Implantation of Glucose Sensor

It is important to avoid exerting pressure on the implantation site during sensor implantation. The implantation procedure is as follows: (1) place the sensor in the sensor inserter and set the sensor inserter leg against the skin at a 45° angle; (2) place the forefinger and middle finger of one hand on the sensor inserter leg to maintain it at a correct angle; (3) press the white button on the sensor inserter and implant the sensor; (4) check that the sensor has been inserted properly through the skin; (5) hold the sensor in place and gently slide

W. Lu · Y. Bao (✉)
Department of Endocrinology and Metabolism, Shanghai Clinical Center for Diabetes, Shanghai Diabetes Institute, Shanghai Jiao Tong University Affiliated Sixth People's Hospital, Shanghai, China
e-mail: yqbao@sjtu.edu.cn

W. Jia (ed.), *Continuous Glucose Monitoring*, https://doi.org/10.1007/978-981-10-7074-7_4

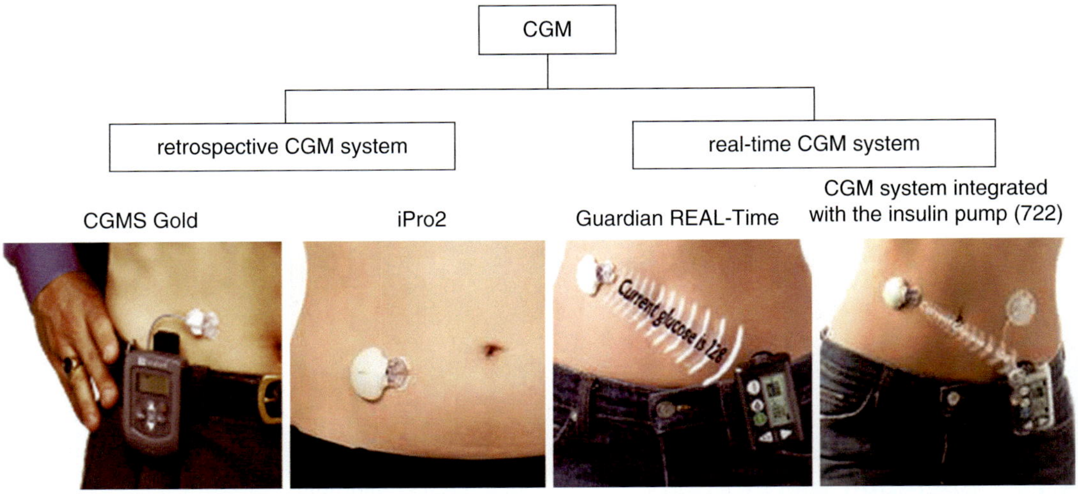

Fig. 4.1 Classification of Medtronic's CGM systems

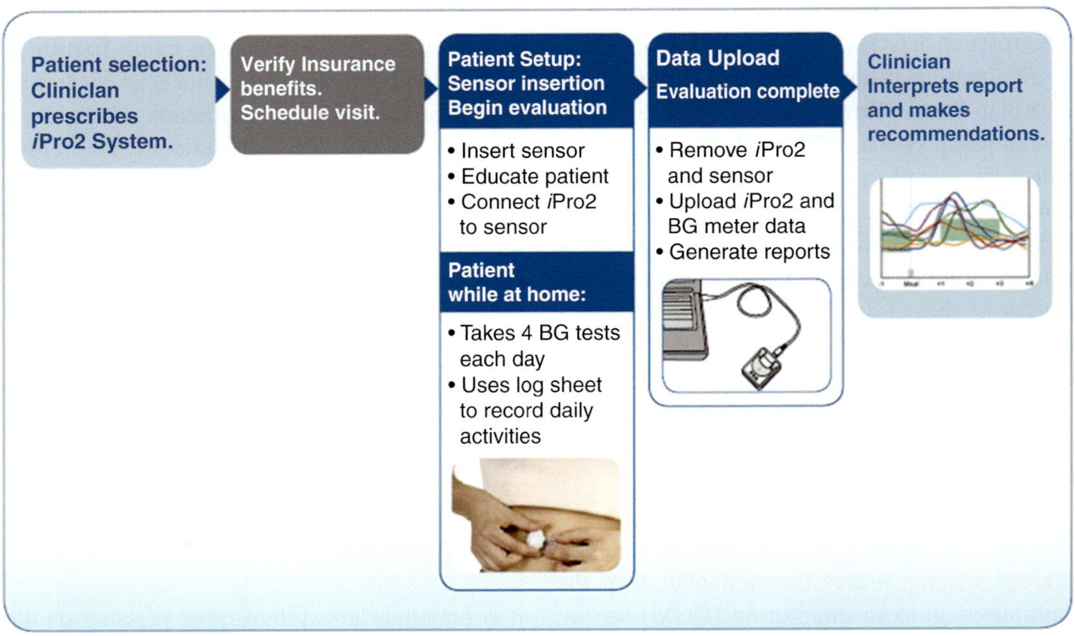

Fig. 4.2 Steps with the iPro2 System

the inserter away from the sensor; (6) remove the paper from the adhesive pad; (7) hold the sensor with two fingers on its base and gently remove the introducer needle at a 45° angle, avoiding rotation of the introducer needle; (8) dispose the introducer needle into a sharps container; and (9) check for redness, bleeding, pain, tenderness, etc. If bleeding occurs, the sensor does not have to be removed; just apply pressure to stop bleeding by using a piece of gauze dressing.

4.4 Sensor Initialization and Calibration

Initialization should be allowed for 60–120 min between implantation of the sensor and the first blood glucose measurement. During this period, the sensor is fixed in subcutaneous tissue, and it is gradually infiltrated with surrounding interstitial fluid, so that it can respond to glucose level in the interstitial fluid. The retrospective CGM sensor

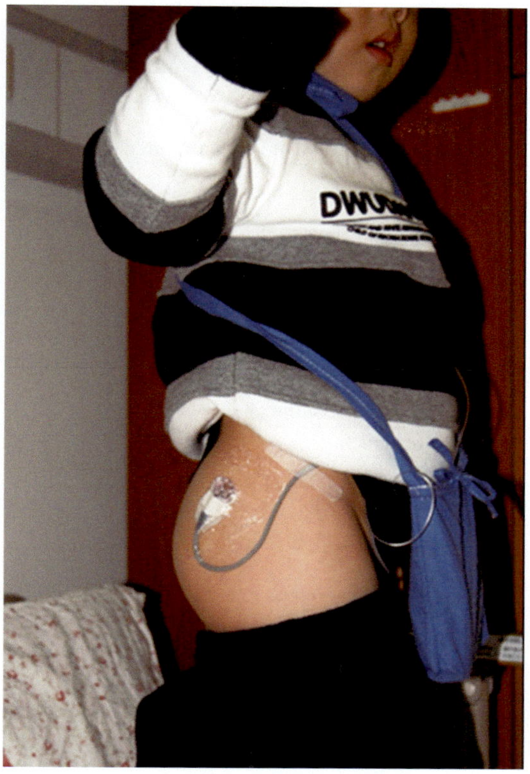

Fig. 4.3 The recommended sensor implantation site for children with type 1 diabetes

has 1-h period of initialization, and the real-time CGM sensor has 2-h period of initialization. Some sensors may even require a longer initialization duration. Only a new sensor needs initialization, and a sensor must not be initialized repeatedly. Abdominal obesity patients are sometimes prone to present a low electrical current signal after implantation of a sensor. Instead of immediate initialization, the user can hold the sensor with his/her fingers and gently press and rub the sensor to make full contact with the subcutaneous tissue fluid, until a stable signal is achieved.

Calibration of the sensor three to four times a day is recommended, with an interval of no more than 12 h; otherwise, the glucose monitoring is interrupted (Fig. 4.4). Typically, the best times to calibrate are before meals and before bedtime when glucose levels are stable. Calibration immediately after exercise, within 2–3 h after meals or within 1.5–2 h after infusion of high-dose insulin, should all be avoided. In the case of real-time CGM, the sensor should be calibrated at 2 h after sensor implantation, at 6 h after the first calibration, and then at least once every 12 h thereafter. It is also recommended that the sensor should be

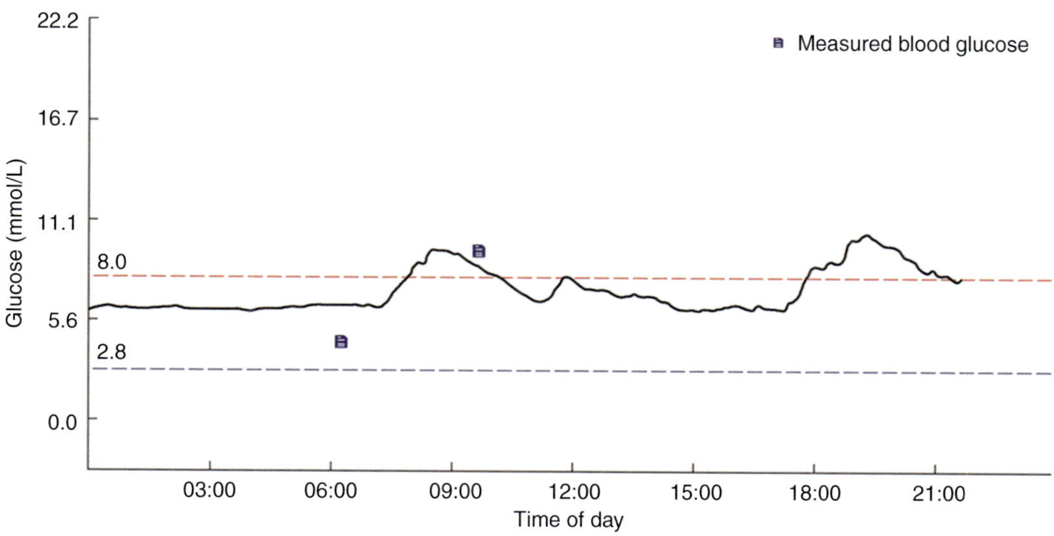

Fig. 4.4 Interrupted retrospective CGM caused by failure to enter a meter glucose value for calibration over a 12-h period

Table 4.1 Implantation and calibration of Medtronic real-time CGM sensor

	Events	Suggestions
Program 1: Implantation of sensor in the morning		
The 1st day		
08:30 a.m.	Implant sensor, inform precautions	Sensor infiltration more than 15 min
09:00 a.m.	Connect to the transmitter, green light flashes	
11:00 a.m.	The 1st calibration	Calibration after display [METER BG NOW] before lunch
05:00 p.m.	The 2nd calibration	Before dinner
10:00 p.m.	The 3rd calibration	Before bedtime
The 2nd–3rd day		
07:00 a.m.	The 1st calibration Download data and generate report	Before breakfast Complete before the rounds
11:00 a.m.	The 2nd calibration	Before lunch
05:00 p.m.	The 3rd calibration	Before dinner
10:00 p.m.	The 4th calibration	Before bedtime
Program 2: Implantation of sensor in the afternoon		
The 1st day		
02:00 p.m.	Implant sensor, inform precautions	Sensor infiltration more than 15 min
02:30 p.m.	Connect to the transmitter, green light flashes	
04:30 p.m.	The 1st calibration	Calibration after display [METER BG NOW] before dinner
10:00 p.m.	The 2nd calibration	Before bedtime
The 2nd–3rd day		
07:00 a.m.	The 1st calibration Download data and generate report	Before breakfast Complete before the rounds
11:00 a.m.	The 2nd calibration	Before lunch
05:00 p.m.	The 3rd calibration	Before dinner
10:00 p.m.	The 4th calibration	Before bedtime

calibrated during times when glucose levels are stable and there are no “arrows” shown on the display (Table 4.1).

4.5 Troubleshooting

For the continuous electrical current signal (ISIG, acronym for interstitial signal, i.e., the electrical current) and the sensor voltage (VCTR), the current signal transmitted by the sensor to the glucose recorder can be viewed on the ISIG display. When the sensor works normally, the ISIG value ranges from about 10 to 200 nA, and the VCTR value is approximately 0.4–1.6 V. When the ISIG value drops below 1.0 nA, a DISCONNECT alarm appears. After calibration with a fingerstick glucose value, if the ratio of glucose measurements divided by the ISIG exceeds 1.5–15.0, a calibration error (CAL ERR) alarm appears (Table 4.2).

We have analyzed the CGM alarms in 2171 cases of diabetes patients wearing a retrospective CGM (CGM Gold) and found that CAL ERR alarm is the most common type of alarm (11.0%), with others being less common, for example, 1.4% disconnection alarms, 5 cases of high voltage alarms, and 1 case of a low battery power alarm. Incorrect selection of the implantation site and improper preservation or use of the sensor are main causes that lead to unstable current signal and calibration error alarms [3]. CGM sensors should be stored in the refrigerator at 2–10 °C; otherwise sensor ineffectiveness or inaccuracy of blood glucose monitoring results could occur. The sensor

Table 4.2 Alarm message for Medtronic real-time CGM (Paradigm 722) insulin pump system

Display	Causes	Solutions
8:35A METER BG NOW Sensor reading invalid Enter meter BG now ESC, ACT to clear	A calibration is needed to receive sensor glucose readings	Enter a meter blood glucose now
1:05P METER BG BY 7:23 p This is a reminder to enter meter BG soon ESC, ACT to clear	A calibration reminder to enter a meter blood glucose at a set time point	Enter a meter blood glucose to eliminate [METER BG NOW] alarm
11:17A HIGH 200 MG/DL Glucose is higher than user specified limit ESC, ACT to clear	Sensor glucose value is equal to or higher than user specified high limit	Confirm it using your blood glucose meter. Treat if necessary based on actual situation
12:05A LOW 40 MG/DL Glucose is lower than user specified limit ESC, ACT to clear	Sensor glucose value is equal to or lower than user specified low limit	Confirm it using your blood glucose meter. Treat if necessary based on actual situation
3:36P CAL ERROR Invalid sensor data or invalid BG value See user guide ESC, ACT to clear	The ratio of blood glucose measurements to current value is not between 1.5 and 15.0	Recalibrate when the glucose level is stable
10:05A BAD SENSOR Replace Sensor See user guide ESC, ACT to clear	Sensor problem	1. During initialization, wait for full infiltration of sensor, then restart 2. If it is caused by two consecutive CAL ERRs, please replace the sensor 3. If this alarm appears alone, check with tester
8:35A SENSOR END Replace Sensor See user guide ESC, ACT to clear	The sensor reaches the maximum service life of 72 h	Replace sensor
12:52P SENSOR ERROR Sensor failed self- test See user guide ESC, ACT to clear	Sensor error	1. Clear it if during initialization or only one reminder 2. If two or more reminders, replace sensor
11:17A LOST SENSOR Pump no longer getting Sensor data. See user guide ESC, ACT to clear	Lost sensor signal	1. Check that the sensor is still inserted in the skin and the transmitter and sensor are still connected 2. Use the "Find Lost Sensor" function to find the sensor 3. If it occurs repeatedly during initialization, turn off the sensor for 2 h before turning on

(continued)

Table 4.2 (continued)

Display	Causes	Solutions
9:42A WEAK SIGNAL Sensor too far away from pump See user guide ESC, ACT to clear	Communication between pump and transmitter has been lost up to the limit time (by Missed Data setting)	Move insulin pump closer to the transmitter
12:00A LOW TRANSMTR Replace transmitter now ESC, ACT to clear	Low battery of transmitter	Disconnect and charge the transmitter
8:35A BAD TRANSMTR Replace transmitter now ESC, ACT to clear	No power of transmitter	Immediately charge the transmitter for about 8 h until the green light on transmitter does not flash

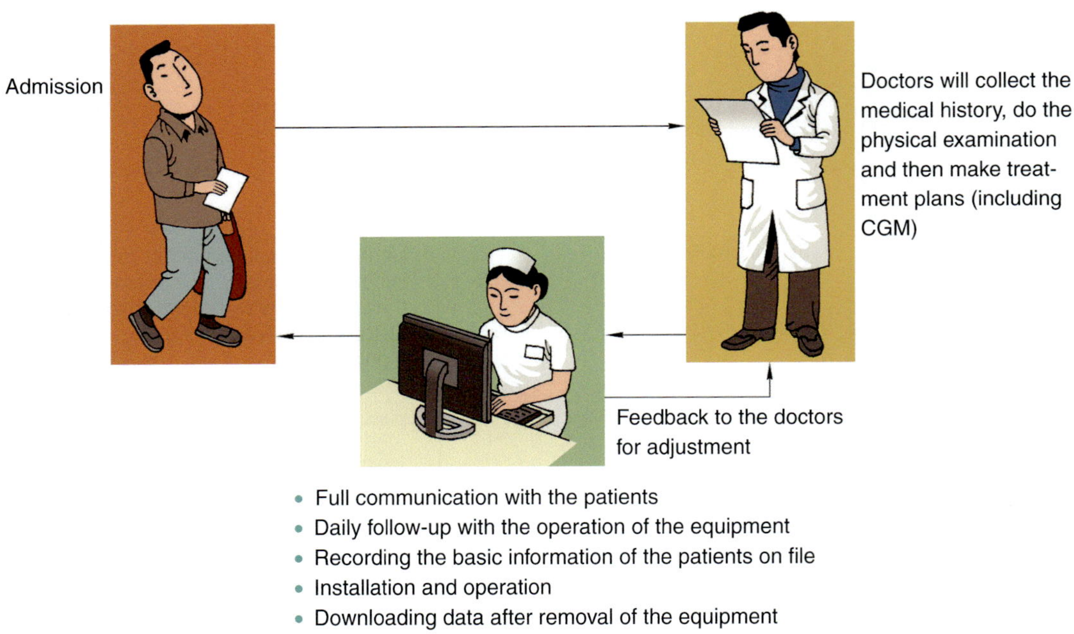

Fig. 4.5 The workflow of CGM system installation carried out by specialized, full-time nurses

should be placed at room temperature for at least 10 min after removal from refrigerator to restore the activity of glucose oxidase (GOD). According to our experience from clinical practice, appropriate extension of the time facilitates normal operation of the sensor and reduces the occurrence of alarms. Also, the sensor should be recalibrated whenever an alarm appears. The CGM system does not record monitoring results until calibration with the finger-stick glucose value is eligible, that is, the ratio of glucose measurements divided by ISIG within 1.5–15.0 (Table 4.2).

With experience from more than 10 years of clinical practice, we recommend that CGM systems should be operated, maintained, and managed by specialized, full-time nurses and be stored or placed separately (Fig. 4.5), which is conducive to patient education and avoidance of the causes for alarms during operation, ensuring successful usage of CGM systems.

Statement on Consent for Participation

All the clinical trials carried out by the authors in this book have been reported to the Ethics Committee of Shanghai Jiao Tong University Affiliated Sixth People's Hospital already and were in accordance with the Good Clinical Practice and Standards of China Association for Ethical Studies (approval number: 2007-45).

References

1. Lu W, Zhou J, Bao YQ, Li M, Yu HY, Zhang L, Jia WP. Nursing care of 2 children with type 1 diabetes during continuous glucose monitoring. Chin J Nurs. 2009;44:713–4. https://doi.org/10.3761/j.issn.0254-1769.2009.08.015.
2. Zheng XP, Shao Y, Zou CC, Liang L. Application and nursing of continuous glucose monitoring system in children with type 1 diabetes. Chin J Nurs. 2008;43:235–6. https://doi.org/10.3761/j.issn.0254-1769.2008.03.018.
3. Lu W, Zhou J, Bao YQ, Lu FD, Jia WP. Analysis of the failure cause of continuous glucose monitoring system and nursing care. Chin J Nurs. 2008;43:561–2. https://doi.org/10.3761/j.issn.0254-1769.2008.06.033.

5 Methods for Interpreting Continuous Glucose Monitoring Graphs

M. Li and Y. Bao

Through the interpretation of glucose profiles and graphs obtained by continuous glucose monitoring (CGM), clinicians and patients can mutually communicate and analyze the short-term glycemic profiles of patients. The CGM measurements only reflect the blood glucose information for several days, and they do not represent long-term glucose profiles. Therefore, the first principle for interpretation of CGM data is not to expand the time window. The second principle is to emphasize the trend and regularity of glucose fluctuations (rather than individual, specific glucose values) and to find suspicious events that cause abnormal glucose fluctuations (such as relationship between abnormal hyperglycemia and snacks or hypoglycemia and excessive exercise, etc.). As shown in Fig. 5.1, the CGM data of a newly diagnosed type 2 diabetes patient shows a typical blood glucose feature of "three peaks and one valley," that is, glucose peaks after three meals and glucose valley at nighttime, and postprandial hyperglycemia is most prominent following breakfast. Figure 5.2 shows data for a case of a special type of diabetes due to pancreatectomy for the treatment of pancreatic cancer. The CGM result does not show a typical "three peaks and one valley" feature, and postprandial hyperglycemia is most prominent from after lunch until bedtime. The third principle is to interpret CGM results in an understandable pattern, for instance, statistical reports or charts (Fig. 5.3), which facilitates good communication between clinicians and patients.

CGM technology can be divided into two categories as the retrospective and the real-time CGM [1]. This chapter introduces the interpretation of both the retrospective and real-time CGM data both from the aspect of theory and clinical practice.

5.1 Basic Principles for Interpretation of a Retrospective CGM Report

The interpretation of retrospective CGM data should be conducted in three steps: first, analysis of nocturnal glucose; second, analysis of preprandial blood glucose; and third, analysis of postprandial blood glucose. In each step, hypoglycemia is observed first, followed by hyperglycemia, and the data are analyzed to find specific causes and to guide treatment adjustment [2]. The reasons for observation of hypoglycemia first are the following: (1) for patients with diabetes, hypoglycemia is an important and potentially life-threatening event that needs to be given priority for treatment; and (2) if the patients experience both hypoglycemic and hyperglycemic events, the relationship between them should

M. Li · Y. Bao (✉)
Department of Endocrinology and Metabolism, Shanghai Clinical Center for Diabetes, Shanghai Diabetes Institute, Shanghai Jiao Tong University Affiliated Sixth People's Hospital, Shanghai, China
e-mail: yqbao@sjtu.edu.cn

W. Jia (ed.), *Continuous Glucose Monitoring*, https://doi.org/10.1007/978-981-10-7074-7_5

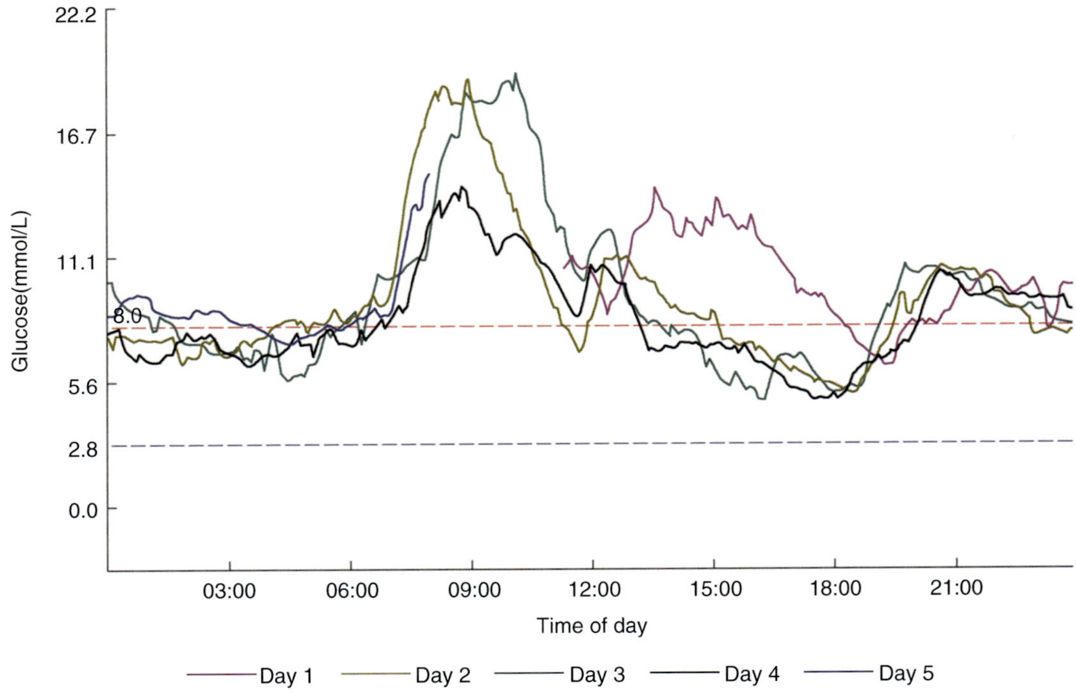

Fig. 5.1 The CGM profiles of a newly diagnosed type 2 diabetes patient whose postprandial hyperglycemia is most prominent following breakfast. Notes: The graph represents an overlay of CGM readings for multiple days, and each curve reflects the glucose trend over a single day. The graph can be used to analyze the trend and regularity of blood glucose fluctuations in the patient

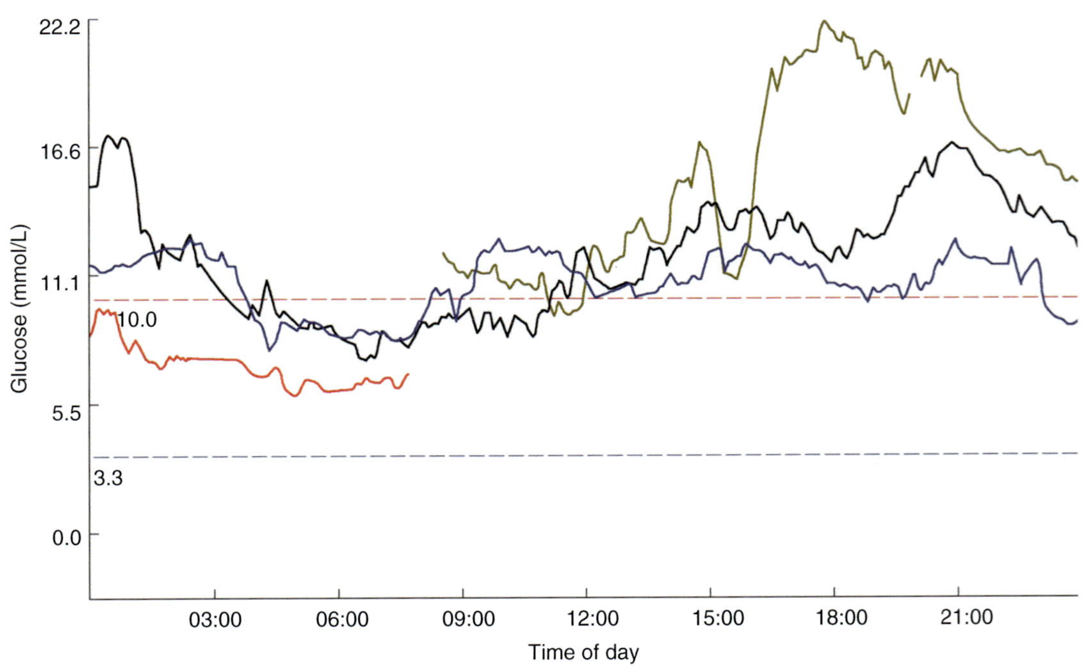

Fig. 5.2 The CGM profiles of a patient with diabetes induced by pancreatectomy performed as treatment for pancreatic cancer whose postprandial hyperglycemia is most prominent from after lunch until bedtime

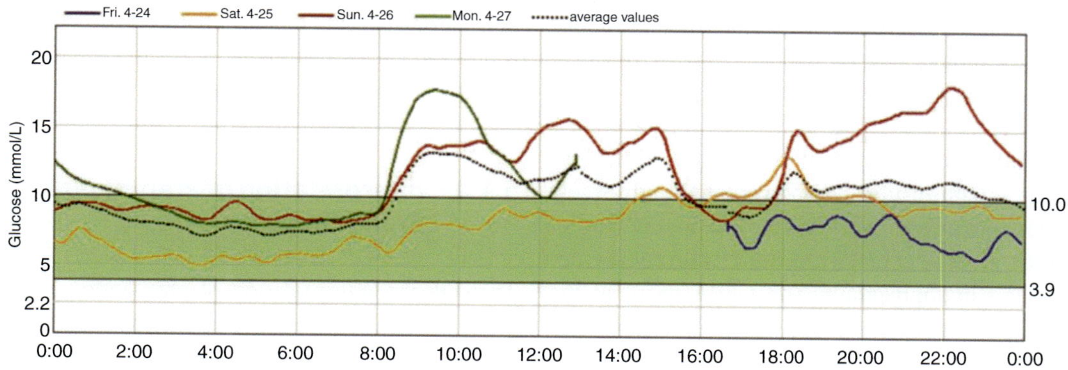

	Fri 4-24	Sat 4-25	Sun 4-26	Mon 4-27	Average values/total
The number of the values from the sensor	88	288	288	156	820
Upper limit	9.0	13.1	18.3	17.8	18.3
Lower limit	5.7	4.9	8.1	7.9	4.9
The Average value	7.6	8.2	12.0	10.8	10.0
SD	0.9	2.0	3.0	3.1	3.1
MAD%	9.8	14.1	9.6	2.5	9.7
Correlation coefficient	N/A	0.89	0.94	1.00	0.95
Number of the adjustment	3	5	5	3	16
Notes					

X: Judging based on the clinical experience S: No data from the sensor C:No data adjusted

	Fri 4-24	Sat 4-25	Sun 4-26	Mon 4-27	Average values/total
Total number of the glycemic excursion	0	2	2	1	5
Number of the upward excursion	0	2	2	1	5
Number of the downward excursion	0	0	0	0	0
Above the upper limit of AUC	0.00	0.17	2.50	1.61	1.24
Below the lower limit of AUC	0.00	0.00	0.00	0.00	0.00

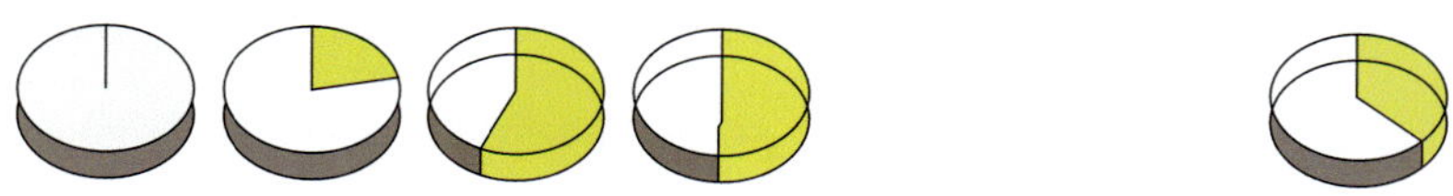

	Fri 4-24	Sat 4-25	Sun 4-26	Mon 4-27	Average values/total
>10.0	0:00 0%	5:10 22%	13:40 57%	6:35 51%	25:25 37%
3.9~10.0	7:20 100%	18:50 78%	10:20 43%	6:25 49%	42:55 63%
<3.9	0:00 0%	0:00 0%	0:00 0%	0:00 0%	0:00 0%

Fig. 5.3 The CGM graphs and statistical reports of the Medtronic retrospective iPro2 system of a patient with type 2 diabetes

be analyzed, and hyperglycemia should be reevaluated once hypoglycemia is corrected.

5.1.1 Interpretation of Nocturnal Blood Glucose

Nocturnal blood glucose is defined as the blood glucose levels during the period from the time of the last meal or snack in the evening to the morning (usually from midnight to 06:00 a.m.) [3].

First, a specific range of blood glucose levels during nighttime should be defined. Hypoglycemia is defined as blood glucose decreases to below the low limit, and hyperglycemia is defined as blood glucose rises to above the high limit. The target blood glucose range can be personalized according to different individuals. Once hypoglycemia occurs, further work-up should be pursued to determine the causes of the hypoglycemia event, for example, overdose of insulin during nighttime, little food uptake, or excessive exercise after dinner. If hyperglycemia happens, the above causes should also be reviewed [4]. A practical example is presented below.

Case 1 An elderly woman with type 1 diabetes treated with insulin pump presented with excessive glycemic variability. Her self-monitoring of blood glucose (SMBG) showed recurrent asymptomatic hypoglycemia. The CGM result at the first day after admission is shown in Fig. 5.4.

Analysis of CGM data shows that the patient had recurrent hypoglycemia and the coexistence of hypoglycemia and hyperglycemia but without obvious hypoglycemic symptoms. According to the priority rule mentioned above, hypoglycemia should be treated first when hypoglycemia and hyperglycemia coexist. Therefore, the basal rate of the insulin pump was decreased by 0.05 U/h at night, and the patient was recommended to eat an appropriate amount of snack before bedtime. The follow-up CGM result (Fig. 5.5) shows that nocturnal hypoglycemia was corrected.

5.1.2 Interpretation of Preprandial Blood Glucose

Through the interpretation of preprandial blood glucose, clinicians can analyze the effects of insulin injection or other hypoglycemic drugs before the last meal, the effects of meal intake, and the effects of exercise after last meal on blood glucose changes.

Similarly, the first step is to define a range of target preprandial blood glucose values and then to analyze the causal relationship between various factors (such as drugs) and preprandial blood glucose changes. Preprandial blood glucose is interpreted in an order of breakfast, lunch, and dinner

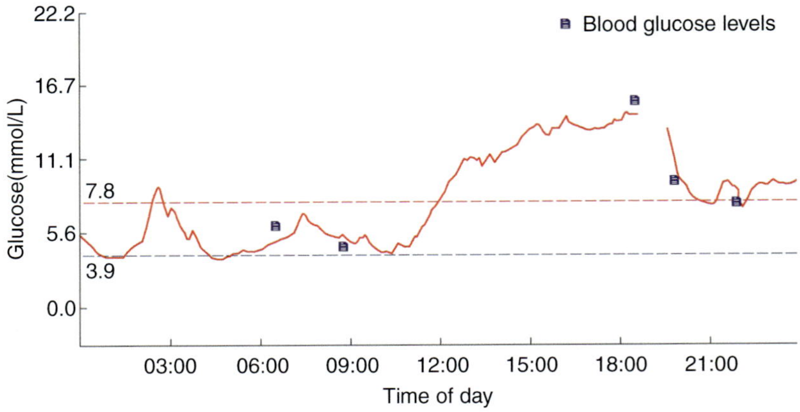

Fig. 5.4 Case 1: CGM profiles of an elderly patient with type 1 diabetes at the first day of admission. Notes: blood glucose levels

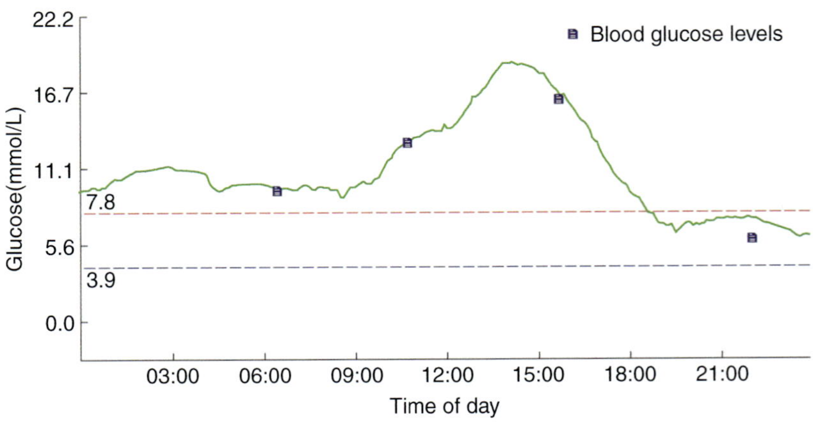

Fig. 5.5 Case 1: CGM profiles reflecting improved nocturnal hypoglycemia after adjustment of the basal dose on the insulin pump. Notes: blood glucose levels

(or the habit of a clinician). First, check if there exists preprandial hypoglycemia, and analyze the possible causes if it exists, for example, an overdose of insulin before last meal, residual insulin activity, the length, amount and ingredients of the last meal, exercise, or other events. Second, similar causes should be reviewed if there exists preprandial hyperglycemia. Finally, in the case of hyperglycemia before breakfast, the dawn phenomenon should be taken into consideration.

Case 2 A patient with a 20-year history of diabetes was treated with subcutaneous premixed insulin injection (twice daily). The CGM data at admission reveals an overall elevated blood glucose during the daytime (Fig. 5.6).

According to the CGM results, we increased the dosage of premixed insulin before breakfast in order to control daytime hyperglycemia. The follow-up CGM result shows significant improvement in blood glucose during the daytime, especially for preprandial blood glucose, for which the target goal was achieved (Fig. 5.7).

5.1.3 Interpretation of Postprandial Blood Glucose

In recent years, it has been found that postprandial hyperglycemia is significantly associated with chronic complications of diabetes and is an independent risk factor for macrovascular and microvascular complications [5, 6]. Postprandial hyperglycemia therefore increasingly attracts special attention by clinicians. The impact of acute postprandial glycemic fluctuations on endothelial function in diabetic patients is also of concern [7]. Postprandial blood glucose is defined as the blood glucose changes within 3 h

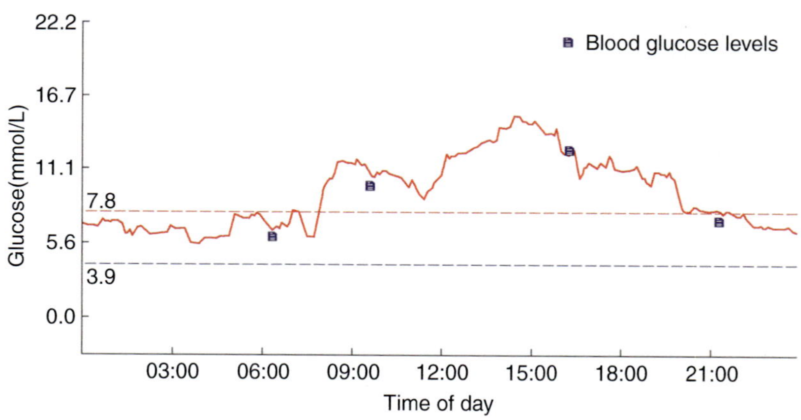

Fig. 5.6 Case 2: CGM profiles reflecting overall daytime hyperglycemia in a patient with a 20-year history of diabetes. Notes: blood glucose levels

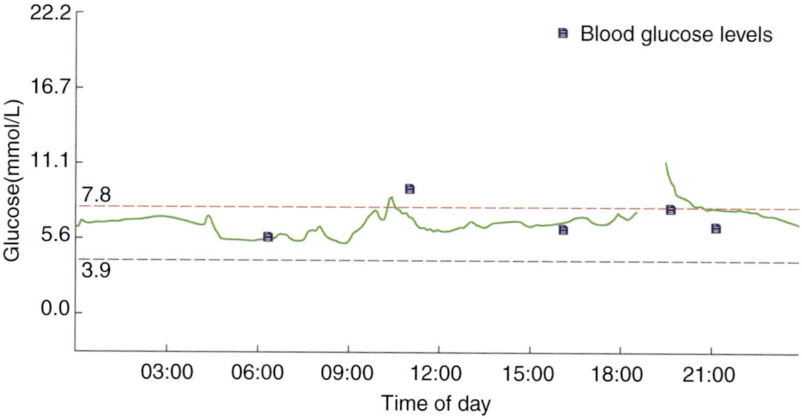

Fig. 5.7 Case 2: CGM profiles reflecting improved daytime hyperglycemia after adjustment of the insulin regimen. Notes: blood glucose levels

after a meal. Factors affecting the changes in postprandial blood glucose are the following: use of insulin or oral hypoglycemic drugs before a meal, the amount and ingredients of the meal, and exercise and other events after the meal.

Similarly, postprandial blood glucose should be interpreted in an order of breakfast, lunch, and dinner, to determine whether a postprandial hypoglycemia or hyperglycemia event occurs and to analyze a causal relationship between various factors and any glycemic events that exist. If postprandial hypoglycemia occurs (2–3 h after meal), the usage of insulin and medication before meal should be revalued, such as the time of drug taken, the dosage, type and formulation of medication and insulin, exercises, and gastrointestinal function. If the postprandial blood glucose peak is >10.0 mmol/L, the time of drug action, the dosage, type and formulation of medication, the accuracy of medication prescription, as well as the amount and composition of food should be considered.

Case 3 A patient with a 6-year history of diabetes was treated with acarbose and insulin glargine. The admission CGM results showed postprandial hyperglycemia that was most dramatic after breakfast and dinner (Fig. 5.8).

According to the CGM profile, the hypoglycemic regimen was adjusted to insulin aspart 30 before all three meals, and the postprandial blood glucose was significantly improved (Fig. 5.9).

5.2 Basic Principles for Interpretation of a Real-Time CGM Report

The basic principles for interpretation of a real-time CGM report are similar to those for retrospective CGM data. The real-time CGM system can reflect the immediate blood glucose information (including point and trend of blood glucose

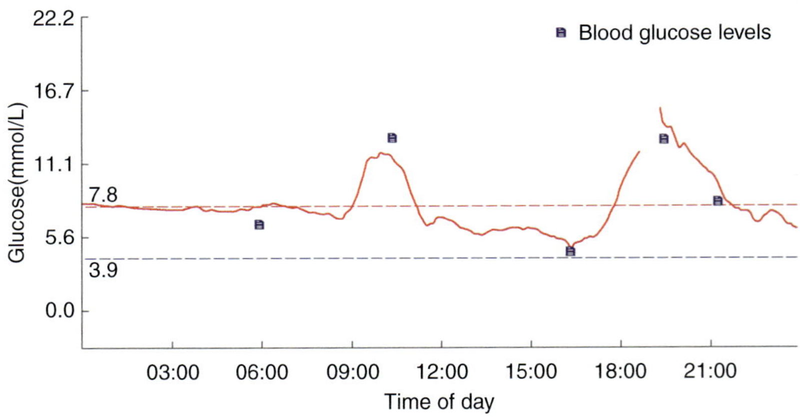

Fig. 5.8 Case 3: CGM profiles reflecting postprandial hyperglycemia in a patient with a 6-year history of diabetes. Notes: blood glucose levels

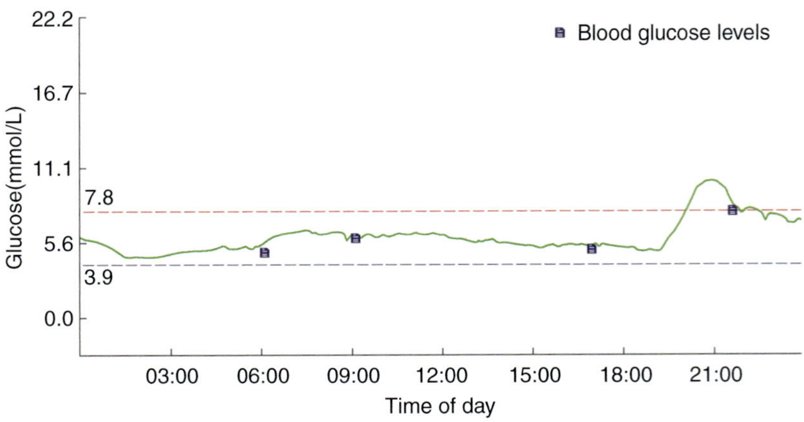

Fig. 5.9 Case 3: CGM profiles reflecting improved daytime hyperglycemia after adjustment of the insulin regimen. Notes: Blood glucose levels

levels) and has hyperglycemia and hypoglycemia alarm or predictive alert features. When it is integrated to an insulin pump, it allows timely intervention of rapid blood glucose fluctuations and hyperglycemia or hypoglycemia events, thus achieving better management of blood glucose for diabetic patients, especially those with type 1 diabetes. As a new technology, medical staff should have the ability to interpret real-time CGM results. It should be noted that real-time CGM data can be used to guide diabetes treatment only when the following criteria are met: (1) the real-time CGM system has been worn for at least 12 h; (2) the real-time CGM system has been adequately calibrated, i.e., calibration with a glucose meter value at least once every 12 h with a good match between CGM sensor glucose values and meter glucose values (difference <15%); (3) the patient presents stable immediate blood glucose values, without a sharp rise or drop in blood glucose; and (4) the real-time CGM readings have no false alarms.

According to the results of glucose monitoring over a period of time, the real-time CGM system can be used to demonstrate a trend curve reflecting blood glucose changes (Fig. 5.10). Clinicians can then interpret the glucose monitoring results and accordingly adjust the treatment regimen (Fig. 5.11) [8]. Two practical examples are presented below.

Case 4 A middle-aged patient with type 2 diabetes mellitus was admitted due to poor glycemic control. The patient was then treated with intensive insulin pump therapy and monitored with real-time CGM. The real-time CGM data from the first day on insulin pump therapy showed that the patient had high glucose levels during the period after breakfast until dinner time and a relatively normal glucose level at nighttime (Fig. 5.12). The next day, the doses of insulin before breakfast and lunch and the basal rate of the insulin pump during the breakfast-to-dinner period were increased accordingly. The CGM data showed that the patient's daytime blood glucose was improved after adjustment of the antihyperglycemic regimen (Fig. 5.13).

Case 5 A young patient with type 1 diabetes had good glycemic control and was on long-term insulin pump therapy. He was admitted to screen for diabetes-related complications. The real-time CGM data showed that the patient had good glycemic control on the second day after admission (Fig. 5.14), but he experienced postprandial hyperglycemia after breakfast on the third day (Fig. 5.15). The patient mentioned that he ate a snack when he felt hungry during the checkup after breakfast. The patient was given additional high-dose insulin.

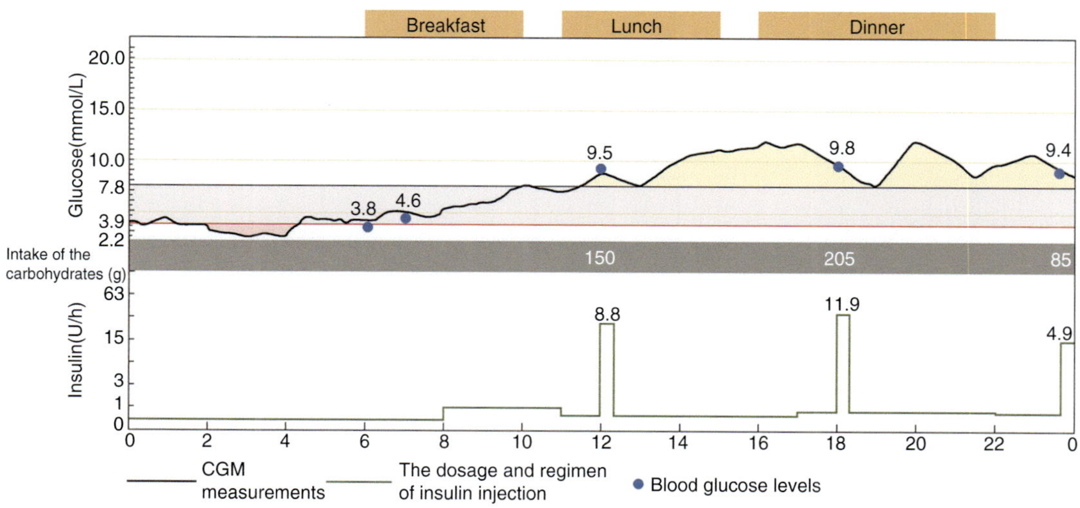

Fig. 5.10 Comprehensive analysis of CGM profiles and adjustment of insulin pump settings using Carelink software

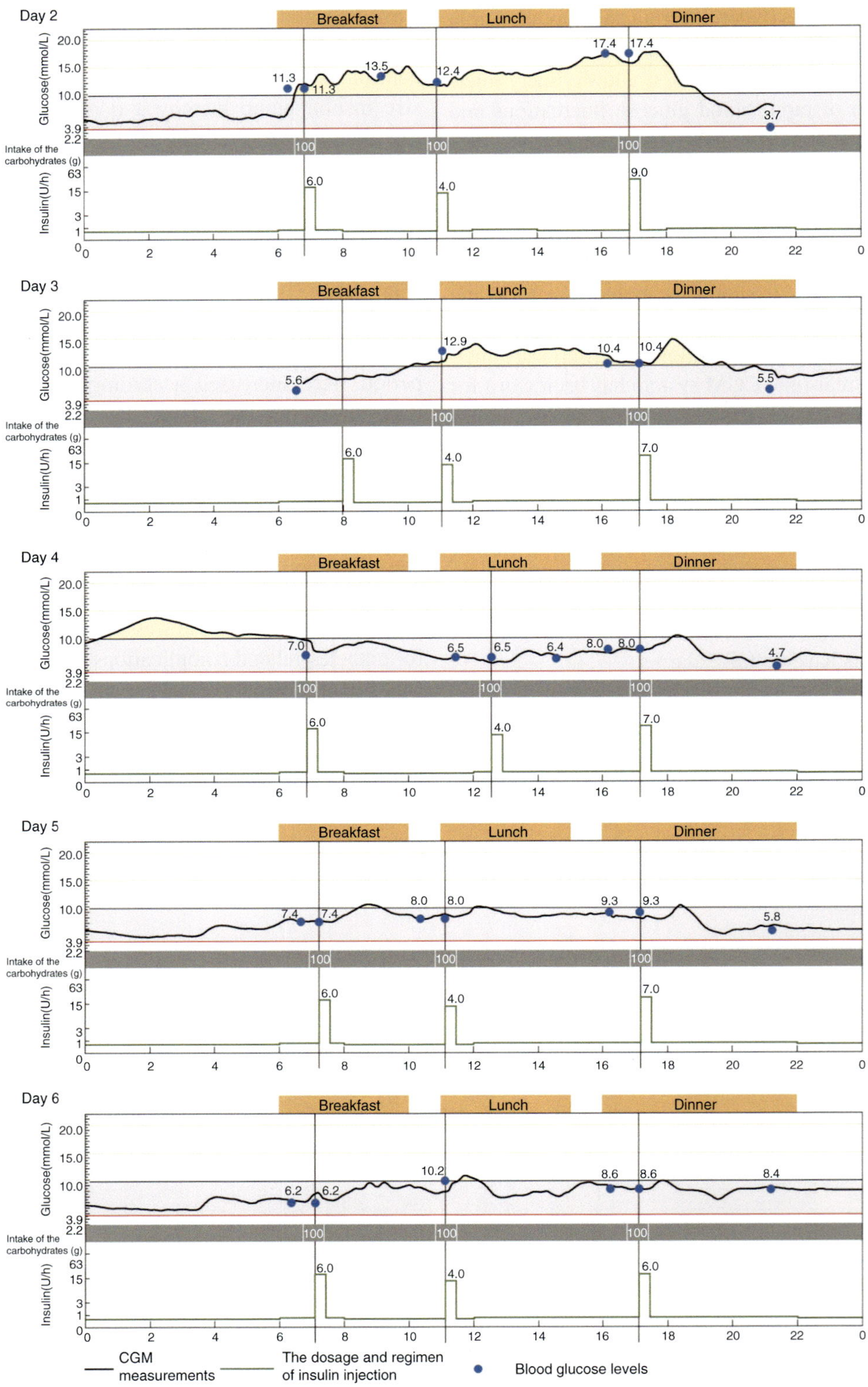

Fig. 5.11 CGM profiles of a 14-year-old type 1 diabetes patient with poor glycemic control [HbA_{1c} 10.2% (88 mmol/mol)]. After 1 week, glycemic control was improved after adjustment of insulin pump settings according to CGM glucose values

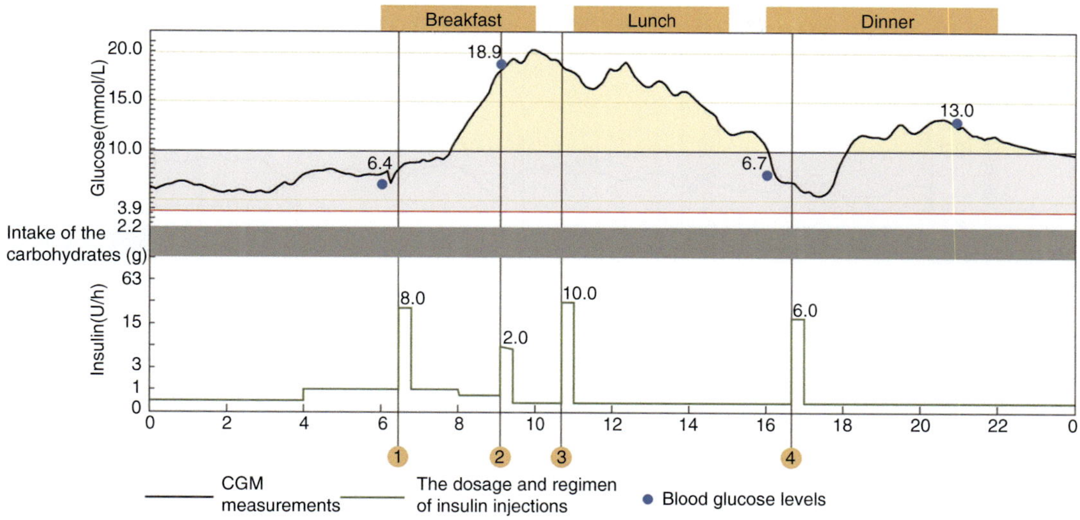

Fig. 5.12 Case 4: Real-time CGM profiles and insulin pump settings for a middle-aged type 2 diabetes patient on the first day of insulin pump therapy

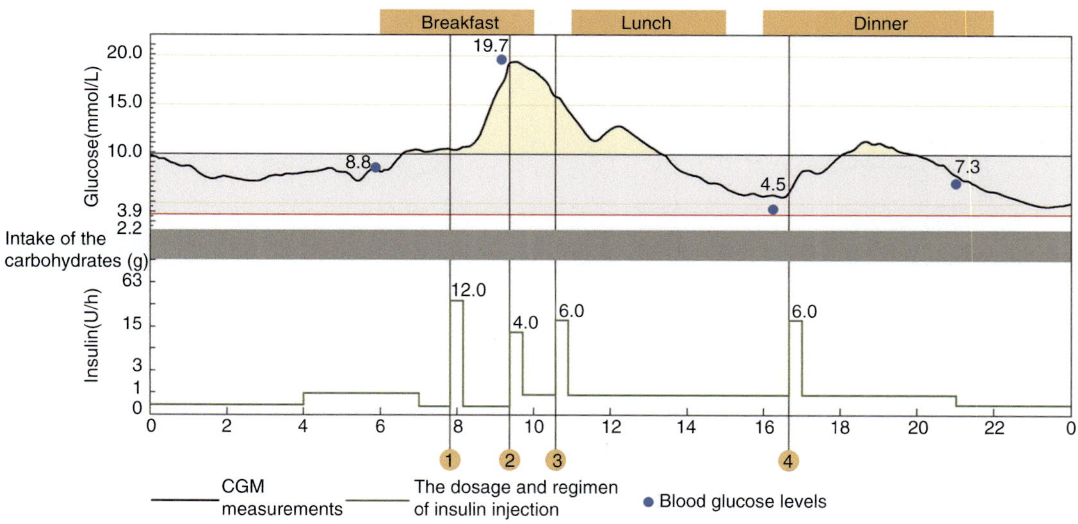

Fig. 5.13 Case 4: Real-time CGM profiles reflecting improved glucose control on the second day of insulin pump therapy after adjustment of insulin pump settings

Through the above two examples, we can find that the real-time CGM system has certain advantages in reflecting the immediate blood glucose level and predictive alerts for abnormal glucose values. In particular, patients can make full use of the high or low glucose alarm function, which is helpful for implementing timely interventions and thus reducing blood glucose fluctuations and maintaining stable blood glucose control, especially for the prevention of hypoglycemia [9].

On the real-time CGM display, the user can view 3-h, 12-h, and 24-h trends in blood glucose changes, and the data can be downloaded to generate charts, graphs, and alarm information. The 3-h trend graph is used for the analysis of preprandial and postprandial blood glucose, the 12-h trend graph for the analysis of nocturnal blood glucose, and the 24-h trend graph for the analysis of a full day of blood glucose levels. Similar to that for retrospective CGM, interpretation of a

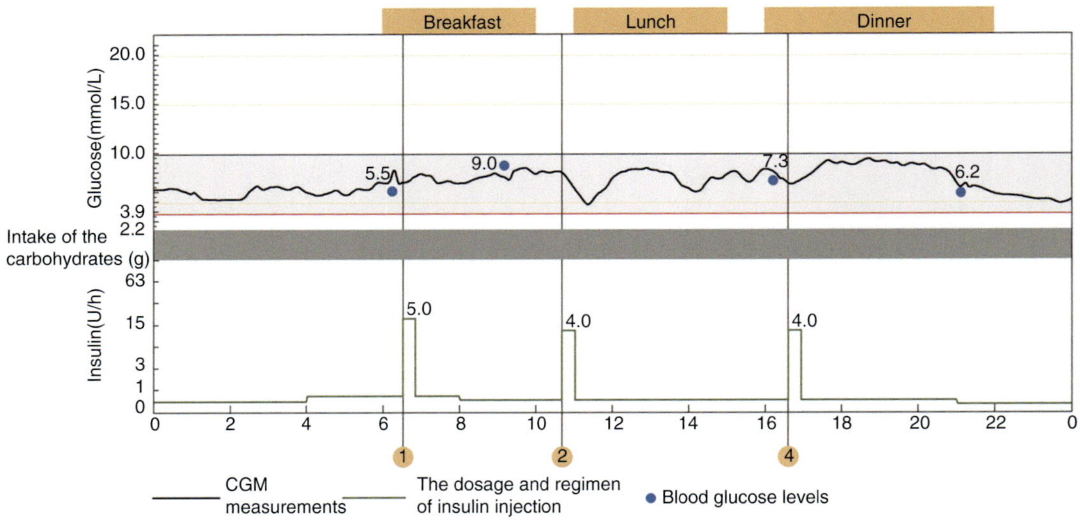

Fig. 5.14 Case 5: Real-time CGM profiles and insulin pump settings for a young type 1 diabetes patient with good glycemic control on the second day on insulin pump therapy

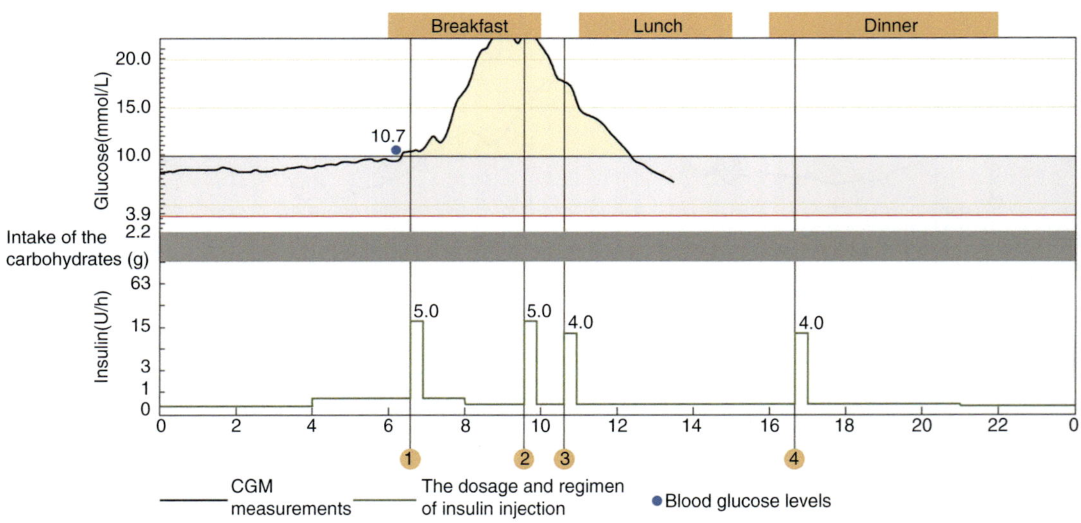

Fig. 5.15 Case 5: Real-time CGM profiles reflecting prominent postprandial hyperglycemia following breakfast and a decrease in glucose values achieved by an injection of a high dose of insulin on the third day on insulin pump therapy

real-time CGM report can be divided into three periods according to the analysis of events that may affect blood glucose: nighttime (the period least affected by food or exercise), the premeal period (at least 3 h after the last meal), and the post-meal period (within 3 h after the meal, divided into the early 90 min and late 90 min).

On the real-time CGM system display, the trends in blood glucose change are indicated by arrows, which represent the direction and speed of blood glucose changes over the past 20 min. A single up/down arrow (↑/↓) indicates that the patient's blood glucose level has increased/decreased by 1.1–2.2 mmol/L in the previous 20 min. Double up/down arrows (↑↑/↓↓) indicate that the patient's blood glucose level has risen/fallen by 2.2 mmol/L or more in the previous 20 min. The predictive alerts indicate that the blood glucose may reach or exceed the preset high or low limit within 5–30 min (depending on the time set

Table 5.1 Tips for "arrows" on real-time CGM systems and recommended measures

Arrows	Clinical significance	Nighttime	Premeal (at least 3 h after last meal)	Post-meal (early 90 min/late 90 min after a meal)
↓	Predictive of hypoglycemia	Take measures	Possibly normal	Take measures/possibly normal
↓↓	Predictive of hypoglycemia	Take prompt measures	Take measures	Take measures/possibly normal
↑	Predictive of hyperglycemia	Possibly normal	Possibly normal	Possibly normal/take measures
↑↑	Predictive of hyperglycemia	Take measures	Possibly normal	Possibly normal/take measures

Notes: Possibly normal, no need to take any measures and just continue regular monitoring; take measures, pay close attention to the trend in blood glucose changes, immediately recheck blood glucose reading using a glucose meter; take prompt measures, recheck blood glucose reading with a glucose meter, correct hypoglycemia with glucose solution or hyperglycemia with insulin if necessary

by users, which can be set as 5, 10, 15, 20, 25, or 30 min) if no intervention is applied. Tips for the "arrows" on the real-time CGM displayer and recommended measures are shown in Table 5.1.

For interpretation of real-time CGM results, it should also be noted that one should (1) focus on the trend in blood glucose changes while proficiently mastering the meanings of the "arrows" and predictive alerts; (2) once the "arrows" and predictive alerts are encountered, comprehensive judgment should be made on the basis of clinical situation, and also overcorrection and "stacking" insulin should be avoided; and (3) analysis of CGM data over a long period helps to identify the regularity and trend of blood glucose changes and accordingly optimize the treatment regimen.

In short, CGM provides a set of intuitive, detailed CGM data and graphs for medical staff and patients. To interpret a CGM report, the clinician should have a general understanding of the glycemic features of the patient and then comprehensively analyze the CGM glucose data and graphs based on the "three-step" method in combination with the events that may impact blood glucose levels, such as food intake and exercise. Both perspectives of the clinicians and patients should be fully and carefully discussed, thus achieving the optimization of hypoglycemic regimen.

Statement on Consent for Participation

All the clinical trials carried out by the authors in this book have been reported to the Ethics Committee of Shanghai Jiao Tong University Affiliated Sixth People's Hospital already and were in accordance with the Good Clinical Practice and Standards of China Association for Ethical Studies (approval number: 2007-45).

References

1. Chinese Diabetes Society. Chinese clinical guideline for continuous glucose monitoring (2012). Chin Med J. 2012;125:4167–74.
2. Chinese Diabetes Society. Clinical application guide of blood glucose monitoring in China (Edition 2015). Chin J Diabetes Mellitus. 2015;7:603–13. https://doi.org/10.3760/cma.j.issn.1674-5809.2015.10.004.
3. Blevins TC, Bode BW, Garg SK, Grunberger G, Hirsch IB, Jovanovič L, Nardacci E, Orzeck EA, Roberts VL, Tamborlane WV, Rothermel C, AACE Continuous Glucose Monitoring Task Force. Statement by the American Association of Clinical Endocrinologists consensus panel on continuous glucose monitoring. Endocr Pract. 2010;16:730–45. https://doi.org/10.4158/EP.16.5.730.
4. Klonoff DC, Buckingham B, Christiansen JS, Montori VM, Tamborlane WV, Vigersky RA, Wolpert H, Endocrine Society. Continuous glucose monitoring: an endocrine society clinical practice guideline. J Clin Endocrinol Metab. 2011;96:2968–79. https://doi.org/10.1210/jc.2010-2756.
5. Ceriello A, Davidson J, Hanefeld M, Leiter L, Monnier L, Owens D, Tajima N, Tuomilehto J, International Prandial Glucose Regulation Study Group. Postprandial hyperglycaemia and cardiovascular complications of diabetes: an update. Nutr Metab Cardiovasc Dis. 2006;16:453–6. https://doi.org/10.1016/j.numecd.2006.05.006.
6. Au SC, Tang SM, Rong SS, Chen LJ, Yam JC. Association between hyperglycemia and retinopathy of prematurity: a systemic review and meta-analysis. Sci Rep. 2015;5:9091. https://doi.org/10.1038/srep09091.

7. Fiorentino TV, Prioletta A, Zuo P, Folli F. Hyperglycemia-induced oxidative stress and its role in diabetes mellitus related cardiovascular diseases. Curr Pharm Des. 2013;19:5695–703. https://doi.org/10.2174/1381612811319320005.
8. Jia WP. Information changes recognition: clinical use of continuous glucose monitoring system. Zhonghua Yi Xue Za Zhi. 2009;89:649–50. https://doi.org/10.3760/cma.j.issn.0376-2491.2009.10.001.
9. Zhou J, Jia WP. Further improvement of continuous glucose monitoring's clinical application in Chinese subjects. Zhonghua Yi Xue Za Zhi. 2010;90:2953–5.

6 Definition and Clinical Significance of Continuous Glucose Monitoring Parameters

Y. F. Mo and W. Jia

6.1 Parameters Reflecting Mean Blood Glucose (MBG) and Their Clinical Significance

The parameters reflecting MBG include:

1. Twenty-four-hour MBG: mean of daily continuous 24-h blood glucose measured by continuous glucose monitoring (CGM), reflecting overall blood glucose level.
2. Pre-meal 1-h MBG: the average blood glucose within 1–60 min before three meals, reflecting the preprandial blood glucose level.
3. Post-meal 3-h MBG: the average blood glucose within 1–180 min after three meals, reflecting the characteristics of postprandial blood glucose, that is, the impact of food intake on blood glucose.
4. Percentage of time (PT): the frequency and total time of blood glucose values above, below, and within the target range (presented by pie chart and statistics). For example, analysis of the PTs spent at glucose >10.0 mmol/L, 3.9–10.0 mmol/L, and <3.9 mmol/L can better reflect the characteristics of blood glucose changes. It is easy to understand and is suitable for diabetes education. Our retrospective study using the CGM system demonstrated that the intraday PT spent on the blood glucose between 2.8 and 7.8 mmol/L was 99% in individuals with normal glucose regulation, whereas the PTs spent with a blood glucose >7.8 mmol/L and >11.1 mmol/L were 96% and 62%, respectively, in patients with newly diagnosed type 2 diabetes mellitus [1].
5. Area under the curve (AUC): the area between the target blood glucose curve and CGM measurement curve. This is a comprehensive statistical method for analyzing the time and extent of blood glucose changes. However, its clinical significance is relatively difficult to understand for patients. The calculation method and clinical significance of the main parameters are shown in Table 6.1 [2].

Y. F. Mo · W. Jia (✉)
Department of Endocrinology and Metabolism, Shanghai Clinical Center for Diabetes, Shanghai Diabetes Institute, Shanghai Jiao Tong University Affiliated Sixth People's Hospital, Shanghai, China
e-mail: wpjia@sjtu.edu.cn

6.2 Parameters Reflecting Glycemic Variability and Their Clinical Significance

6.2.1 Parameters Reflecting Intraday Glycemic Variability

The main parameters include standard deviations of blood glucose (SDBG), coefficient of variation (CV), largest amplitude of glycemic excursion (LAGE), mean amplitude of glycemic excursion (MAGE), *M*-value, and others (Table 6.2).

W. Jia (ed.), *Continuous Glucose Monitoring*, https://doi.org/10.1007/978-981-10-7074-7_6

Table 6.1 Summary of main glycemic parameters in CGM [2]

Parameters	Name	Calculation method	Features/clinical significance
Glycemic level	MBG	Mean of daily continuous 24-h blood glucose	Reflects the overall blood glucose level
	Pre-meal 1-h MBG	MBG within 1–60 min before three meals	Reflects the characteristics of preprandial or postprandial blood glucose, that is, the impact of food intake on blood glucose
	Post-meal 3-h MBG	MBG within 1–180 min after three meals	
	PT	Frequency and total time of blood glucose values above, below, and within the target range (presented by pie chart and statistics)	Emphasizes on reflecting the characteristics of blood glucose changes, which is simple and easy to understand, suitable for diabetes education
	AUC	Area between the target blood glucose curve and CGM measurement curve	A comprehensive statistical method for analyzing the time and extent of blood glucose changes
Glycemic variability	SDBG	Standard deviation of blood glucose measurements during CGM	Reflects overall deviation from the mean, without discriminating major and small fluctuations
	LAGE	Difference between maximum and minimum blood glucose concentrations within a day	Reflects the range of glucose fluctuations
	MAGE	Mean of amplitude of glucose excursions (more than one SDBG) based on the direction of the first qualifying AGE	Truly reflects the degree of glycemic excursions rather than discrete features by removal of small amplitudes that do not exceed a certain threshold
	MODD	Mean of the absolute difference between paired blood glucose values in two consecutive 24-h periods	Assesses the degree of inter-day glucose fluctuations and reflects the repeatability of daily blood glucose

Notes: *MBG* mean blood glucose, *PT* percentage of time, *AUC* area under the curve, *SDBG* standard deviation of blood glucose, *LAGE* largest amplitude of glycemic excursion, *MAGE* mean amplitude of glycemic excursion, *MODD* mean of daily differences

Table 6.2 Summary of glycemic variability measures in CGM

Parameter	Definition	Formula	Variables
SDBG	Standard deviation of blood glucose	$\sqrt{\frac{\Sigma\left(G-\bar{G}\right)^2}{N-1}}$	G = glucose measured N = number of observations
CV	Coefficient of variation	$\frac{\text{SDBG}}{\bar{G}}$	$\bar{G}$ = mean of glucose measured
LAGE	Difference between maximum and minimum blood glucose concentration within a day	$G_{\max} - G_{\min}$	$G_{\max}$ = maximum glucose measured $G_{\min}$ = minimum glucose measured
MAGE	Valid glycemic excursion is defined as more than 1 SDBG during 24-h CGM. Amplitude of glycemic excursion is calculated based on the direction of first valid excursion. MAGE is the average value of all AGEs	$\text{MAGE} = \Sigma\frac{\lambda}{x} \quad \text{if } \lambda > v$	λ = blood glucose changes from peak to nadir x = number of observations v = 1 SD of mean glucose for a 24-h period

Table 6.2 (continued)

Parameter	Definition	Formula	Variables
M-value	Mean of the logarithmic transformation of the deviation from a reference or target glucose value	$M = \frac{\sum_{t=t_1}^{t_k} \left\|10 \times \log \frac{G_t \times 18}{\text{IGV}}\right\|^3}{N}$	G = glucose measured N = total number of readings K = total number of observations IGV = ideal glucose value
J-index	Square of the sums of MBG and SDBG	$J = 0.324 \times (\text{MBG} + \text{SDBG})^2$	MBG = mean glucose levels SDBG = SD of glucose levels
CONGA*n*	Standard deviation of differences between each observed blood glucose reading and the reading recorded *n* hour(s) previously	$\text{CONGA} = \sqrt{\frac{\sum_{t=t_1}^{t_k} (D_t - \bar{D})^2}{k-1}}$	k = number of observations D_t = difference between glucose readings at time n and at n hour(s) previously $\bar{D}$ = mean of D_t
MAG	Mean absolute change (increase and decrease) in glucose concentration per unit of time	$\text{MAG} = \frac{\sum_{n=1}^{N-1} (G_n - G_{n+1})}{T}$	G = glucose measured N = number of observations T = observation time (h)
MODD	Mean of the absolute difference between paired blood glucose values in two consecutive 24-h periods	$\text{MODD} = \frac{\sum_{t=t_1}^{t_k} \|G_t - G_{t-1440}\|}{k}$	k = number of observations with an observation 24-h ago G = glucose measured t = time (in min)
ADRR	Mean of the logarithmic transformation of glucose measurements translated into risk of hyperglycemia or hypoglycemia	$\text{ADRR} = \frac{1}{N}\sum_{t=1}^{N} [\text{LR} + \text{HR}]$ $x_i = 1.509 \times \{[\ln(G_i)]^{1.084} - 5.381\}$	N = number of readings LR = risk value attributed to low glucose HR = risk value attributed to high glucose x_i = glucose value after conversion
LBGI	Mean of the logarithmic transformation of glucose measurements translated into risk of hypoglycemia	$\text{LBGI} = \frac{1}{N}\sum_{t=1}^{N} \text{rl}(x_i)$ $x_i = 1.794 \times \{[\ln(G_i)]^{1.026} - 1.861\}$	N = number of readings rl = risk value associated with a low glucose (if $x_i < 0$) x_i = glucose value after conversion G = glucose measured (mmol/L)
HBGI	Mean of the logarithmic transformation of glucose measurements translated into risk of hyperglycemia	$\text{HBGI} = \frac{1}{N}\sum_{t=1}^{N} \text{rh}(x_i)$ $x_i = 1.794 \times \{[\ln(G_i)]^{1.026} - 1.861\}$	N = number of readings rh = risk value associated with a high glucose (if $x_i > 0$) x_i = glucose value after conversion G = glucose measured (mmol/L)

(continued)

Table 6.2 (continued)

Parameter	Definition	Formula	Variables
GRADE	Weighted risk score from the hypoglycemic, euglycemic, hyperglycemic range	GRADE = median $(425 \times \{\log[\log(G_n)] + 0.16\}^2)$	G = glucose measured (mmol/L)
LI	The formula processes three glucose values to calculate a lability value, then moves to the next three glucose values, and so on. The LI is the mean of these values	$\mathrm{LI} = \sum_{n=1}^{N-1} \frac{(G_n - G_{n+1})^2}{(t_{n+1} - t_n)}$	G = glucose measured (mmol/L) N = number of observations t = observation time (h)

6.2.1.1 SDBG

Standard deviation (SD) is a commonly used discrete index in statistics. In clinical practice and scientific studies, mean ± SD is often used to reflect discrete features of normally distributed data. SDBG is an important and simple parameter for assessing blood glucose variability for both self-monitoring of blood glucose (SMBG) and CGM measurements [3]. Moberg et al. [4] analyzed the distribution of SDBG in 100 patients with type 1 diabetes mellitus by using measures of SMBG. The results indicated that the SDBG levels were normally distributed, and the glucose variation recorded before dinner predominantly contributed to the total glucose variability. Krinsley et al. [5] conducted a study of blood glucose variability in critically ill patients in the surgical intensive care unit. A total of 3252 critically ill patients were admitted between 1999 and 2007. They found that increased glycemic variability conferred a strong independent risk of mortality in critically ill patients. Similar findings were also reported by Egi et al. [6]. Through analyzing SDBG in patients with type 1 diabetes mellitus, Kuenen et al. [7] found that SDBG affected the association between MBG and glycated hemoglobin A_{1c} (HbA_{1c}); that is, for the same MBG, the greater the SDBG, the higher the HbA_{1c}. In addition, an 11-year follow-up study of SMBG data in type 1 diabetes patients showed that SDBG was associated with diabetic peripheral neuropathy, suggesting that glycemic variability may be important in the development of peripheral neuropathy in diabetes patients [8].

In recent years, some scholars have suggested that SDBG can be further divided into subtypes. For instance, Rodbard et al. [9] described several methods to characterize glycemic variability: (1) "SDBG total", which is the SD for all of the data from CGM; (2) "within-day variability," which is a measure of the variability within a given day, i.e., from midnight to midnight; (3) "between day-within time points variability"; (4) "between daily means variability"; (5) "between time points variability" of the glucose profile averaged over several days; and (6) "within series variability" for a time segment of any arbitrary length. These parameters cover the measurements of intraday glycemic variability and inter-day glycemic variability. They show good correlation with traditional parameters like MAGE and mean of daily differences (MODD) and, thus, could be applied to assess glycemic variability in diabetes patients in future researches.

6.2.1.2 CV

The CV of blood glucose reflects the amount of variation or dispersion from the MBG.

$$\mathrm{CV} = (\mathrm{SDBG} / \mathrm{MBG}) \times 100\%$$

The CV is calculated from the ratio of SDBG to MBG, which is a simple and easy variable. The CV is closely related to hypoglycemia episodes and is not affected by the average blood glucose level. Rodbard et al. [10] suggested that the CV can be used as a simple parameter to reflect and compare glycemic control among different populations. For example, glucose variability can be defined as excellent, good, fair, and poor, respectively, based on the quartiles for percentage of coefficient of variation (%CV) (25th, 50th, and

75th percentiles). Besides, there's no hypoglycemia events in the %CV <20% group.

Due to easy calculation, the CV has been widely used to assess glycemic variability not only in CGM but also in in-hospital glucose monitoring and SMBG. Šoupal et al. [11] conducted a retrospective study in type 1 diabetes patients and found that after 2 weeks of CGM, CVs were found to be higher in patients with microvascular complications than in those without complications. Jun et al. [12] performed a study in a total of 110 type 2 diabetes patients who underwent 3-day CGM and completed cardiovascular autonomic neuropathy tests. Through calculation of the CV, SDBG, and MAGE, they found that the CV in CGM was significantly higher in patients with autonomic neuropathy, and, in multivariate analysis, CV, but neither SD nor MAGE, was independently correlated with the presence of cardiovascular autonomic neuropathy. Subramaniam et al. [13] reported a study of 1461 type 2 diabetes patients underwent coronary artery bypass grafting surgery and found that the postoperative CV of blood glucose was associated with adverse outcomes (i.e., postoperative death, myocardial infarction, infection, pneumonia, pericardial tamponade, etc.). Takeishi et al. [14] retrospectively analyzed the cases of 620 diabetes patients admitted to the hospital for various infections. Based on parameters including the CV, mean glucose concentrations during hospital stay, and reactive inflammatory biomarkers, they found that hypoglycemia and CV were associated with mortality in diabetes patients with infections. Currently, CV, SDBG, and interquartile range (IQR) are classified as three important parameters reflecting glycemic variability [15].

6.2.1.3 LAGE

The LAGE is the difference between the maximum and minimum blood glucose concentrations within a day, which is equivalent to a range in statistics. The LAGE depends on the highest and lowest blood glucose levels, so it cannot be used to reflect precise glycemic information in CGM. It only represents the single, biggest fluctuation in blood glucose within a day.

6.2.1.4 MAGE

In order to accurately reflect intraday glycemic variability in diabetes patients, Service et al. [16] put forward the parameter MAGE. The idea of MAGE is to adopt a "filtering" method to remove small amplitudes that do not exceed a certain threshold, in order to truly reflect the degree of blood glucose fluctuations rather than discrete features. The formula for MAGE calculation is $\sum \lambda / x$ (when $\lambda > \nu$).

The λ is the difference between the maximum and minimum values of glycemic fluctuations for each valid fluctuation; x is the number of valid fluctuations; and ν depends on the purpose of the study, generally taking a SDBG from 24-h glucose data.

The calculation steps are as follows:

1. Calculate 24-h SDBG.
2. Calculate the amplitude of glucose excursion (AGE). The AGE is the difference in blood glucose from the direction of the peak to the nadir, and it is regarded valid only when the ascending or descending excursion is more than one SDBG away from the mean. The first valid AGE direction is used as the standard to calculate the AGE value.
3. Calculate MAGE, which is the mean value of all AGE values.

As Fig. 6.1 illustrates:

1. The SDBG was 5.2 mmol/L. We used one SDBG to measure whether it is a qualified excursion.
2. The first descending excursion of glucose was calculated as 18.50 mmol/L − 11.56 mmol/L = 6.94 mmol/L, and the ascending excursion of glucose was 17.89 mmol/L − 11.56 mmol/L = 6.33 mmol/L. Both are regarded as qualified AGEs with an excursion exceeding 5.2 mmol/L. Given the direction depends on the first glucose excursion, all AGE measurements were descending excursions.

   For the second glycemic excursion, although the ascending excursion exceeded 5.2 mmol/L, its descending excursion was less

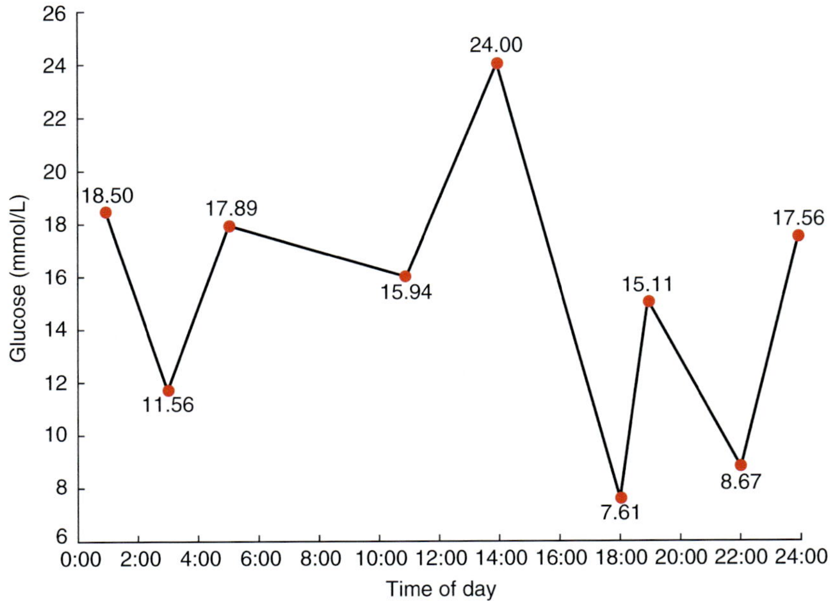

Fig. 6.1 Calculation example of MAGE. The 24-h SMBG chart of a patient with type 1 diabetes mellitus [17] (Reprint with permission from Chinese Journal of Diabetes Mellitus)

than 5.2 mmol/L (17.89 mmol/L − 15.94 mmol/L = 1.95 mmol/L). Thus, it was not a qualified AGE.

Both the third and fourth glycemic excursions were qualified AGEs. The third and fourth descending excursions were 24.00 mmol/L − 7.61 mmol/L = 16.39 mmol/L and 15.11 mmol/L − 8.67 mmol/L = 6.44 mmol/L, respectively.

3. MAGE = (6.94 mmol/L + 16.39 mmol/L + 6.44 mmol/L)/3 = 9.92 mmol/L [17].

It can be seen that the MAGE is characterized by removal of small amplitudes that do not exceed a certain threshold, and thus, it truly reflects the degree of glycemic excursions rather than discrete features. Selection of the "threshold" largely depends on the statistic needs, such as 0.5 SDBG, 1 SDBG, and 1.5 SDBG. Usually, 1 SDBG is selected, due to blood glucose fluctuation usually exceeds 1 SDBG after eating in normal individuals.

Figure 6.2 illustrates the MAGE results for one case of newly diagnosed type 2 diabetes and for one case of a normal individual (diagnosed by oral glucose tolerance test) calculated on the basis of the statistical principles described above.

Service et al. [16] initially compared data for three normal individuals, three diabetes patients with stable glycemic control, and eight diabetes patients with poor glycemic control and found that diabetes patients had a significant higher MAGE than normal individuals and that the MAGE in diabetes patients with poor glycemic control was significantly greater than that for those with stable glycemic control, suggesting that a high MAGE is an important feature of blood glucose instability. Subsequently, Service et al. [18] suggested that the control of glycemic fluctuation with MAGE is an important measure for blood glucose management. They also reported that MAGE was associated with SDBG and *M*-value in type 2 diabetes patients receiving intensive insulin therapy. Our previous studies have shown that MAGE levels are significantly higher in newly diagnosed type 2 diabetes patients than in those with normal glucose regulation. The increase in MAGE in newly diagnosed type 2 diabetes mellitus is mainly attributed to the changes in postprandial and nocturnal blood glucose fluctuations.

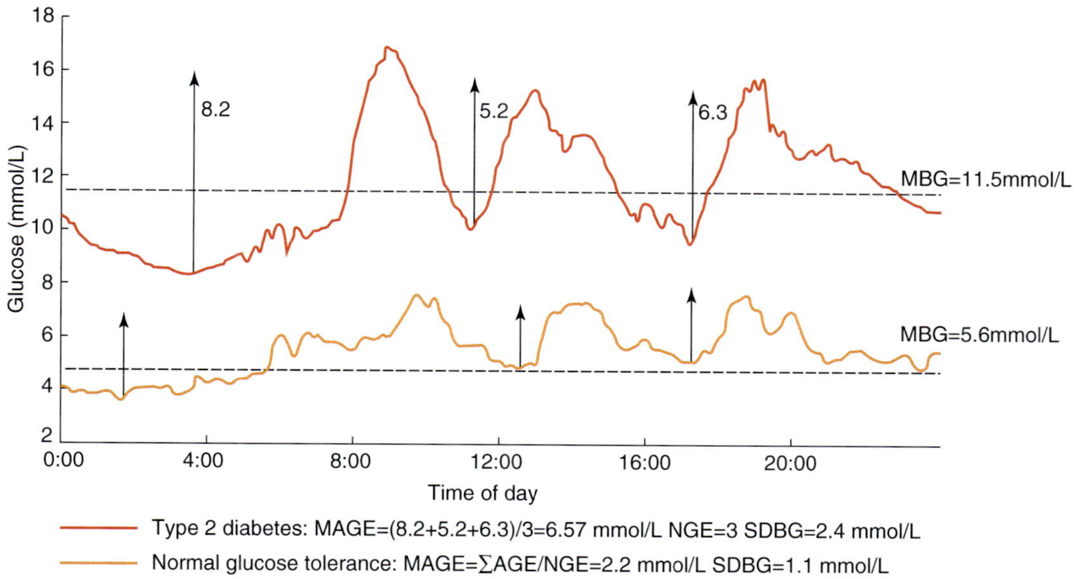

Fig. 6.2 Calculation of MAGE during CGM. The results of one case of newly diagnosed type 2 diabetes mellitus and one case of a normal individual Notes: *MBG* mean blood glucose, *SDBG* standard deviation of blood glucose, *NGE* numbers of glucose excursions, *MAGE* mean amplitude of glycemic excursion, *AGE* amplitude of glycemic excursion

6.2.1.5 *M*-value

The *M*-value was first proposed by Schlichtkrull et al. [19] in the 1960s and subsequently modified by Mirouze et al. [20], and it is also known as *M*-value of Schlichtkrull. It is the mean of the logarithmic transformation of the deviation from a reference or target glucose value (usually, taking MBG over a 24-h period for normal individuals, e.g., 5 mmol/L) plus an amplitude correction factor. If taking the target glucose value of 5 mmol/L, for instance, the formula is

$$\text{corrected } M \text{ value} = \sum\left|10\times\log\left(\text{BG}/5\right)\right|^3 / N + W/20$$

In the formula, *N* is total number of glucose readings, and *W* is LAGE. The *M*-value actually reflects both the overall blood glucose level and glycemic variability. It gives greater emphasis to hypoglycemia. For instance, the choice of 5 mmol/L as the reference value yields an *M*-value of 27.3 for both 2.5 and 10.0 mmol/L glucose measurements. Saisho et al. [21] have reported that *M*-value was correlated with SDBG and the mean glucose. There are studies on the association between the *M*-value and diabetic complications. Oyibo et al. [22] explored the relationship between glycemic variability and painful neuropathy in type 1 diabetes patients using a CGM system. The results demonstrated that in addition to elevated blood glucose levels, diabetes patients with painful peripheral neuropathy had a significantly increased *M*-value.

6.2.1.6 *J*-index

The *J*-index is also used for CGM, and it is calculated by the formula:

$$\text{J} = 0.324\times\left(\text{MBG}+\text{SDBG}\right)^2 \\ \left(\text{glucose in mmol/L}\right)$$

The *J*-index reflects the MBG and glycemic variability [23]. However, it has not yet been widely applied.

6.2.1.7 Continuous Overlapping Net Glycemic Action over an *n*-Hour Period (CONGA*n*)

CONGA*n* is a parameter designed for measuring glycemic variability in CGM, and *n* can vary from 1 to 24 h. It has the advantages of reflecting glycemic variability at different time periods [24]. Taking CONGA-2 and CONGA-4, for instance, the SDBG from the difference between the current glucose and the glucose 2 or 4 h previously is determined. CONGA-2, which reflects rapid, small glycemic swings occurring over a short-time interval, is particularly suitable for monitoring diabetes patients with stable glycemic control [25]. Some researchers have suggested that CONGA*n* is a more objective parameter reflecting blood glucose fluctuations. It is also proposed that the average value of CONGA*n* with n = (1–24) can be calculated to measure glycemic variability [26]. Some studies have explored the relationship between CONGA*n* and diabetic complications. However, the A1C-Derived Average Glucose (ADAG) study demonstrated that measurements of glycemic variability including CONGA*n* had non-significant associations with cardiovascular disease risks in both type 1 and 2 diabetes patients [27].

6.2.1.8 Mean Absolute Glucose (MAG)

Hermanides et al. [28] first put forward the concept of MAG, which is the mean absolute change (increase and decrease) in glucose concentration per unit of time. The parameter reflects all blood glucose fluctuations, including physiological glucose fluctuations. Kohnert et al. [29] analyzed CGM data from 815 diabetes patients and calculated the MAG using 5-min, 60-min, and 7-point glucose profile sampling intervals. The results showed strong linear correlations between MAG change and classical markers including SDBG, MAGE, and CONGA*n*, suggesting MAG as an indicator for assessing glycemic variability. In a reanalysis study of hyperglycemia and its effect after acute myocardial infarction on cardiovascular outcomes in patients with type 2 diabetes mellitus (HEART2D), the researchers showed that the decrease in intraday glycemic variability after insulin therapy by targeting the MAG, calculated from 7-point SMBG profiles, did not result in a reduction in cardiovascular outcomes [30]. Of course, some scholars argued that by using only the change in MAG to assess glycemic variability, the data in that study were not convincing enough to judge the possible impact of glycemic variability on the development or progression of macrovascular complications in type 2 diabetes [31].

6.2.2 Parameters Reflecting Inter-day Glycemic Variability

The main parameters include the CV of fasting plasma glucose (CV-FPG) and MODD.

6.2.2.1 CV-FPG

The CV-FPG is a simple parameter for assessing inter-day glycemic variability. The %CV is the ratio of the SD to the mean. It can eliminate the influence caused by different mean levels on variation. Mooy et al. [32] reported CV-FPG values of 14%, 16%, and 20% for individuals with normal glucose tolerance, impaired glucose tolerance, and newly diagnosed type 2 diabetes, respectively. Gimeno-Orna et al. [33] reported that the CV-FPG was an independent risk factor for diabetic retinopathy in 130 type 2 diabetes patients previously without retinopathy after a follow-up of 5.2 years. Similar results were later confirmed in a Japanese population [34]. A study of 5008 patients with type 2 diabetes found that the CV-FPG was a predictor of 5-year all-cause mortality and cardiovascular mortality [35]. The Verona Diabetes Study showed that the CV-FPG within 3 years of follow-up was an independent predictor of cardiovascular mortality [36]. Buscemi et al. [37] measured brachial artery flow-mediated dilation, carotid intima-media thickness (IMT), and glycemic variability using 48-h continuous subcutaneous glucose monitoring in 3 groups of 75 subjects, that is, those without metabolic syndrome and those with metabolic syndrome with or without newly diagnosed type 2 diabetes. Their results revealed that glycemic variability was associated with endothelial function even in nondiabetic subjects.

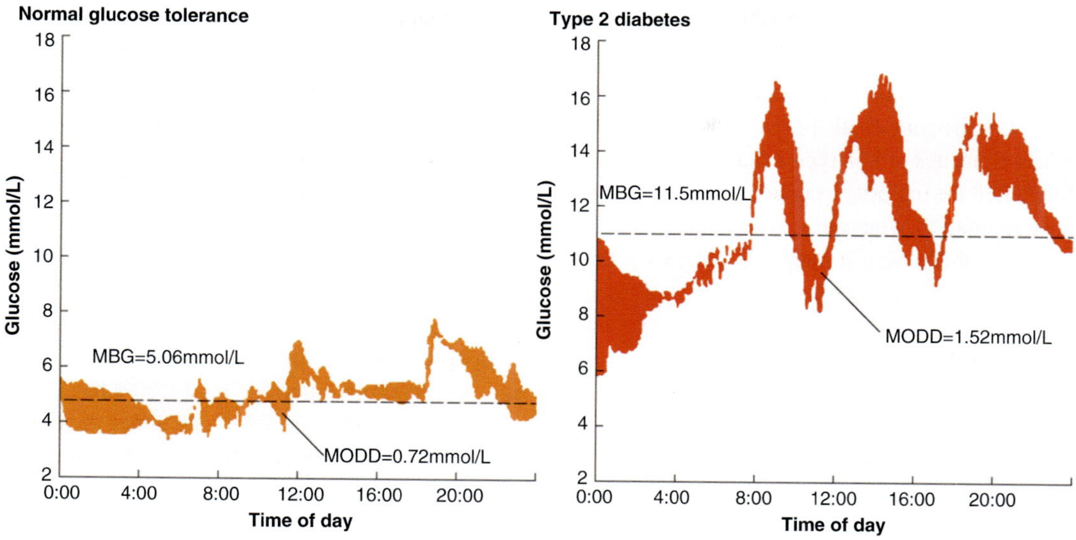

Fig. 6.3 Calculation of MODD during CGM. Notes: *MBG* mean blood glucose, *MODD* mean of daily differences. Note: The figures above are CGM profiles including one subject of newly diagnosed type 2 diabetes mellitus and one subject of normal glucose tolerance for 2 consecutive days (24 h), and the colored areas represent the MODD that needed to be calculated

6.2.2.2 MODD

MODD refers to the mean of the absolute difference between paired blood glucose values in two consecutive 24-h periods. It reflects the consistency and stability of day-to-day blood glucose patterns (Fig. 6.3). Different daily lifestyle patterns including irregular mealtimes and eating habits may influence the MODD. Thus, recording of glucose data and lifestyle patterns together during the CGM period is necessary for calculating the MODD. The study from Alemzadeh et al. [38] showed that the MODD from CGM data was significantly increased in patients with type 1 diabetes. Colombel et al. [39] observed 25 type 1 diabetes patients receiving multiple daily insulin injections and found that a regimen using lispro combined with multiple neutral protamine hagedorn insulin (NPH) compared to a standard multiple daily insulin injections using soluble insulin regimen (20–30 min before each meal and NPH at bedtime) reduced the MODD, with generally similar overall glycemic control.

6.2.3 Parameters Reflecting Postprandial Glycemic Variability

The main parameters include postprandial glucose excursion (PPGE), mean postprandial maximum glucose (MPMG), incremental area under the curve of postprandial glucose (AUCpp), and others.

6.2.3.1 PPGE

The PPGE is the difference between the postprandial blood glucose peak and the corresponding pre-meal glucose concentration [40]. The blood glucose concentration in individuals with normal glucose tolerance generally reaches a peak (usually not exceeding 7.8 mmol/L) within 1 h after eating and returns to the pre-meal level within 2–3 h, and the corresponding PPGE is about 2.0 mmol/L [41, 42]. We have compared the features of postprandial glucose state in individuals with normal glucose regulation and those with type 2 diabetes. The postprandial glucose state in type 2 diabetes mellitus is characterized by a delay of the postprandial glucose peak and excessive glucose excursion for a long time after the ingestion of a meal. Postprandial hyperglycemia was most pronounced after breakfast [42]. Bonora et al. [43] evaluated the blood glucose profiles of 856 type 2 diabetes patients and found that the majority of patients had an excessive postprandial glucose excursion (PPGE >2.2 mmol/L), even among 2/3 patients with an HbA_{1c} <7% (53 mmol/mol).

6.2.3.2 MPMG

MPMG is the mean of maximum postprandial blood glucose levels after three meals over a period of 24 h. Chon et al. [44] calculated a few glycemic parameters in 39 patients who achieved the glycemic target of an HbA_{1c} <7% (53 mmol/mol). The MPMG was 10.34 ± 1.84 mmol/L, and the MPMG was positively correlated with the level of fructosamine.

6.2.3.3 AUCpp

Usually, AUCpp is calculated by the trapezoidal method as the area under the postprandial blood glucose curve above the baseline value (Fig. 6.4). AUCpp can be divided into early (0–2 h) and late (2–5 h) phases. AUCpp can be used to comprehensively assess the characteristics of postprandial blood glucose. Moreover, it has been widely used in the studies exploring the relationship between FPG, postprandial blood glucose, and HbA_{1c}. Monnier et al. [45] carried out a study of a total of 290 type 2 diabetes patients to analyze the exact contributions of postprandial and fasting glucose increments to overall hyperglycemia. Plasma glucose concentrations were determined at fasting (08:00 a.m.) and during postprandial and postabsorptive periods (at 11:00 a.m., 02:00 p.m., and 05:00 p.m.). The areas under the curve above FPG and plasma glucose >6.1 mmol/L were calculated. The relative contribution of postprandial glucose excursions was predominant in patients with fairly good blood glucose control, whereas the contribution of fasting hyperglycemia increased gradually as the severity of diabetes worsened. These results thus provide a unifying explanation for the discrepancies observed in previous studies. We retrospectively reviewed the data of 41 normal individuals and 60 newly diagnosed type 2 diabetes patients by CGM for 3 consecutive days. The relative contri-

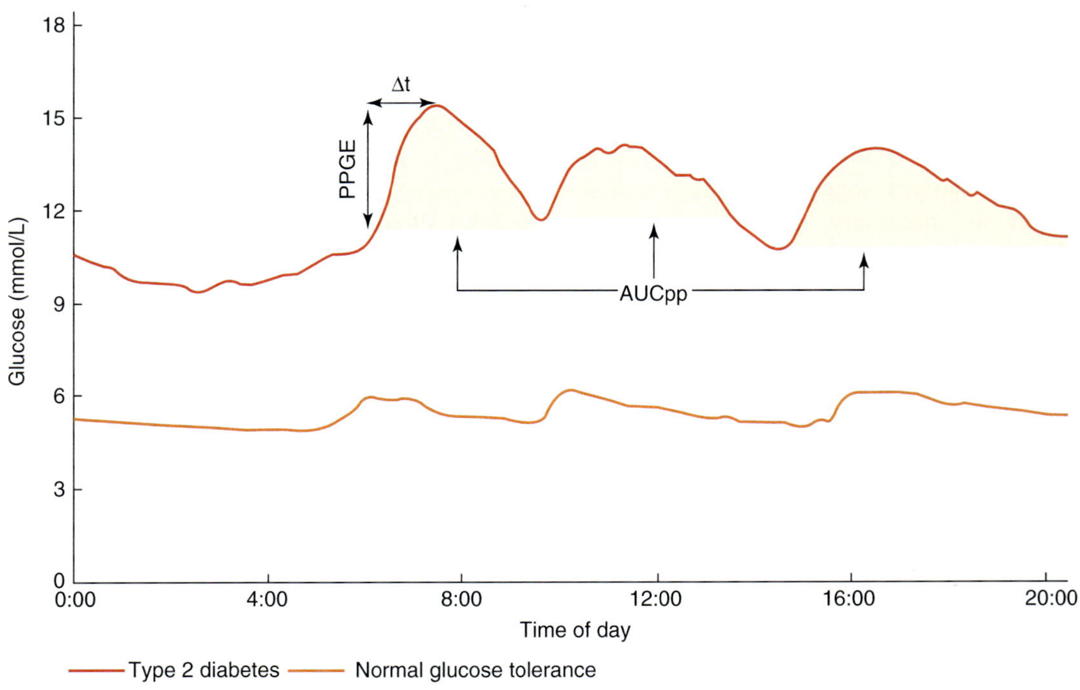

Fig. 6.4 Calculation of parameters affecting postprandial blood glucose fluctuations [42] (Reprint with permission from National Medical Journal of China). Notes: *PPGE* range of postprandial blood glucose concentrations, $\triangle t$ peak time, *AUCpp* incremental area under the curve of postprandial glucose

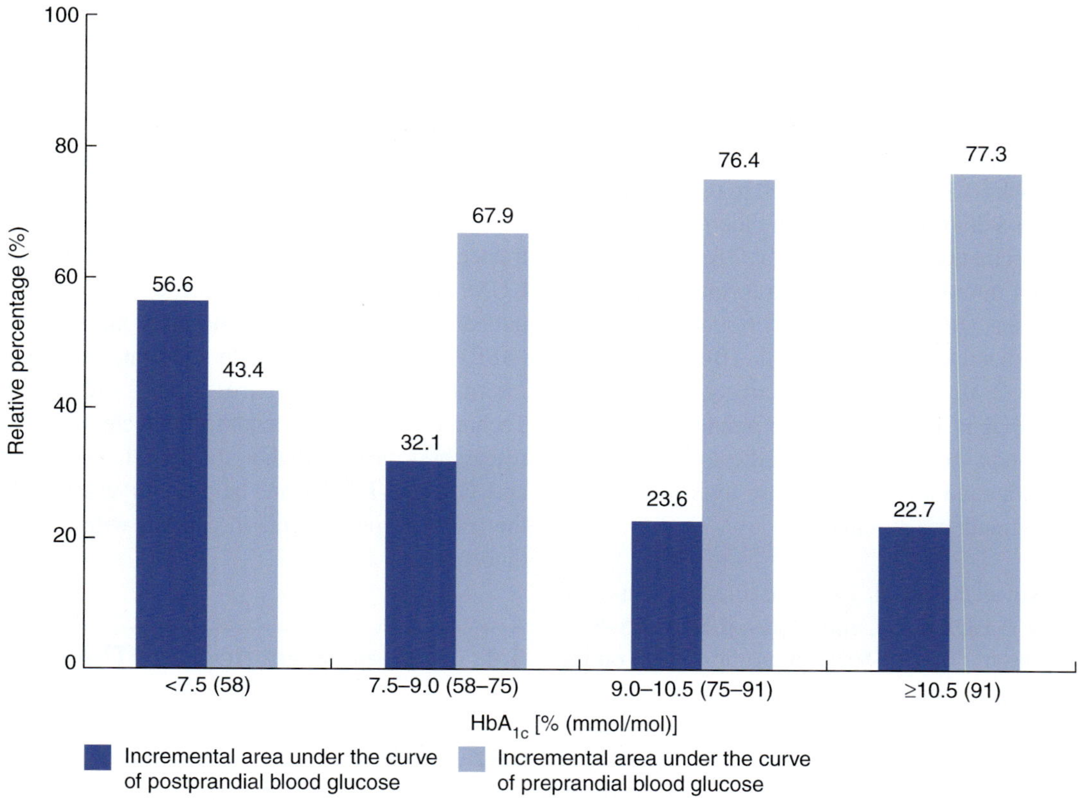

Fig. 6.5 The relative contribution of preprandial and postprandial hyperglycemia to total hyperglycemia in 60 newly diagnosed type 2 diabetes patients [42] (Reprint with permission from National Medical Journal of China)

bution of postprandial hyperglycemia to overall diurnal hyperglycemia was about 1/3 in Chinese type 2 diabetes patients. Postprandial hyperglycemia contributed even more when the HbA_{1c} level was below 7.5% (58 mmol/mol), whereas the relative contribution of postprandial hyperglycemia to overall hyperglycemia decreased progressively as HbA_{1c} increased and accounted for 1/4 when the HbA_{1c} ≥9% (75 mmol/mol) (Fig. 6.5) [42].

6.3 Parameters Reflecting the Risk of Hypoglycemia

6.3.1 Low Blood Glucose Index (LBGI)

The LBGI is a comprehensive score proposed by Kovatchev et al. in the 1990s. It can reflect the frequency and severity of hypoglycemia occurring within 1 month and be used to predict the risk of severe hypoglycemia in the next 3–6 months [46–50], with severe hypoglycemia defined as hypoglycemia leading to coma, epileptic seizure, or unconsciousness that requires medical help for recovery. Similar to the *M*-value, the LBGI was calculated through the logarithmic transformation of blood glucose measurements as below:

1. Convert the blood glucose measurements based on the formula:

$$\text{Trans}(\text{BG}) = 1.794 \times \left\{\left[\text{In}(\text{BG})\right]^{1.026} - 1.861\right\}$$
$$(\text{BG range } 1.1 - 33.3\,\text{mmol/L})$$

2. Calculate the Risk (BG) on the basis of the Trans (BG). If Trans (BG) <0, then Risk

(BG) = 10 × [Trans (BG)]^2; if Trans (BG) ≥0, Risk (BG) = 0.
3. LBGI is the mean of all Risk (BG). From the above, when BG >6.25 mmol/L, Risk (BG) = 0; and when BG is 1.10–6.25 mmol/L, Risk (BG) ranges from 100 to 0. For example, for a diabetes patient with blood glucose measurements of 2.6 mmol/L, 7.8 mmol/L, and 4.4 mmol/L, based on the formula above, the Trans (BG) values are −1.6, 0.4, and −0.66, respectively, and the Risk (BG) values are 25.6, 0, and 4.4, respectively. Finally, the LBGI is 10. It should be pointed out that to obtain the LBGI, measurements from at least four random blood glucose tests per day for 1 month are required.

Kovatchev et al. [47] classified patients into low- (LBGI <2.5), moderate- (LBGI 2.5–5.0), and high- (LBGI >5.0) risk groups based on the analysis of odds for future severe hypoglycemia. Over the following 6 months, low-, moderate-, and high-risk patients reported 0.4, 2.3, and 5.2 severe hypoglycemia episodes, respectively ($P < 0.001$). Another study found that the LBGI can be used to predict severe hypoglycemic events by using real-time dynamic insulin pumps and that the ratio of the LBGI to the high blood glucose index (HBGI) is more helpful in reducing the magnitudes of blood glucose fluctuations [51]. In addition, Peña et al. [52] found that the glycemic risk assessment in diabetes equation (GRADE) and LBGI were significantly associated with flow-mediated dilatation in adolescents with type 1 diabetes, suggesting that hypoglycemia, rather than glucose fluctuation, during CGM relates to impaired vascular endothelial function in children with type 1 diabetes.

6.3.2 Hypoglycemic (HYPO) Score and Lability Index (LI)

These two glucose parameters were proposed by Ryan et al. in 2004 and are mainly used to reflect repeated severe hypoglycemia episodes and the instability of glycemic control [53]. HYPO scores were defined based on the frequency, severity, and degree of unawareness of hypoglycemia. The LI was calculated from 4-week blood glucose measurements of patients. At the 49th Annual Meeting of the European Diabetes Association (2013), Pappas et al. pointed out that through using the HYPO scores suggestive of hypoglycemia episodes when undergoing real-time CGM monitoring in type 1 diabetes patients treated with insulin pumps, 3-month real-time CGM could improve glycemic control of the patients, without affecting the body mass index (BMI) and hypoglycemia. In addition, at the 5th International Conference on Advanced Technologies & Treatments for Diabetes (2012), researchers proposed that the LBGI, GRADE, and GRADE-HYPO are helpful for evaluating the risk of hypoglycemia in patients with type 1 diabetes.

6.4 Other Parameters and Their Clinical Significance

6.4.1 *Q*-Score

Augstein et al. [54] constructed a new metric (*Q*-Score) for assessing blood glucose fluctuations by incorporating five primary factors, namely, central tendency, hyperglycemia, hypoglycemia, and intra- and inter-daily variations. Based on *Q*-Score, the patients were classified into groups of "very good," "good," "satisfactory," "fair," and "poor" metabolic control. Thus, the *Q*-Score is a new metric suitable for screening for CGM profiles that require therapeutic action. Further efforts are needed to identify its practical application and to explore its correlation with complications.

6.4.2 GRADE

The GRADE score was first put forward by Hill et al. [55] and is a tool for comprehensive assessment of blood glucose levels. The calculation formula is listed below:

$$\text{GRADE} = \text{median}\left(425 \times \left\{\log\left[\log(\text{BG})\right] + 0.16\right\}^2\right)$$

The GRADE formula converts glucose values to a risk score, calculates the median, and provides the risk attributable to hypoglycemia, euglycemia, and hyperglycemia. As in the study of Hill et al., for type 1 diabetes patients, the GRADE was 8.09 (20, 8, and 72%), whereas for type 2 diabetes patients, the GRADE was 9.97 (2, 7, and 91%). The results suggested that type 1 diabetes patients had more risk of hypoglycemia.

6.5 Reasonable Selection of CGM Parameters in Clinical Application and Their Perspectives

From the above analysis, we see there is a variety of assessment parameters that have their own characteristics and scopes of application. CV and SDBG, as simple parameters, are valuable in practice and are attracting increasing attention. The LAGE, PT, and AUC also partially reflect the characteristics of glycemic variability. The LBGI and *M*-value, which share the same principle, focus on hypoglycemic factors through the logarithmic transformation of glucose profiles. Especially, the LBGI, as a novel metric for assessing the risk of severe hypoglycemia, facilitates the optimization of diabetes management. The MODD can accurately assess daily glucose fluctuations but requires two consecutive whole-day blood glucose profiles. The CV-FPG is a simple and effective glycemic parameter. However, it only reflects the characteristics of daytime FPG fluctuations. In short, a reasonable selection of CGM parameters should be made based on a comprehensive consideration of characteristics of different parameters as well as the purpose of the assessment.

Currently, the CV, SDBG, and IQR are considered the most preferred measures of glycemic variability [15]. Because there is still a lack of a gold standard for glycemic variability, the relationship between glycemic variability and diabetic complications is currently inconclusive. For microvascular disease, evidence related to glucose variability is mainly presented in patients with type 1 diabetes mellitus. For macrovascular diseases, although the HEART2D study suggested that lowering glucose variability does not improve cardiovascular events in patients with type 2 diabetes after acute myocardial infarction, whereas some other studies suggested that blood glucose fluctuations may increase cardiovascular risks in patients with type 2 diabetes. In addition, several studies have shown that glycemic variability was not an independent risk factor for microvascular complications [56–58].

The effect of short-term blood glucose fluctuations on chronic complications of diabetes has been extensively studied. In recent years, the effects of long-term blood glucose fluctuations on the development of diabetic complications have received widespread attention. Long-term blood glucose fluctuations mainly refer to the HbA_{1c} variability for the same patient obtained from multiple HbA_{1c} measurements during follow-up (usually presented as HbA_{1c} standard deviation, HbA_{1c}-SD). At present, investigators have initiated studies on the correlation between HbA_{1c}-SD and the occurrence of microvascular complications (diabetic nephropathy, diabetic retinopathy, etc.) and macrovascular complications (cardio-cerebrovascular diseases) in both types 1 and 2 diabetes patients. Kilpatrick et al. [59] analyzed the data from type 1 diabetes patients in the Diabetes Control and Complications Trial (DCCT) and found that, in addition to the mean HbA_{1c}, the HbA_{1c}-SD was also correlated with the development of diabetic retinopathy or nephropathy. Similarly, the Finnish National Diabetic Nephropathy Research Group (FinnDiane) conducted a follow-up study in type 1 diabetes patients to analyze the incidence of microalbuminuria, end-stage renal disease, and cardiovascular events and found that the HbA_{1c}-SD was associated with the development of microalbuminuria, diabetic nephropathy, and cardiovascular events [60]. Sugawara et al. [61] followed a total of 812 type 2 diabetes patients without microalbuminuria and found that the HbA_{1c}-SD was an independent predictor of microalbuminuria. Rodríguez-Segade et al. [62] conducted a 6-year follow-up study of 2103 patients with type 2 diabetes and found that the HbA_{1c}-SD was an independent predictor of the progression of diabetic nephropathy. Similarly, Hsu et al. [63] reported that the HbA_{1c}-SD was associated with the progression of microalbuminuria after a 2-year follow-up, suggesting that early control of HbA_{1c} fluctuation is of great significance for the prevention of diabetic nephropathy. The Hong Kong Diabetes Registry study revealed that the risk ratios of the HbA_{1c}-SD for chronic kidney disease and cardiovascular disease were 1.16 and 1.27, respectively [64]. Lee et al. [65] found that in 269 type 2 diabetes patients with a mean $HbA_{1c} \geq 7\%$ (53 mmol/mol), the HbA_{1c}-SD was an independent factor for the development of coronary artery disease. However, other studies have demonstrated that the HbA_{1c}-SD has no significant correlation with chronic diabetic complications. Kim et al. [66] determined the carotid IMT in 120 type 2 diabetes patients and concluded that although higher HbA_{1c} variability was associated with carotid IMT progression in type 2 diabetes patients, it was not an independent predictor of carotid IMT progression. In the large, multicenter cohort of type 2 diabetes patients from the Renal Insufficiency and Cardiovascular Events (RIACE) Italian Multicenter, the HbA_{1c}-SD was an independent predictor of macroalbuminuria and stages 3–5 chronic renal disease, but not diabetic retinopathy [67]. In subsequent studies, they found that the HbA_{1c}-SD was not an independent factor of cardiovascular disease [68]. HbA_{1c}-SD, as a representative parameter reflecting long-term blood glucose fluctuations, as well as its correlation with the occurrence and development of diabetic complications will continue to be a hot research topic.

With a deep understanding of glycemic variability, novel and more comprehensive assessment tools and parameters will be designed, so as to better facilitate the prevention and management of diabetes. On the other hand, the popularization and application of CGM in clinical practice will greatly promote the translation of glycemic variability assessment from research to clinical application, potentially making it an important evaluation system for achieving target glycemic control.

Statement on Consent for Participation
All the clinical trials carried out by the authors in this book have been reported to the Ethics Committee of Shanghai Jiao Tong University Affiliated Sixth People's Hospital already and were in accordance with the Good Clinical Practice and Standards of China Association for Ethical Studies (approval number: 2007-45).

References

1. Yu M, Zhou J, Xiang K, Lu H, Ma X, Lu W. The glycemic excursions in normal glucose tolerance individuals revealed by continuous glucose monitoring system. Zhonghua Yi Xue Za Zhi. 2004;84:1788–90. https://doi.org/10.3760/j:issn:0376-2491.2004.21.009.
2. Chinese Diabetes Society. Chinese clinical guideline for continuous glucose monitoring (2012). Chin J Diabetes Mellit. 2012;4:582–90. https://doi.org/10.3760/cma.j.issn.1674-5809.2012.10.003.
3. McCarter RJ, Hempe JM, Chalew SA. Mean blood glucose and biological variation have greater influence on HbA1c levels than glucose instability: an analysis of data from the Diabetes Control and Complications Trial. Diabetes Care. 2006;29:352–5.
4. Moberg E, Kollind M, Lins PE, Adamson U. Estimation of blood-glucose variability in patients with insulin-dependent diabetes mellitus. Scand J Clin Lab Invest. 1993;53:507–14.
5. Krinsley JS. Glycemic variability: a strong independent predictor of mortality in critically ill patients. Crit Care Med. 2008;36:3008–13. https://doi.org/10.1097/CCM.0b013e31818b38d2.
6. Egi M, Bellomo R, Stachowski E, French CJ, Hart G. Variability of blood glucose concentration and short-term mortality in critically ill patients. Anesthesiology. 2006;105:244–52.
7. Kuenen JC, Borg R, Kuik DJ, Zheng H, Schoenfeld D, Diamant M, Nathan DM, Heine RJ, ADAG Study Group. Does glucose variability influence the relationship between mean plasma glucose and HbA1c levels in type 1 and type 2 diabetic patients? Diabetes Care. 2011;34:1843–7. https://doi.org/10.2337/dc10-2217.
8. Bragd J, Adamson U, Bäcklund LB, Lins PE, Moberg E, Oskarsson P. Can glycaemic variability, as calculated from blood glucose self-monitoring, predict the development of complications in type 1 diabetes over a decade? Diabete Metab. 2008;34:612. https://doi.org/10.1016/j.diabet.2008.04.005.
9. Rodbard D. New and improved methods to characterize glycemic variability using continuous glucose monitoring. Diabetes Technol Ther. 2009;11:551–65. https://doi.org/10.1089/dia.2009.0015.

10. Rodbard D. Clinical interpretation of indices of quality of glycemic control and glycemic variability. Postgrad Med. 2011;123:107–18. https://doi.org/10.3810/pgm.2011.07.2310.
11. Šoupal J, Škrha J Jr, Fajmon M, Horová E, Mráz M, Škrha J, Prázný M. Glycemic variability is higher in type 1 diabetes patients with microvascular complications irrespective of glycemic control. Diabetes Technol Ther. 2014;16:198–203. https://doi.org/10.1089/dia.2013.0205.
12. Jun JE, Jin SM, Baek J, Oh S, Hur KY, Lee MS, Lee MK, Kim JH. The association between glycemic variability and diabetic cardiovascular autonomic neuropathy in patients with type 2 diabetes. Cardiovasc Diabetol. 2015;14:70. https://doi.org/10.1186/s12933-015-0233-0.
13. Subramaniam B, Lerner A, Novack V, Khabbaz K, Paryente-Wiesmann M, Hess P, Talmor D. Increased glycemic variability in patients with elevated preoperative HbA1C predicts adverse outcomes following coronary artery bypass grafting surgery. Anesth Analg. 2014;118:277–87. https://doi.org/10.1213/ANE.0000000000000100.
14. Takeishi S, Mori A, Hachiya H, Yumura T, Ito S, Shibuya T, Hayashi S, Fushimi N, Ohashi N, Kawai H. Hypoglycemia and glycemic variability are associated with mortality in non-intensive care unit hospitalized infectious disease patients with diabetes mellitus. J Diabetes Invest. 2016;7:429–35. https://doi.org/10.1111/jdi.12436.
15. Bergenstal RM, Ahmann AJ, Bailey T, Beck RW, Bissen J, Buckingham B, Deeb L, Dolin RH, Garg SK, Goland R, Hirsch IB, Klonoff DC, Kruger DF, Matfin G, Mazze RS, Olson BA, Parkin C, Peters A, Powers MA, Rodriguez H, Southerland P, Strock ES, Tamborlane W, Wesley DM. Recommendations for standardizing glucose reporting and analysis to optimize clinical decision making in diabetes: the Ambulatory Glucose Profile (AGP). Diabetes Technol Ther. 2013;15:198–211. https://doi.org/10.1089/dia.2013.0051.
16. Service FJ, Molnar GD, Rosevear JW, Ackerman E, Gatewood LC, Taylor WF. Mean amplitude of glycemic excursions, a measure of diabetic instability. Diabetes. 1970;19:644–55.
17. Mo YF, Zhou J, Jia WP. The clinical significance and research progress of MAGE as a glycemic variability index. Chin J Diabetes Mellit. 2011;3:259–63. https://doi.org/10.3760/cma.j.issn.1674-5809.2011.03.016.
18. Service FJ, O'Brien PC, Rizza RA. Measurements of glucose control. Diabetes Care. 1987;10:225–37.
19. Schlichtkrull J, Munck O, Jersild M. M-value, an index of blood-sugar control in diabetics. Acta Med Scand. 1965;177:95–102.
20. Mirouze J, Satingher A, Sany C, Jaffiol C. Insulin efficiency coefficient. m coefficient of Schlichtkrull corrected and simplified by the continuous blood glucose recording technic. Diabete. 1963;11:267–73.
21. Saisho Y, Tanaka C, Tanaka K, Roberts R, Abe T, Tanaka M, Meguro S, Irie J, Kawai T, Itoh H. Relationships among different glycemic variability indices obtained by continuous glucose monitoring. Prim Care Diabetes. 2015;9:290–6. https://doi.org/10.1016/j.pcd.2014.10.001.
22. Oyibo SO, Prasad YD, Jackson NJ, Jude EB, Boulton AJ. The relationship between blood glucose excursions and painful diabetic peripheral neuropathy: a pilot study. Diabet Med. 2002;19:870–3. https://doi.org/10.1046/j.1464-5491.2002.00801.x.
23. Wójcicki JM. J″-index. A new proposition of the assessment of current glucose control in diabetic patients. Horm Metab Res. 1995;27:41–2.
24. McDonnell CM, Donath SM, Vidmar SI, Werther GA, Cameron FJ. A novel approach to continuous glucose analysis utilizing glycemic variation. Diabetes Technol Ther. 2005;7:253–63. https://doi.org/10.1089/dia.2005.7.253.
25. Cameron FJ, Donath SM, Baghurst PA. Measuring glycaemic variation. Curr Diabetes Rev. 2010;6:17–26. https://doi.org/10.2174/157339910790442592.
26. Nathan DM, Kuenen J, Borg R, Zheng H, Schoenfeld D, Heine RJ. A1c-Derived Average Glucose Study Group. Translating the A1C assay into estimated average glucose values. Diabetes Care. 2008;31:1473–8. https://doi.org/10.2337/dc08-0545.
27. Borg R, Kuenen JC, Carstensen B, Zheng H, Nathan DM, Heine RJ, Nerup J, Borch-Johnsen K, Witte DR. ADAG Study Group. HbA_1(c) and mean blood glucose show stronger associations with cardiovascular disease risk factors than do postprandial glycaemia or glucose variability in persons with diabetes: the A1C-Derived Average Glucose (ADAG) study. Diabetologia. 2011;54:69–72. https://doi.org/10.1007/s00125-010-1918-2.
28. Hermanides J, Vriesendorp TM, Bosman RJ, Zandstra DF, Hoekstra JB, Devries JH. Glucose variability is associated with intensive care unit mortality. Crit Care Med. 2010;38:838–42. https://doi.org/10.1097/CCM.0b013e3181cc4be9.
29. Kohnert KD, Heinke P, Fritzsche G, Vogt L, Augstein P, Salzsieder E. Evaluation of the mean absolute glucose change as a measure of glycemic variability using continuous glucose monitoring data. Diabetes Technol Ther. 2013;15:448–54. https://doi.org/10.1089/dia.2012.0303.
30. Siegelaar SE, Kerr L, Jacober SJ, Devries JH. A decrease in glucose variability does not reduce cardiovascular event rates in type 2 diabetic patients after acute myocardial infarction: a reanalysis of the HEART2D study. Diabetes Care. 2011;34:855–7. https://doi.org/10.2337/dc10-1684.
31. Monnier L, Colette C. Glycemic variability: can we bridge the divide between controversies? Diabetes Care. 2011;34:1058–9. https://doi.org/10.2337/dc11-0071.
32. Mooy JM, Grootenhuis PA, de Vries H, Kostense PJ, Popp-Snijders C, Bouter LM, Heine RJ. Intra-individual variation of glucose, specific insulin and proinsulin concentrations measured by two oral glucose tolerance tests in a general Caucasian population: the Hoorn Study. Diabetologia. 1996;39:298–305.

33. Gimeno-Orna JA, Castro-Alonso FJ, Boned-Juliani B, Lou-Arnal LM. Fasting plasma glucose variability as a risk factor of retinopathy in Type 2 diabetic patients. J Diabetes Complicat. 2003;17:78–81.
34. Takao T, Ide T, Yanagisawa H, Kikuchi M, Kawazu S, Matsuyama Y. The effect of fasting plasma glucose variability on the risk of retinopathy in type 2 diabetic patients: retrospective long-term follow-up. Diabetes Res Clin Pract. 2010;89:296–302. https://doi.org/10.1016/j.diabres.2010.03.027.
35. Lin CC, Li CI, Yang SY, Liu CS, Chen CC, Fuh MM, Chen W, Li TC. Variation of fasting plasma glucose: a predictor of mortality in patients with type 2 diabetes. Am J Med. 2012;125:416.e9–18. https://doi.org/10.1016/j.amjmed.2011.07.027.
36. Muggeo M, Zoppini G, Bonora E, Brun E, Bonadonna RC, Moghetti P, Verlato G. Fasting plasma glucose variability predicts 10-year survival of type 2 diabetic patients: the Verona Diabetes Study. Diabetes Care. 2000;23:45–50.
37. Buscemi S, Re A, Batsis JA, Arnone M, Mattina A, Cerasola G, Verga S. Glycaemic variability using continuous glucose monitoring and endothelial function in the metabolic syndrome and in Type 2 diabetes. Diabet Med. 2010;27:872–8. https://doi.org/10.1111/j.1464-5491.2010.03059.x.
38. Alemzadeh R, Loppnow C, Parton E, Kirby M. Glucose sensor evaluation of glycemic instability in pediatric type 1 diabetes mellitus. Diabetes Technol Ther. 2003;5:167–73. https://doi.org/10.1089/152091503321827821.
39. Colombel A, Murat A, Krempf M, Kuchly-Anton B, Charbonnel B. Improvement of blood glucose control in Type 1 diabetic patients treated with lispro and multiple NPH injections. Diabet Med. 1999;16:319–24. https://doi.org/10.1046/j.1464-5491.1999.00077.x.
40. Service FJ, Nelson RL. Characteristics of glycemic stability. Diabetes Care. 1980;3:58–62.
41. American Diabetes Association. Postprandial blood glucose. American Diabetes Association. Diabetes Care. 2001;24:775–8.
42. Zhou J, Jia WP, Yu M, Ma XJ, Bao YQ, Lu W. The features of postprandial glucose state in type 2 diabetes mellitus. Zhonghua Yi Xue Za Zhi. 2006;86:970–5. https://doi.org/10.3760/j:issn:0376-2491.2006.14.009.
43. Bonora E, Calcaterra F, Lombardi S, Bonfante N, Formentini G, Bonadonna RC, Muggeo M. Plasma glucose levels throughout the day and HbA(1c) interrelationships in type 2 diabetes: implications for treatment and monitoring of metabolic control. Diabetes Care. 2001;24:2023–9.
44. Chon S, Lee YJ, Fraterrigo G, Pozzilli P, Choi MC, Kwon MK, Chin SO, Rhee SY, Oh S, Kim YS, Woo JT. Evaluation of glycemic variability in well-controlled type 2 diabetes mellitus. Diabetes Technol Ther. 2013;15:455–60. https://doi.org/10.1089/dia.2012.0315.
45. Monnier L, Lapinski H, Colette C. Contributions of fasting and postprandial plasma glucose increments to the overall diurnal hyperglycemia of type 2 diabetic patients: variations with increasing levels of HbA(1c). Diabetes Care. 2003;26:881–5.
46. Kovatchev BP, Cox DJ, Gonder - Frederick LA, Clarke W. Symmetrization of the blood glucose measurement scale and its applications. Diabetes Care. 1997;20:1655–8.
47. Kovatchev BP, Cox DJ, Gonder-Frederick LA, Young-Hyman D, Schlundt D, Clarke W. Assessment of risk for severe hypoglycemia among adults with IDDM: validation of the low blood glucose index. Diabetes Care. 1998;21:1870–5.
48. Cox DJ, Kovatchev BP, Julian DM, Gonder-Frederick LA, Polonsky WH, Schlundt DG, Clarke WL. Frequency of severe hypoglycemia in insulin-dependent diabetes mellitus can be predicted from self-monitoring blood glucose data. J Clin Endocrinol Metab. 1994;79:1659–62. https://doi.org/10.1210/jcem.79.6.7989471.
49. Kovatchev BP, Cox DJ, Kumar A, Gonder-Frederick L, Clarke WL. Algorithmic evaluation of metabolic control and risk of severe hypoglycemia in type 1 and type 2 diabetes using self-monitoring blood glucose data. Diabetes Technol Ther. 2003;5:817–28. https://doi.org/10.1089/152091503322527021.
50. Kovatchev BP, Cox DJ, Gonder-Frederick L, Clarke WL. Methods for quantifying self-monitoring blood glucose profiles exemplified by an examination of blood glucose patterns in patients with type 1 and type 2 diabetes. Diabetes Technol Ther. 2002;4:295–303. https://doi.org/10.1089/152091502760098438.
51. Luo P, Cheng Q, Chen B, Li Y, Wu J, Zhang X, Jiao X, Zhao J, Lv X. Hypoglycemia and blood glucose fluctuations in the application of a sensor-augmented insulin pump. Diabetes Technol Ther. 2013;15:984–9. https://doi.org/10.1089/dia.2013.0078.
52. Peña AS, Couper JJ, Harrington J, Gent R, Fairchild J, Tham E, Baghurst P. Hypoglycemia, but not glucose variability, relates to vascular function in children with type 1 diabetes. Diabetes Technol Ther. 2012;14:457–62. https://doi.org/10.1089/dia.2011.0229.
53. Ryan EA, Shandro T, Green K, Paty BW, Senior PA, Bigam D, Shapiro AM, Vantyghem MC. Assessment of the severity of hypoglycemia and glycemic lability in type 1 diabetic subjects undergoing islet transplantation. Diabetes. 2004;53:955–62.
54. Augstein P, Heinke P, Vogt L, Vogt R, Rackow C, Kohnert KD, Salzsieder E. Q-Score: development of a new metric for continuous glucose monitoring that enables stratification of antihyperglycaemic therapies. BMC Endocr Disord. 2015;15:22. https://doi.org/10.1186/s12902-015-0019-0.
55. Hill NR, Hindmarsh PC, Stevens RJ, Stratton IM, Levy JC, Matthews DR. A method for assessing quality of control from glucose profiles. Diabet Med. 2007;24:753–8. https://doi.org/10.1111/j.1464-5491.2007.02119.x.
56. Lachin JM, Bebu I, Bergenstal RM, Pop-Busui R, Service FJ, Zinman B, Nathan for the DCCT/EDIC Research Group. Association of glycemic variability

in type 1 diabetes with progression of microvascular outcomes in the diabetes control and complications trial. Diabetes Care. 2017;40:777–83. https://doi.org/10.2337/dc16-2426.

57. Kilpatrick ES, Rigby AS, Atkin SL. Effect of glucose variability on the long-term risk of microvascular complications in type 1 diabetes. Diabetes Care. 2009;32:1901–3. https://doi.org/10.2337/dc09-0109.
58. Siegelaar SE, Kilpatrick ES, Rigby AS, Atkin SL, Hoekstra JB, Devries JH. Glucose variability does not contribute to the development of peripheral and autonomic neuropathy in type 1 diabetes: data from the DCCT. Diabetologia. 2009;52:2229–32. https://doi.org/10.1007/s00125-009-1473-x.
59. Kilpatrick ES, Rigby AS, Atkin SL. A1C variability and the risk of microvascular complications in type 1 diabetes: data from the Diabetes Control and Complications Trial. Diabetes Care. 2008;31:2198–202. https://doi.org/10.2337/dc08-0864.
60. Wadén J, Forsblom C, Thorn LM, Gordin D, Saraheimo M, Groop PH, Finnish Diabetic Nephropathy Study Group. A1C variability predicts incident cardiovascular events, microalbuminuria, and overt diabetic nephropathy in patients with type 1 diabetes. Diabetes. 2009;58:2649–55. https://doi.org/10.2337/db09-0693.
61. Sugawara A, Kawai K, Motohashi S, Saito K, Kodama S, Yachi Y, Hirasawa R, Shimano H, Yamazaki K, Sone H. HbA(1c) variability and the development of microalbuminuria in type 2 diabetes: Tsukuba Kawai Diabetes Registry 2. Diabetologia. 2012;55:2128–31. https://doi.org/10.1007/s00125-012-2572-7.
62. Rodríguez-Segade S, Rodríguez J, García López JM, Casanueva FF, Camiña F. Intrapersonal HbA(1c) variability and the risk of progression of nephropathy in patients with Type 2 diabetes. Diabet Med. 2012;29:1562–6. https://doi.org/10.1111/j.1464-5491.2012.03767.x.
63. Hsu CC, Chang HY, Huang MC, Hwang SJ, Yang YC, Lee YS, Shin SJ, Tai TY. HbA1c variability is associated with microalbuminuria development in type 2 diabetes: a 7-year prospective cohort study. Diabetologia. 2012;55:3163–72. https://doi.org/10.1007/s00125-012-2700-4.
64. Luk AO, Ma RC, Lau ES, Yang X, Lau WW, Yu LW, Chow FC, Chan JC, So WY. Risk association of HbA1c variability with chronic kidney disease and cardiovascular disease in type 2 diabetes: prospective analysis of the Hong Kong Diabetes Registry. Diabetes Metab Res Rev. 2013;29:384–90. https://doi.org/10.1002/dmrr.2404.
65. Lee EJ, Kim YJ, Kim TN, Kim TI, Lee WK, Kim MK, Park JH, Rhee BD. A1c variability can predict coronary artery disease in patients with type 2 diabetes with mean a1c levels greater than 7. Endocrinol Metab. 2013;28:125–32. https://doi.org/10.3803/EnM.2013.28.2.125.
66. Kim CS, Park SY, Yu SH, Kang JG, Ryu OH, Lee SJ, Hong EG, Kim HK, Kim DM, Yoo JM, Ihm SH, Choi MG, Yoo HJ. Is A1c variability an independent predictor for the progression of atherosclerosis in type 2 diabetic patients? Korean Diabetes J. 2010;34:174–81. https://doi.org/10.4093/kdj.2010.34.3.174.
67. Penno G, Solini A, Bonora E, Fondelli C, Orsi E, Zerbini G, Morano S, Cavalot F, Lamacchia O, Laviola L, Nicolucci A, Pugliese G, Renal Insufficiency and Cardiovascular Events Study Group. HbA1c variability as an independent correlate of nephropathy, but not retinopathy, in patients with type 2 diabetes: the Renal Insufficiency and Cardiovascular Events (RIACE) Italian multicenter study. Diabetes Care. 2013;36:2301–10. https://doi.org/10.2337/dc12-2264.
68. Penno G, Solini A, Zoppini G, Orsi E, Fondelli C, Zerbini G, Morano S, Cavalot F, Lamacchia O, Trevisan R, Vedovato M, Pugliese G, Renal Insufficiency and Cardiovascular Events (RIACE) Study Group. Hemoglobin A1c variability as an independent correlate of cardiovascular disease in patients with type 2 diabetes: a cross-sectional analysis of the renal insufficiency and cardiovascular events (RIACE) Italian multicenter study. Cardiovasc Diabetol. 2013;12:98. https://doi.org/10.1186/1475-2840-12-98.

7 Reference Values for Continuous Glucose Monitoring Parameters

J. Zhou and W. Jia

The differences between continuous glucose monitoring (CGM) and traditional glucose monitoring methods are as follows: (1) the former is used to obtain continuous and dynamic glycemic profiles of subjects throughout the day (including nocturnal glucose, glucose after various activities, etc.), whereas the latter only represents the glucose concentration at a specific time point. (2) CGM is used to monitor glucose concentration in interstitial fluid, while the latter detects the plasma or whole-blood glucose concentration. Therefore, the reference range for blood glucose in the traditional glucose monitoring system is not suitable for CGM. As shown in Fig. 7.1, normal individuals also have transient blood glucose concentrations ≥7.8 mmol/L or ≤3.9 mmol/L. Without normal reference values, it is impossible to reasonably discriminate the normal CGM results from abnormalities, which will hinder the widespread application of CGM.

J. Zhou · W. Jia (✉)
Department of Endocrinology and Metabolism, Shanghai Clinical Center for Diabetes, Shanghai Diabetes Institute, Shanghai Jiao Tong University Affiliated Sixth People's Hospital, Shanghai, China
e-mail: wpjia@sjtu.edu.cn

7.1 Establishment of Normal Reference Values for Physiological Parameters

The normal values of a physiological parameter can generally be established using the following methods: (1) Based on the characteristics of the distribution of the indicator in normal population, normal reference values are derived from the mean plus two standard deviations (SD) for normally distributed data or the 95th percentile for skewed distributed data. For a single-indicator study, the sample size of each group should be not less than 100 cases, and the sample size should be as large as possible if allowed. For a multi-indicator study, the sample size should be 10–20 times, or no less than 10 times, of the number of indicators [1]. (2) With the "gold standard" as control, normal reference values can be developed by analyzing the relationship between the two through a receiver operating characteristic curve (ROC). (3) Normal reference values are determined by the actual distribution of the indicator as determined by conducting a large sample survey of a natural population. (4) A prospective, follow-up study is carried out to determine normal reference values by analyzing the intrinsic link between the indicator and clinical situation.

W. Jia (ed.), *Continuous Glucose Monitoring*, https://doi.org/10.1007/978-981-10-7074-7_7

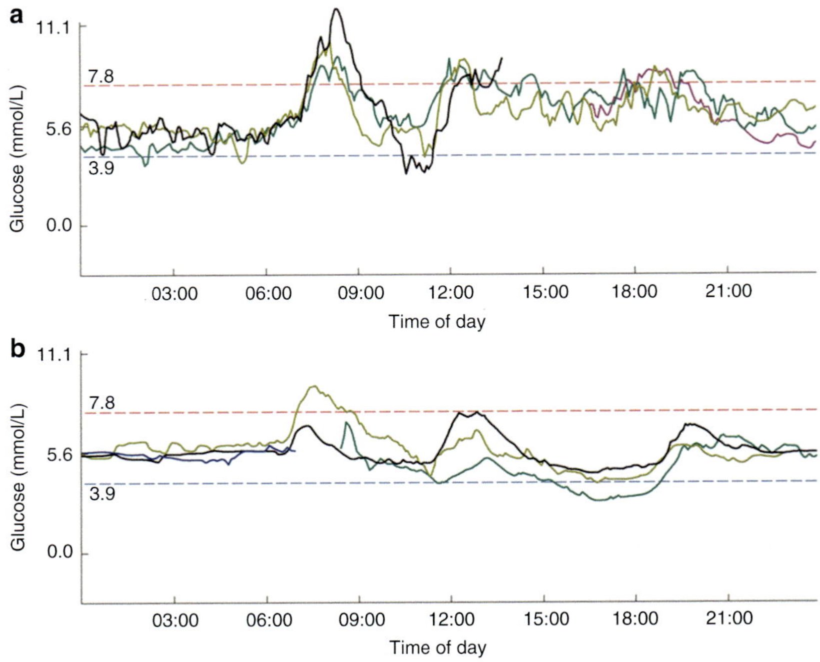

Fig. 7.1 The CGM profiles of one case of type 2 diabetes mellitus (**a**) and one case of an individual with normal glucose regulation identified by oral glucose tolerance test (**b**)

7.2 Establishment of Normal Reference Values for CGM Parameters in the Chinese Population

In the early 1990s, there was a lack of studies on CGM normal reference values, probably because CGM had only been applied clinically for a short time. Using normal values of other physiological indicators (such as ambulatory blood pressure) for reference, it is now considered that reliable CGM normal reference ranges should be based on long-term, prospective follow-up data and large-sample surveys in a healthy population. However, such data are often difficult to obtain. It is feasible to establish the normal reference values for CGM parameters by analyzing CGM measurements in normal subjects.

Our study on normal reference values for CGM parameters was carried out in two steps:

1. First, a preliminary single-center trial utilizing CGM for 3 consecutive days was conducted locally in 48 healthy volunteers in Shanghai, who were 20–59 years of age and had normal glucose regulation identified by oral glucose tolerance test (Fig. 7.2), as the stepping stone for a nationwide multicenter study. The 24-h mean blood glucose level (MBG) was 5.37 ± 0.55 mmol/L, and for 98% (80–100%) of the time, the glucose levels were 3.9–7.8 mmol/L. The mean amplitude of glycemic excursion (MAGE) and mean of daily difference (MODD) were 2.00 ± 0.69 mmol/L and 0.81 ± 0.29 mmol/L, respectively. The blood glucose peaked at 40 (30–45) min, 40 (30–55) min and 52 (35–66) min after breakfast, lunch, and dinner, respectively. The glucose concentrations before three meals were 4.84 ± 0.55 mmol/L, 4.76 ± 0.55 mmol/L, and 4.65 ± 0.49 mmol/L, respectively; and the maximum postprandial glucose concentrations were 6.90 ± 1.29 mmol/L, 6.68 ± 0.88 mmol/L, and 6.85 ± 1.03 mmol/L [2], respectively.
2. A multicenter study was subsequently launched with the aim of establishing preliminary normal reference values for CGM parameters (including those reflecting glycemic level and glycemic variability) in a sample of healthy Chinese subjects with normal glucose regulation, thus providing a theoretical basis for clinical practice.

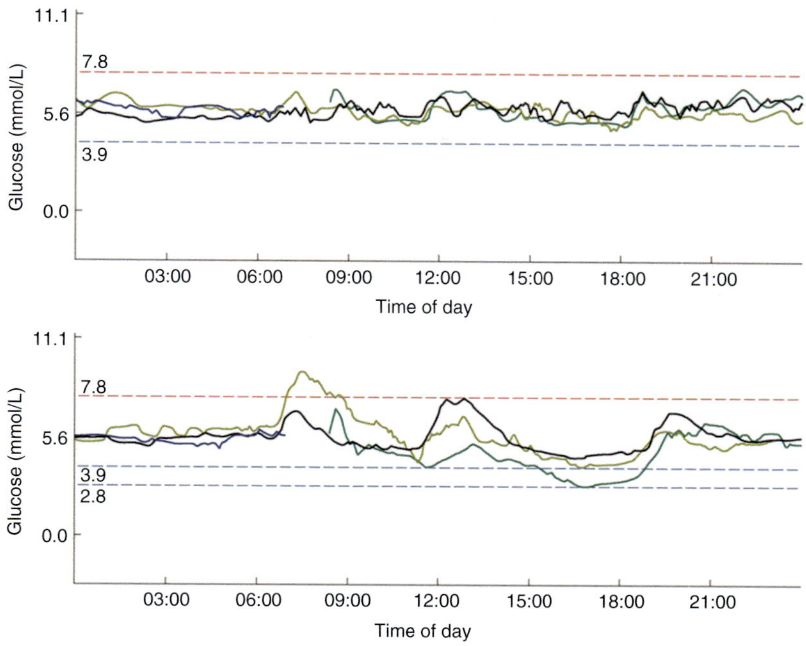

Fig. 7.2 The CGM profiles of two cases of individuals with normal glucose regulation identified by oral glucose tolerance test

We retrospectively reviewed and analyzed 3-day consecutive CGM data from 434 healthy Chinese subjects (20–69 years old, 213 males and 221 females) from 10 hospitals (Shanghai Jiao Tong University Affiliated Sixth People's Hospital; Sir Run Run Shaw Hospital, College of Medicine, Zhejiang University; China-Japan Friendship Hospital; West China Hospital, Sichuan University; the Second Affiliated Hospital of Harbin Medical University; Shanghai Jiao Tong University Affiliated First People's Hospital; the First Affiliated Hospital of Sun Yat-sen University; Fudan University Affiliated Zhongshan Hospital; the First People's Hospital of Foshan; and Ruijin Hospital, Shanghai Jiao Tong University School of Medicine) and established preliminary normal reference ranges for CGM parameters [3]. The inclusion criteria were as follows: (1) no previous medical history of diabetes, hypertension, dyslipidemia, coronary artery disease, or cerebral stroke, (2) fasting glucose monitoring (FPG) <5.6 mmol/L and 2-h plasma glucose (2hPG) <7.8 mmol/L after a 75-g oral glucose tolerance test (OGTT), (3) body mass index (BMI) between 18.5 and 24.9 kg/m^2, (4) triglycerides <1.7 mmol/L and high-density lipoprotein cholesterol ≥1.04 mmol/L, and (5) systolic blood pressure <140 mmHg and diastolic blood pressure <90 mmHg.

In order to maintain the consistency of the data, the research group strengthened the quality control. The training program was carried out at the project start-up meeting, and the CGM use manual was provided. During the study, in addition to contact by telephone, e-mail, and text messages, working conferences were regularly held for training, discussing details and plans, and project summary.

The results showed that subject distribution among age groups was similar: 23.5% were 20–29 years, 20.7% were 30–39 years, 19.8% were 40–49 years, 18.4% were 50–59 years, and 17.6% were 60–69 years. The interstitial glucose values retrieved from the CGM were positively correlated with their corresponding finger stick capillary blood glucose concentrations (r = 0.822). From 434 healthy subjects, a total of 379,308 CGM readings were obtained, and the mean absolute relative difference (MARD) was 9.0 ± 8.4% (Fig. 7.3).

The 24-h MBG for 434 healthy subjects was 5.77 ± 0.57 mmol/L, and the coefficient of variance of MBG over a 24-h period among 10 hospitals was 3.25%, suggestive of a variation within reasonable limits among hospitals.

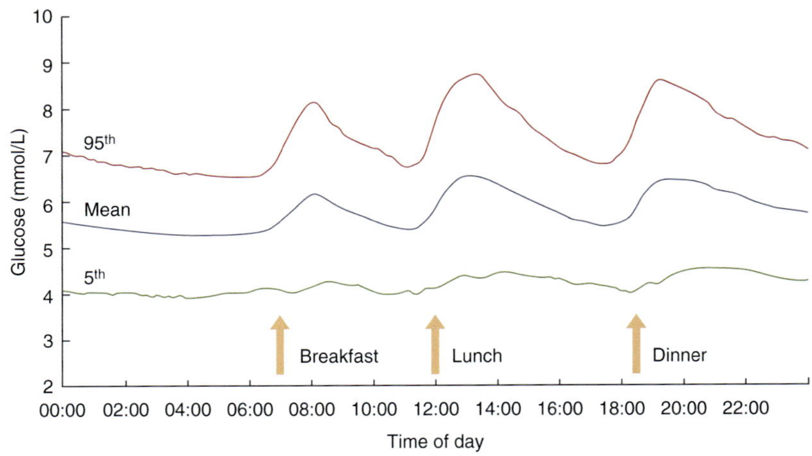

Fig. 7.3 The CGM profiles of subjects with normal glucose regulation. Note: The three curves represent the mean and fifth and 95th percentiles of 24-h blood glucose measurements in normal individuals. The arrows indicate the times of three meals during a day [3] (Reprint with permission from Diabetes Care)

Table 7.1 The 24-h MBG, PT7.8, and PT3.9 of 434 normal subjects of different ages

	Male				Female				
Age (years)	20–39	40–59	60–69	All	20–39	40–59	60–69	All	All
n	93	80	40	213	99	86	36	221	434
24-h MBG	5.63	5.85	5.96	5.78	5.63	5.77	6.07	5.76	5.77
SD	0.60	0.56	0.58	0.60	0.51	0.58	0.50	0.55	0.57
P5	4.57	4.76	4.91	4.68	4.70	4.62	5.29	4.70	4.70
P10	4.76	4.96	5.30	4.90	4.80	4.98	5.40	5.01	4.95
P50	5.70	5.92	6.00	5.80	5.70	5.80	6.18	5.75	5.80
P90	6.45	6.50	6.64	6.50	6.20	6.55	6.72	6.50	6.50
P95	6.56	6.80	6.90	6.70	6.40	6.60	6.84	6.60	6.61
PT7.8									
Mean	3.12	4.24	6.50	4.17	2.93	3.80	7.40	4.0	4.08
SD	4.96	5.98	7.08	5.89	4.47	5.15	8.05	5.75	5.76
P5	0	0	0	0	0	0	0	0	0
P10	0	0	0	0	0	0	0	0	0
P50	0.50	1.75	5.50	1.50	0.50	1.50	5.75	1.00	1.00
P90	9.3	13.0	17.0	12.8	9.0	11.4	21.3	12.5	12.5
P95	14.0	17.5	24.0	17.0	11.5	14.8	22.6	19.0	17.1
PT3.9									
Mean	3.68	1.60	2.50	2.68	1.87	2.40	2.01	2.10	2.38
SD	7.25	4.81	4.95	6.07	3.59	5.61	3.42	4.46	5.31
P5	0	0	0	0	0	0	0	0	0
P10	0	0	0	0	0	0	0	0	0
P50	0	0	0	0	0	0	0	0	0
P90	9.3	4.0	10.9	9.0	6.0	7.2	9.10	7.00	8.0
P95	14.0	8.90	14.4	12.0	11.5	14.0	11.2	11.0	11.6

Note: *MBG* mean blood glucose, *SD* standard deviations, *PT7.8* the time percentage of blood glucose ≥7.8 mmol/L, *PT3.9* the time percentage of blood glucose ≤3.9 mmol/L, *P5*, *P10*, *P50*, *P90*, and *P95* represent percentile values

Among the 434 subjects, the nighttime MBG was lower than the daytime MBG (5.48 ± 0.63 mmol/L vs. 5.91 ± 0.63 mmol/L, $P < 0.001$) by (9 ± 7)%. The percentages of time spent with glucose ≥7.8 mmol/L (PT7.8) and glucose ≤3.9 mmol/L (PT3.9) were 4.1 ± 5.8% and 2.4 ± 5.3%, respectively. There were no significant differences found between men and women regarding the 24-h MBG, PT7.8, and PT3.9 ($P > 0.05$). The 95th percentiles of 24-h MBG, PT7.8, and PT3.9 were 6.61 mmol/L for 24-h MBG, 17.1% for PT7.8, and 11.6% for PT3.9 (Table 7.1). In 434

Table 7.2 MAGE and SDBG of 434 normal subjects of different ages [4] (Reprint from Med Sci Monit)

	Male				Female				
Age (years)	20–39	40–59	60–69	All	20–39	40–59	60–69	All	All
n	93	80	40	213	99	86	36	221	434
MAGE (mmol/L)									
Mean	1.80	1.99	2.16	1.94	1.84	1.95	2.37	1.97	1.96
SD	0.76	0.90	0.84	0.86	0.87	0.94	1.14	0.96	0.91
P5	0.76	0.83	0.84	0.82	0.97	0.72	0.81	0.84	0.84
P10	0.97	1.04	0.92	1.00	1.06	0.87	1.16	1.01	1.01
P50	1.62	1.74	2.03	1.76	1.60	1.72	2.10	1.68	1.73
P90	2.91	3.28	3.37	3.12	2.79	3.41	3.82	3.49	3.26
P95	3.35	3.60	3.69	3.67	3.73	4.08	4.23	4.01	3.86
SDBG (mmol/L)									
Mean	0.75	0.79	0.89	0.79	0.76	0.76	0.94	0.79	0.79
SD	0.32	0.33	0.33	0.33	0.29	0.31	0.36	0.32	0.32
P5	0.35	0.30	0.35	0.35	0.40	0.32	0.34	0.36	0.35
P10	0.40	0.40	0.40	0.40	0.45	0.38	0.48	0.45	0.40
P50	0.70	0.75	0.88	0.75	0.70	0.75	0.98	0.75	0.75
P90	1.20	1.29	1.30	1.25	1.15	1.20	1.44	1.29	1.25
P95	1.38	1.44	1.59	1.43	1.30	1.43	1.60	1.40	1.40

Note: *MAGE* mean amplitude of glycemic excursion, *SD* standard deviations, *SDBG* standard deviations of blood glucose, P5, P10, P50, P90, and P95 represent percentile values

subjects, the maximum and minimum daily blood glucose levels were 8.01 ± 1.29 mmol/L and 4.27 ± 0.63 mmol/L, respectively. The intraday largest amplitudes of glycemic excursion and MAGE were 3.74 ± 1.41 mmol/L and 1.96 ± 0.91 mmol/L, respectively. The standard deviation of blood glucose (SDBG) was 0.79 ± 0.32 mmol/L. The 95th percentiles of MAGE and SDBG were 3.86 mmol/L and 1.40 mmol/L, respectively (Table 7.2).

7.2.1 CGM Parameters (24-h MBG, PT7.8, and PT3.9) Were Evaluated in Relation to Sex and Age in Subjects with Normal Glucose Regulation

24-h MBG showed a weak positive correlation with age ($r = 0.243$ for man, $r = 0.277$ for women; both $P < 0.001$). PT7.8 also showed a weak positive correlation with age ($r = 0.251$ for man, $P < 0.001$; $r = 0.175$ for women, $P = 0.009$). But PT3.9 showed no such association ($P > 0.05$). Analyses for different age subgroups revealed an increased 24-h MBG level for men aged >40 years ($P < 0.01$) and for women aged >60 years ($P < 0.01$). PT7.8 was increased in both male and female subjects aged >60 years ($P < 0.01$). There was no significant difference in the PT3.9 level among the three age subgroups ($P > 0.05$). No significant differences in 24-h MBG, PT7.8 and PT3.9 were observed between men and women within any of the age subgroups ($P > 0.05$, Fig. 7.4).

7.2.2 CGM Parameters (MAGE and SDBG) Were Evaluated in Relation to Sex and Age in Subjects with Normal Glucose Regulation

MAGE showed a weak positive correlation with age ($r = 0.18$ for man, $r = 0.16$ for women; both $P < 0.05$). SDBG also showed a weak positive correlation with age ($r = 0.17$ for man, $r = 0.15$ for women; both $P < 0.05$). Analyses for different age subgroups revealed significant increases in MAGE and SDBG in subjects aged >60 years among all age subgroups (all $P < 0.05$). No significant differences in MAGE and SDBG between men and women were observed within any of the age groups ($P > 0.05$).

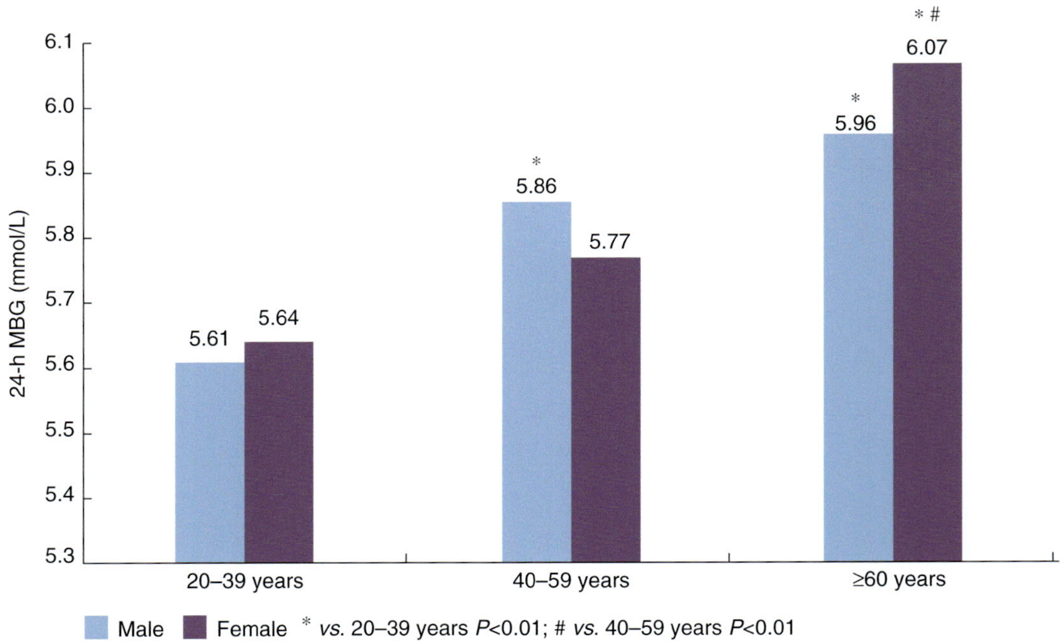

Fig. 7.4 Intergroup comparison of 24-h MBG in 434 normal subjects stratified by sex and age

7.2.3 Reproducibility of CGM Evaluation Was Assessed

A reproducibility test of CGM was carried out in 20 subjects, of whom two men and two women were randomly selected from each of the five age subgroups (20–29, 30–39, 40–49, 50–59, and 60–69 years) at 8–12 weeks after the initial measurements (Fig. 7.5). The average age was 43 ± 16 years (range 22–68); BMI was 22.2 ± 1.8 kg/m^2. No significant differences were observed in terms of 24-h MBG, PT7.8, PT3.9, MAGE, and SDBG parameters between the first time and second time CGM tests (all $P > 0.05$).

7.3 Comparison of Chinese Normal Reference Values for CGM Parameters with International Values

In our study of 434 normal individuals aged 20–69 years old, we found that the 24-h MBG was 5.8 mmol/L by CGM, and the daytime and nighttime MBG were 5.9 and 5.5 mmol/L, respectively. The results were similar to those of a study performed by Mazze et al. [5] who used the FreeStyle Navigator CGM system in 32 normal subjects for 28 days. The 24-h MBG was 5.7 ± 0.4 mmol/L, and the daytime and nighttime MBG concentrations were 5.8 ± 0.4 mmol/L and 5.4 ± 0.3 mmol/L, respectively. In our study, we observed that approximately 60% of subjects experienced blood glucose exceeding 7.8 mmol/L, and blood glucose lower than 3.9 mmol/L was detected in 41% of subjects. A few subjects even experienced a transient (lasting about 30 min) glucose elevation (>11.1 mmol/L) and drop (<2.8 mmol/L). The Juvenile Diabetes Research Foundation (JDRF)-CGM Study Group used CGM to analyze the glucose profiles of 118 subjects with normal glucose regulation (8–65 years old, 83 males and 35 females) from 10 clinical centers. They found that normal subjects had blood glucose exceeding 7.8 mmol/L or lower than 3.9 mmol/L; but in general, 93% of the time, their glucose concentrations were within the range of 4.0–7.7 mmol/L. Moreover, the study demonstrated good reproducibility of CGM in normal individuals, suggesting that this monitoring system had high reliability.

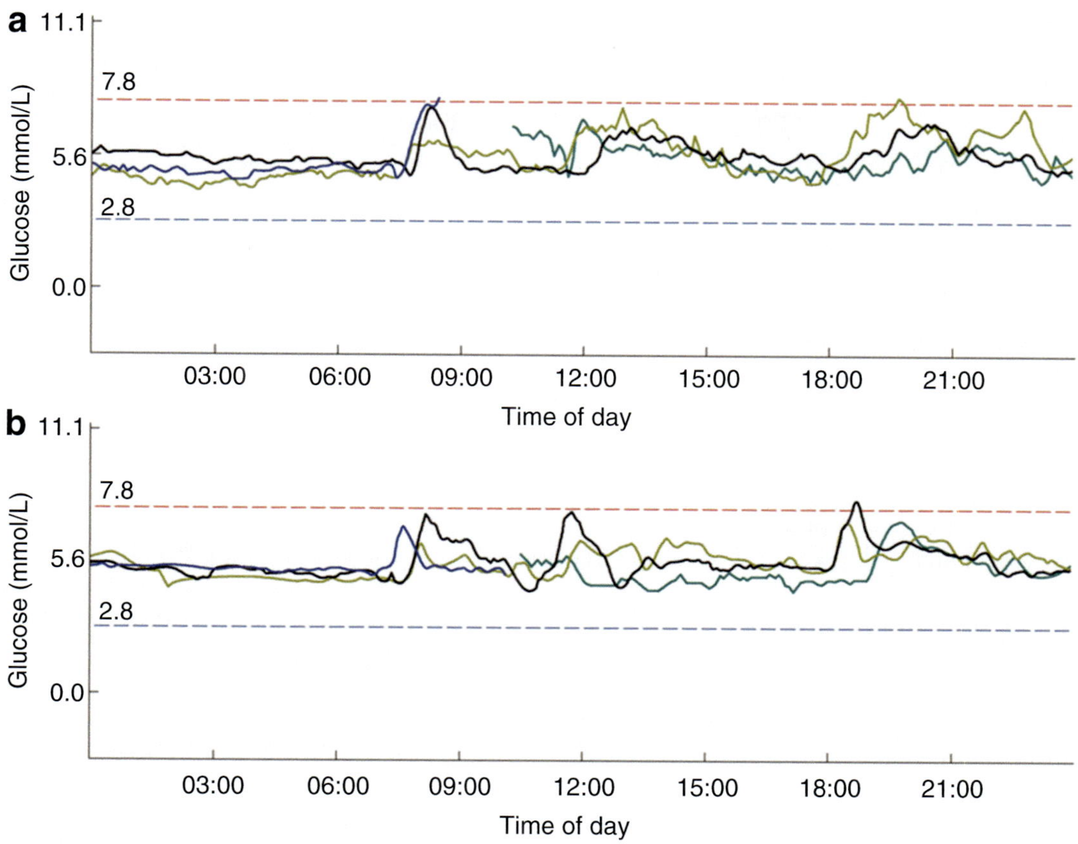

Fig. 7.5 Reproducibility of CGM evaluation. Note: (**a**) first CGM; (**b**) second CGM

The study of CGM in normal individuals has been a hot field of research in recent years. An in-depth understanding of the characteristics of normal blood glucose fluctuations and establishment of normal reference values is essential for clinical application and research using CGM, as well as for the further development of subcutaneous closed-loop systems [6]. Therefore, in addition to our research group, several domestic and international institutions have also carried out relevant research work (Table 7.3). The investigators in the Oxford Centre for Diabetes, Endocrinology, and Metabolism, University of Oxford, analyzed the glucose profiles of 70 subjects with normal glucose regulation (44 American Caucasian, 13 American Hispanic, 7 Asian, and 6 African American) and reported normative ranges for SDBG (0–3.0 mmol/L), MODD (0–3.5 mmol/L), and MAGE (0–2.8 mmol/L). The authors of that article pointed out that measurements of CGM normative ranges in normal subjects added to the body of knowledge regarding normal values, allowing for better identification of abnormalities [7]. Tsujino et al. [8] measured glucose profiles of 24 Japanese subjects (16 males and 8 females) for 4 days by using CGM and found that the 24-h MBG was 5.6 mmol/L and the corresponding SDBG was 0.9 mmol/L. Their study emphasized the significance of CGM in the diagnosis and treatment of postprandial glucose fluctuations in individuals with normal glucose regulation. In 2010, JDRF reported CGM data from 74 subjects with normal glucose tolerance (9–65 years old). The percentages of time (PTs) spent with a blood glucose ≤3.3 mmol/L and >7.8 mmol/L were 0.2% and 0.4%, respectively, and blood glucose was within the range of 4.0–7.7 mmol/L for a PT of 91%. These findings were consistent with some other studies [9, 10]. In addition, it

Table 7.3 Summary of CGM studies in individuals with normal glucose regulation

Author	Publication time	Journal	Sample size	Population	24-h MBG (mmol/L)	SDBG (mmol/L)	MAGE (mmol/L)
Mazze et al.	2008	Diabetes Technol Ther	32	American	5.7	1.0	/
Zhou et al.	2009	Diabetes Care	434	Chinese	5.8	0.8	2.0
Tsujino et al.	2009	Diabetes Technol Ther	24	Japanese	5.6	0.9	/
JDRF-CGM	2010	Diabetes Care	74	American	5.5	/	/
Hill et al.	2011	Diabetes Technol Ther	70	American Caucasian (n=44) American Hispanic (n=13) Asian (n=7) African (n=6)	5.1	1.5	1.4
Xu et al.	2012	Natl Med J China	40	Chinese	6.0	0.9	1.9
Wijsman et al.	2013	Aging Cell	84	Dutchman	4.9–5.4	0.6–0.7	/

Note: *MBG* mean blood glucose, *JDRF-CGM* Juvenile Diabetes Research Foundation Continuous Glucose Monitoring Dataset

has been reported that the 24-h MBG, daytime MBG, and nighttime MBG were 5.4 mmol/L, 5.5 mmol/L, and 5.3 mmol/L, respectively [11]. In a study in the Netherlands that included 58 individuals of different ages with normal glucose regulation, the 24-h MBG was 4.9–5.4 mmol/L, and the daytime and nighttime blood glucose levels were 4.9–5.5 mmol/L and 4.8–5.2 mmol/L, respectively. Moreover, blood glucose levels increased with age [9]. In 2012, Xu et al. [12] analyzed 40 cases with normal glucose regulation (23 males and 17 females) and reported a 24-h MBG of 6.0 ± 0.7 mmol/L, SDBG of 0.9 ± 0.1 mmol/L, MAGE of 1.9 ± 0.8 mmol/L, MODD of 1.1 ± 0.1 mmol/L, and PT 7.8 of 21.7% (5.2 h).

As indicated by the relationship between CGM parameters with age and sex in our study, 24-h MBG is independent of sex but increases with age. There was a significant increase in the 24-h MBG in men aged >40 years and women aged >60 years. We also recommend a unified cutoff point for normal reference values for the CGM parameters, similar to the normal glucose tolerance cutoff points recommended by the American Diabetes Association (ADA) [13] or World Health Organization (WHO) [14]. Therefore, through a multicenter study, we recommend a 24-h MBG value <6.6 mmol/L, PT7.8 <17% (4 h), PT3.9 <12% (3 h), MAGE <3.9 mmol/L, and SDBG <1.4 mmol/L as CGM normal reference ranges for the Chinese population [3, 4] (Table 7.4).

Table 7.4 The reference values for CGM parameters (in 24 h) in Chinese adults with normal glucose regulation [15] (Reprint with permission from Chinese Journal of Diabetes Mellitus)

	Parameters	Normal reference
Glycemic level	MBG	<6.6 mmol/L
	PT 7.8	<17% (4 h)
	PT 3.9	<12% (3 h)
Glycemic variability	SDBG	<1.4 mmol/L
	MAGE	<3.9 mmol/L

Note: *MBG* mean blood glucose, *PT7.8* the time percentage of blood glucose ≥7.8 mmol/L, *PT3.9* the time percentage of blood glucose ≤3.9 mmol/L, *SDBG* standard deviations of blood glucose, *MAGE* mean amplitude of glycemic excursions

Moreover, through subsequent analysis of CGM data from the national multicenter study conducted from 2007 to 2009, we found a significant positive correlation between 24-h MBG and

Table 7.5 The relationship between HbA_{1c} and 24-h MBG during CGM [16] (Reprint from PLoS One)

HbA_{1c} [% (mmol/mol)]	24-h MBG (mmol/L)
5.0 (31)	5.4 (4.7–6.2)
6.0 (42)	6.6 (5.8–7.4)
6.5 (48)	7.2 (6.4–8.1)
7.0 (53)	7.8 (6.9–8.7)
8.0 (64)	9.0 (8.1–10.0)
9.0 (75)	10.2 (9.2–11.2)
10.0 (86)	11.4 (10.3–12.5)
11.0 (97)	12.5 (11.5–13.7)
12.0 (108)	13.8 (12.6–15.0)

glycated hemoglobin A_{1c} (HbA_{1c}) ($r = 0.735$, $P < 0.001$). The linear regression equation between 24-h MBG and HbA_{1c} was as follows:

$$\text{24-h MBG} = 1.198 \times HbA_{1c} - 0.582$$
$$\left(R^2 = 0.670, P < 0.001\right)$$

When the HbA_{1c} was 6.0% (42 mmol/mol), 6.5% (48 mmol/mol), and 7.0% (53 mmol/mol), the corresponding 24-h MBG values were 6.6 mmol/L, 7.2 mmol/L, and 7.8 mmol/L, respectively, during CGM [16] (Table 7.5).

In addition, in 2008, A1c-Derived Average Glucose Study Group also analyzed 507 subjects and investigated the relationship between the HbA_{1c} and average glucose (AG) values. Linear regression equation was showed as follows:

$$\text{AG}(\text{mg}/\text{dl}) = 28.7 \times HbA_{1c} - 46.7$$
$$\left(R^2 = 0.84, P < 0.0001\right)$$

And the linear regression equations did not differ significantly across subgroups based on age, sex, diabetes type, race/ethnicity, or smoking status [17].

Statement on Consent for Participation

All the clinical trials carried out by the authors in this book have been reported to the Ethics Committee of Shanghai Jiao Tong University Affiliated Sixth People's Hospital already and were in accordance with the Good Clinical Practice and Standards of China Association for Ethical Studies (approval number: 2007-45).

References

1. Chen B, Li LP, Li K. Lecture 11: how to determine the range of reference values. Zhonghua Yu Fang Yi Xue Za Zhi. 2002;36:355–7. https://doi.org/10.3760/j:issn:0253-9624.2002.05.023.
2. Zhou J, Jia WP, Yu M, Yu HY, Bao YQ, Ma XJ, Lu W, Hu C, Xiang KS. The reference values of glycemic parameters for continuous glucose monitoring and its clinical application. Zhonghua Nei Ke Za Zhi. 2007;46:189–92. https://doi.org/10.3760/j.issn:0578-1426.2007.03.005.
3. Zhou J, Li H, Ran X, Yang W, Li Q, Peng Y, Li Y, Gao X, Luan X, Wang W, Jia W. Reference values for continuous glucose monitoring in Chinese subjects. Diabetes Care. 2009;32:1188–93. https://doi.org/10.2337/dc09-0076.
4. Zhou J, Li H, Ran X, Yang W, Li Q, Peng Y, Li Y, Gao X, Luan X, Wang W, Jia W. Establishment of normal reference ranges for glycemic variability in Chinese subjects using continuous glucose monitoring. Med Sci Monit. 2011;17:CR9–13. https://doi.org/10.12659/MSM.881318.
5. Mazze RS, Strock E, Wesley D, Borgman S, Morgan B, Bergenstal R, Cuddihy R. Characterizing glucose exposure for individuals with normal glucose tolerance using continuous glucose monitoring and ambulatory glucose profile analysis. Diabetes Technol Ther. 2008;10:149–59. https://doi.org/10.1089/dia.2007.0293.
6. Freckmann G, Hagenlocher S, Baumstark A, Jendrike N, Gillen RC, Rössner K, Haug C. Continuous glucose profiles in healthy subjects under everyday life conditions and after different meals. J Diabetes Sci Technol. 2007;1:695–703. https://doi.org/10.1177/193229680700100513.
7. Hill NR, Oliver NS, Choudhary P, Levy JC, Hindmarsh P, Matthews DR. Normal reference range for mean tissue glucose and glycemic variability derived from continuous glucose monitoring for subjects without diabetes in different ethnic groups. Diabetes Technol Ther. 2011;13:921–8. https://doi.org/10.1089/dia.2010.0247.
8. Tsujino D, Nishimura R, Taki K, Miyashita Y, Morimoto A, Tajima N. Daily glucose profiles in Japanese people with normal glucose tolerance as assessed by continuous glucose monitoring. Diabetes Technol Ther. 2009;11:457–60. https://doi.org/10.1089/dia.2008.0083.
9. Wijsman CA, van Heemst D, Hoogeveen ES, Slagboom PE, Maier AB, de Craen AJ, van der Ouderaa F, Pijl H, Westendorp RG, Mooijaart SP. Ambulant 24-h glucose rhythms mark calendar and biological age in apparently healthy individuals. Aging Cell. 2013;12:207–13. https://doi.org/10.1111/acel.12042.

10. Derosa G, Salvadeo SA, Mereu R, D'Angelo A, Ciccarelli L, Piccinni MN, Ferrari I, Gravina A, Maffioli P, Tinelli C. Continuous glucose monitoring system in free-living healthy subjects: results from a pilot study. Diabetes Technol Ther. 2009;11:159–69. https://doi.org/10.1089/dia.2008.0101.
11. Borg R, Kuenen JC, Carstensen B, Zheng H, Nathan DM, Heine RJ, Nerup J, Borch-Johnsen K, Witte DR, ADAG Study Group. Real-life glycaemic profiles in non-diabetic individuals with low fasting glucose and normal HbA1c: the A1C-derived average glucose (ADAG) study. Diabetologia. 2010;53:1608–11. https://doi.org/10.1007/s00125-010-1741-9.
12. Xu W, Zhu YH, Yan JH, Yang XB, Zhang GC, Zeng LY, Weng JP. Characteristics of real-life glucose profiles monitored by continuous glucose monitoring system in persons with normal glucose tolerance. Zhonghua Yi Xue Za Zhi. 2012;92:1820–3. https://doi.org/10.3760/cma.j.issn.0376-2491.2012.26.007.
13. Genuth S, Alberti KG, Bennett P, Buse J, Defronzo R, Kahn R, Kitzmiller J, Knowler WC, Lebovitz H, Lernmark A, Nathan D, Palmer J, Rizza R, Saudek C, Shaw J, Steffes M, Stern M, Tuomilehto J, Zimmet P, Expert Committee on the Diagnosis and Classification of Diabetes Mellitus. Follow-up report on the diagnosis of diabetes mellitus. Diabetes Care. 2003;26:3160–7.
14. Alberti KG, Zimmet PZ. Definition, diagnosis and classification of diabetes mellitus and its complications. Part 1: diagnosis and classification of diabetes mellitus provisional report of a WHO consultation. Diabet Med. 1998;15:539–53. https://doi.org/10.1002/(SICI)1096-9136(199807)15:7<539::AID-DIA668>3.0.CO;2-S.
15. Chinese Diabetes Society. Chinese clinical guideline for continuous glucose monitoring (2012). Chin J Diabetes Mellitus. 2012;4:582–90. https://doi.org/10.3760/cma.j.issn.1674-5809.2012.10.003.
16. Zhou J, Mo Y, Li H, Ran X, Yang W, Li Q, Peng Y, Li Y, Gao X, Luan X, Wang W, Xie Y, Jia W. Relationship between HbA1c and continuous glucose monitoring in Chinese population: a multicenter study. PLoS One. 2013;8:e83827. https://doi.org/10.1371/journal.pone.0083827.
17. Nathan DM, Kuenen J, Borg R, Zheng H, Schoenfeld D, Heine RJ, A1c-Derived Average Glucose Study Group. Translating the A1C assay into estimated average glucose values. Diabetes Care. 2008;31:1473–8. https://doi.org/10.2337/dc08-0545.

8 Clinical Applications of Continuous Glucose Monitoring Reports and Management Systems

L. Zhang and W. Jia

Continuous glucose monitoring (CGM) technology has been gradually popularized in clinical practice. CGM data can be used to calculate CGM parameters and generate CGM graphs and reports using computer software, helping clinicians to understand the trend and regularity of changes in blood glucose of patients, so as to effectively guide adjustment of treatment regimens and optimization of blood glucose control.

8.1 Standardization of CGM Reports

8.1.1 Contents of the Standardized CGM Report

There are three main types of CGM systems, manufactured by Medtronic Inc. (USA), Dexcom Inc. (USA), and Abbott Company (USA). Due to the different CGM devices, software packages, and statistical methods, CGM reports vary in their contents and formats. In 2008, the US International Diabetes Center (IDC) provided a CGM report format, known as the CGM ambulatory glucose profile (AGP), and elaborated on the contents of the report [1]. In 2012, the expert consensus led by the IDC put forward the standardization of CGM report on the basis of AGP [2]. Standardized AGP should include the following: target range of blood glucose control, blood glucose control level, glycemic variability parameters, and analysis of hypoglycemia and hyperglycemia.

8.1.1.1 Target Range of Blood Glucose Control

The recommended target range of blood glucose control is 3.9–10.0 mmol/L (70–180 mg/dL). It has been reported that if 50% of time is spent within the target range of blood glucose, the glycated hemoglobin A_{1c} (HbA_{1c}) level is generally about 7% (53 mmol/mol) [3]. The CGM report should include the percentage of time (PT) in which blood glucose is within the target range. The parameter PT should be displayed in a prominent position to help patients and clinicians understand the overall control of blood glucose.

8.1.1.2 Blood Glucose Control Level

It is recommended to use daily mean blood glucose (MBG) to assess blood glucose control. The HbA_{1c} value estimated on the basis of MBG should also be included in the report.

8.1.1.3 Glycemic Variability

The use of the standard deviation of blood glucose (SDBG) is recommended to assess glycemic variability. The SDBG is easy to obtain and is associated with multiple glycemic variability parameters. It is a useful tool for assessing intraday blood glu-

L. Zhang · W. Jia (✉)
Department of Endocrinology and Metabolism, Shanghai Clinical Center for Diabetes, Shanghai Diabetes Institute, Shanghai Jiao Tong University Affiliated Sixth People's Hospital, Shanghai, China
e-mail: wpjia@sjtu.edu.cn

W. Jia (ed.), *Continuous Glucose Monitoring*, https://doi.org/10.1007/978-981-10-7074-7_8

cose variability [4]. The coefficient of variance (CV) is calculated from the ratio of SDBG to MBG. It is more stable than MBG and HbA_{1c}, and can reflect the blood glucose fluctuation more effectively, but it is not easy to be displayed in images [5]. The interquartile range is the difference between the upper and lower quartiles. It is easy to be calculated and displayed by images,and it can reflect the glycemic variablity as well [6].

8.1.1.4 Analysis of Hypoglycemia

The blood glucose value ≤3.9 mmol/L (70 mg/dL) is recommended as the cutoff value of hypoglycemia. This criterion is consistent with the definition of hypoglycemia in the 2017 American Diabetes Association (ADA) guidelines for the diagnosis and treatment of diabetes [7]. Based on recommendations from the International Hypoglycaemia Study Group, serious, clinically significant hypoglycemia is now defined as glucose <3.0 mmol/L (54 mg/dL), while the glucose alert value is defined as ≤3.9 mmol/L (70 mg/dL) [8]. Hypoglycemia was defined as a blood glucose less than the threshold value for more than 10 min. The CGM report describes the number and duration of hypoglycemia events.

8.1.1.5 Analysis of Hyperglycemia

The blood glucose values >10.0 mmol/L (180 mg/dL), >13.9 mmol/L (250 mg/dL), and >22.2 mmol/L (400 mg/dL) are recommended as the thresholds for assessing various degrees of hyperglycemia. Also, the PT should be calculated for analysis of hyperglycemia.

8.1.2 Chinese Version of CGM Report

The AGP report can be generated by "CapturAGP" software on the basis of CGM data. Currently, since "CapturAGP" is complex and its Chinese version is not available, the *Chinese Clinical Guideline for Continuous Glucose Monitoring (2012)* recommended the contents and format of a Chinese CGM report [9], including three parts (Table 8.1): (1) general items (basic information of the subject, clinical diagnosis, inspection date, medical staff signature, and report date), (2) CGM data (daily MBG; SDBG; minimum and maximum blood glucose; PTs spent with glucose ≥7.8 mmol/L, ≥10.0 mmol/L, and ≥11.1 mmol/L; and PTs spent with glucose ≤3.9 mmol/L and ≤2.8 mmol/L), and (3) CGM tips (including blood glucose results throughout the monitoring period).

The Chinese version of the CGM report is more concise than the AGP, presenting CGM data in tables, including the target range of blood glucose control, blood glucose control level, glycemic variability parameters, and PTs spent with hypoglycemia and hyperglycemia (Table 8.1).

8.2 Software for Calculating Glycemic Variability Parameters

8.2.1 Commonly Used Glycemic Variability Parameters

Abnormal fluctuations in blood glucose are closely related to chronic complications of diabetes [10]. Therefore, blood glucose fluctuations are also an important part of diabetes management. Application of CGM technology allows for the collection of more glucose data, facilitating accurate assessment of glycemic variability. The clinical parameters reflecting glycemic variability include SDBG, largest amplitude of glycemic excursion (LAGE), *M*-value, mean amplitude of glycemic excursion (MAGE), high blood glucose index (HBGI), low blood glucose index (LBGI), lability index (LI), average daily risk range (ADRR), *J*-index, continuous overlapping net glycemic action over an n-hour period (CONGA*n*), glycemic risk assessment in diabetes equation (GRADE), mean absolute glucose (MAG), mean of daily differences (MODD), and others [11]. The algorithms for these parameters are shown in Table 6.2. Studies have shown that with more time of CGM mornitoring, the percentage error among glycemic variability parameters is reduced. For example, the percentage error of SDBG can be reduced to 10% with the use of CGM for 12 consecutive days [12].

Table 8.1 CGM report [9] (Reprint with permission from Chinese Journal of Diabetes Mellitus)

Name: ____ Sex: ____ Age: ____ Examination Date: ____					
Department: ____ Ward: ____ Bed: ____Hospitalization No./Outpatient No.: ____					
Clinical diagnosis: ____					
Item	Normal reference value (24 h)	Date	Date	Date	Date
Sensor glucose measurement times	–				
Mean sensor glucose (mmol/L)	<6.6				
Standard deviation (mmol/L)	<1.4				
Maximum (mmol/L)	–				
Minimum (mmol/L)	–				
Duration ≥11.1 mmol/L (hour:minute)	–				
Duration ≥10.0 mmol/L (hour:minute)	–				
Duration ≥7.8 mmol/L (hour:minute)	<4 h (17%)				
Duration ≤3.9 mmol/L (hour:minute)	<3 h (12%)				
Duration ≤2.8 mmol/L (hour:minute)	–				
CGM parameters:					
Total sensor glucose measurements:					
Mean absolute difference (MAD): ______%					
Average sensor glucose: ______ mmol/L					
Sensor glucose standard deviation: ______ mmol/L					
Highest sensor glucose value and lowest sensor glucose value: ______ mmol/L and ______ mmol/L					
Times when sensor glucose ≥7.8 mmol/L, ≥10.0 mmol/L, and ≥11.1 mmol/L: ____ h ____ min (__%),____ h ____ min (__%), ____ h ____ min (__%)					
Times when sensor glucose ≤3.9 mmol/L and ≤2.8 mmol/L: ____ h____ min (__%), ____ h____ min (__%)					
Reporter: ____________ Auditor: ____________Report date: ____________					

8.2.2 Software for Calculating Glycemic Variability Parameters

The calculation process for glycemic variability parameters is cumbersome and error-prone, whereas the use of computer software is more rapid and accurate. Therefore, there are a number of calculation software programs available for calculating glycemic variability parameters in clinical and research applications. In 2011, the Oxford Centre for Diabetes developed "EasyGV" software for calculating glycemic variability of blood glucose. This software is developed based on Excel VBA and is able to assess a variety of glycemic variability parameters, including SDBG, *M*-value, MAGE, ADRR, LI, *J*-index, LBGI, and MODD. The software is currently available at http://www.phc.ox.ac.uk/research/technology-outputs/EasyGV. With "EasyGV," researchers have analyzed CGM results from 70 healthy subjects, calculated glycemic variability parameters, and put forward a normal reference range for each parameter [13].

In 2011, Polish scholars developed the Internet-based calculation software for glycemic variability parameters, namely, "GlyCulator" [14]. The software runs on the website and can directly analyze the files containing the CGM data (files with suffix of .xls or .fst). "GlyCulator" can analyze a variety of glycemic parameters including SDBG, *M*-value, MAGE, ADRR, LI, *J*-index, and CONGA*n*.

8.2.3 Calculation Software for MAGE

Because MAGE is reasonably designed and it has good correlation with oxidative stress and chronic complications of diabetes, it was recognized as a "golden standard" reflecting glycemic variability

[15]. However, manual calculation of MAGE is cumbersome and error-prone. Thus, many investigators have developed software that automatically calculates MAGE values for convenient application.

In 2011, the German researchers developed the software "Calculator of MAGE" [16]. The software is designed based on Delphi 6, and it is able to calculate MAGE values for subjects from CGM data. The calculation method of the software is similar to a manual calculation method. Through plotting the CGM graph, the software seeks the amplitude of glucose excursions more than 1 SDBG to obtain the MAGE value. The software was used to analyze the CGM data of 474 outpatients to calculate MAGE values, which were compared to manually calculated MAGE values. The results showed that the two MAGEs were highly correlated in diabetes patients ($r = 0.960$, $P < 0.001$). A Bland–Altman scatter plot showed excellent agreement between the two MAGE methods.

In 2011, the Australian researchers developed another software program, the "Automated Algorithm of MAGE," for calculating MAGE [17]. The software provides two algorithms that can both be used to calculate MAGE. One algorithm creates a moving average with exponentially smoothing weights and filters out glucose excursions >1 SDBG to calculate MAGE. The other algorithm is designed to compare three consecutive glucose measurements. If three consecutive observations are in the same direction (increasing or decreasing sequence), then the second or middle observation is of no interest. Using this algorithm, glycemic excursions are filtered out, and then a SDBG value is used to eliminate noncountable excursions and finally calculate MAGE value. Owing to a great relationship between the direction of the first countable excursion and the "rule" for the remainder excursions, the software used "MAGE+" to represent upward excursions, "MAGE−" to represent downward excursions, and "MAGEavg" to represent the mean of upward and downward excursions.

Due to differences in the algorithms of various softwares, the results of glycemic variability parameters by softwares may also differ. Taking MAGE as an example, researchers have compared the agreement of four MAGE software programs, "EasyGV," "GlyCulator," "Calculator of MAGE," and "Automated Algorithm of MAGE" [18]. The results showed significant differences in MAGE values calculated by different software programs ($P < 0.01$). Specifically, "GlyCulator" returned the highest MAGE, and "EasyGV" gave the lowest MAGE; "Calculator of MAGE" and "Automated Algorithm of MAGE" returned the intermediate MAGE values. Correlation analysis showed that "Calculator of MAGE" and "Automated Algorithm of MAGE" had the best correlation ($r = 0.999$), whereas "EasyGV" and "GlyCulator" had worse correlation ($r = 0.787$). The correlations of "EasyGV" with "Calculator of MAGE" ($r = 0.873$) and "Automated Algorithm of MAGE" ($r = 0.871$) were observed, which were similar to the correlations of "GlyCulator" with "Calculator of MAGE" ($r = 0.909$) and "Automated Algorithm of MAGE" ($r = 0.910$). Therefore, it is better to manually recheck the software results of glycemic parameters combined with CGM graphs prior to using in scientific research and clinical application.

8.2.4 Main Controversy in Glycemic Variability Parameters

The conflicting results for glycemic variability parameters are derived from uncertain definitions and inconsistent algorithms. Taking MAGE as an example, the algorithm needs to be standardized in the following aspects:

1. The selection of the starting time point may affect the MAGE result. In the MAGE algorithm, the chronological CGM data are used, with common starting time points at 12:00 a.m., 07:00 a.m., 12:00 p.m., 04:00 p.m., etc. Since the starting time point is manually selected, analysis at different starting time points may lead to differences in the direction of the first excursion. Because all glucose excursions that have the same direction with the first qualifying excursion are included for calculation of MAGE, the selection of the first

excursion will affect the MAGE calculation result.

2. Direction of glucose excursions is another possible controversy. In the MAGE algorithm, "Calculator of MAGE" software calculates all glucose excursions that have the same direction as the first qualifying excursion. However, "EasyGV" software calculates the mean of all glucose excursions, irrespective of upward or downward directions. "Automated Algorithm of MAGE" calculates the upward excursions as "MAGE+" and the downward excursions as "MAGE−" and finally relies on manual selection based on CGM graphs. The different amplitudes between upward and downward excursions lead to the differences in MAGE results.
3. Whether starting or ending points are included in the calculation may also affect the MAGE calculation. Starting-point and end-point blood glucose levels are "unfinished" fluctuations in blood glucose, which may overestimate or underestimate the magnitude of blood glucose fluctuations. Thus, they are excluded by some calculation software programs, for example, "EasyGV." However, exclusion of starting-point and end-point blood glucose may lead to loss of some glycemic information; thus, these data are selectively included for calculation by some software programs, such as "Automated Algorithm of MAGE." For "Calculator of MAGE" software, users can decide whether the starting-point or end-point blood glucose data are included by the settings of the software.

8.3 CGM Software in China

8.3.1 MAGE Software

8.3.1.1 Algorithm and Features of MAGE Software

"EasyGV" and other software programs are only available in English, which do not fit the habits of Chinese users. In 2011, we first developed the "Parameter calculating continuous glucose monitoring—Calculation software of MAGE" ("MAGErun," Software Copyright No. 2011SR089489). The software was based on C++ language and can be used to obtain MAGE values by calculating CGM data. The software is user-friendly and easy to operate. It is able to process multiple sets of data at the same time and can also calculate the MODD value. It has been widely used in scientific research and clinical practice. Subsequently, we independently developed the CGM Reporting Management System ("CGMreport," Software Copyright Registration No. 2012SR049264; see below). Then in 2013, the two software systems were integrated and upgraded to generate the CGM Reporting Management System V2.0 (Software Copyright Registration No. 2014SR034309). In 2015, the V2.0 was upgraded to V3.0, allowing for support of real-time CGM systems, including automatic reporting capabilities, calculation of glycemic variability parameters, and plotting fusion diagram of glucose data (Fig. 8.1).

The algorithm used by the software to calculate MAGE is as follows: the starting time point for MAGE analysis is generally chosen as 00:00, and 24-h glycemic variability from 00:00 to 23:59 is analyzed. First, three consecutive blood glucose measurements are analyzed from the starting point. If they are in the same direction, the second or middle observation is ignored; if different, the middle observation is retained. Then from the second value, another three consecutive measurements are analyzed, and so on. The glycemic excursions are screened after multiple cycles, and then the glycemic excursions are filtered out by 1 SDBG value. The MAGE is calculated based on all glucose excursions that have the same direction as the first qualifying excursion. The algorithm requires continuous monitoring of blood glucose without interruption for a long time; otherwise, the glycemic information is lost, and a calculation error is generated.

8.3.1.2 How to Use the Software

The CGM data must be input prior to use of the software. First, open the template file MAGE.xls (an Excel spreadsheet file) in the template directory. Then, replace with CGM measurement data

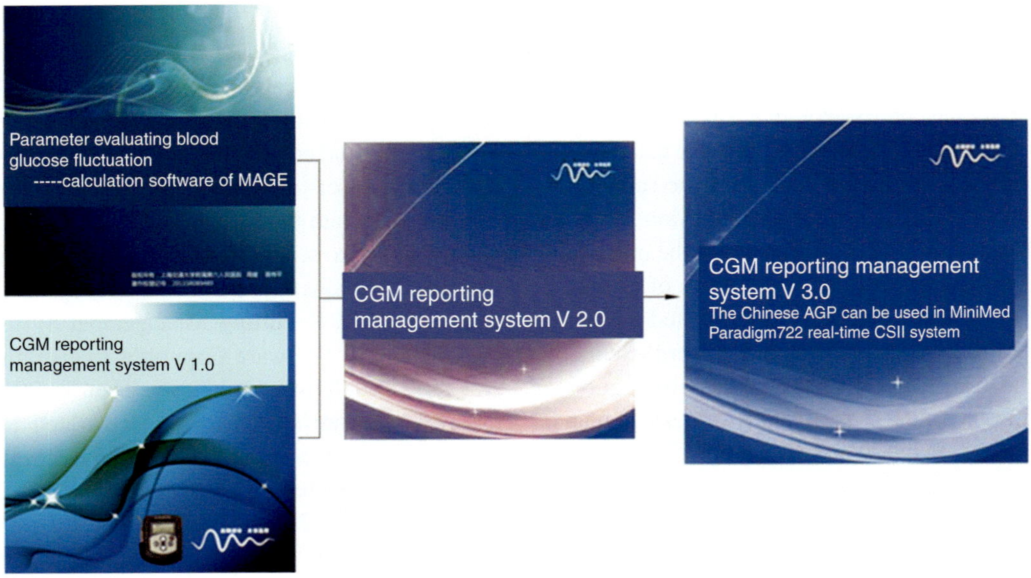

Fig. 8.1 The CGM Report Management System developed by the Department of Endocrinology and Metabolism, Shanghai Jiao Tong University Affiliated Sixth People's Hospital

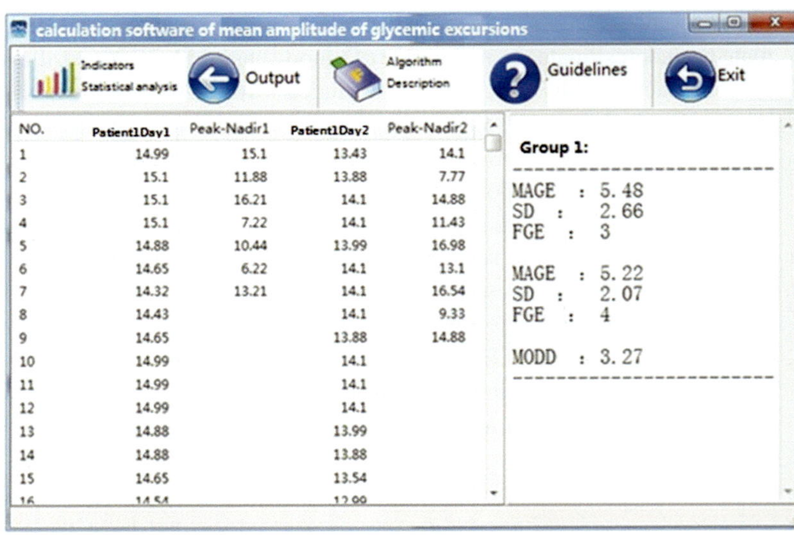

Fig. 8.2 The calculation interface of "MAGErun" software and calculation results

in the table. The first row in the table (BG1) corresponds to the first CGM value, the second row (BG2) corresponds to the second CGM value, and so on until all CGM data are input. Then, the .xls file is saved and exited after the completion of data input.

After the data input is completed, run MAGErun.exe to access the system. First, make sure that the MAGE.xls file is closed, and then click the [Indicators statistical analysis] button. The system will automatically calculate MAGE and SDBG values in each column and MODD values of two adjacent columns from the input data (Fig. 8.2). Check if the results are correct, and click [Output] to export the results to an Excel file.

8.3.1.3 Clinical Application of the Software

The software has been utilized to analyze the CGM data of 434 normal subjects from 10 centers in China. It was found that SDBG <1.4 mmol/L and MAGE <3.9 mmol/L can be used as the normal reference values for assessing glycemic variability in the Chinese population [19]. In another study, we used the software to calculate the MAGE values of 216 patients with type 2 diabetes and to analyze correlation of the MAGE value with carotid intima-media thickness (IMT). The results showed that MAGE was positively correlated with carotid IMT ($r = 0.365$, $P < 0.01$), demonstrating that glycemic variability may be associated with atherosclerosis [20]. The software has been widely popularized throughout China, providing a great convenience for clinical research involving CGM.

8.3.2 CGM Report Management System

8.3.2.1 Structure of the Software

Since "CapturAGP" and "MiniMed Solution" only have English version, CGM operators need to read the English report and then translate and copy the data to a Word file in a Chinese version when reporting the CGM results. This process is time-consuming, laborious, and not conducive to clinicians' timely and accurate understanding of blood glucose information and fluctuations in patients. Moreover, with the increasing amount of CGM data, it is difficult to manage CGM reports and effectively analyze CGM data. To this end, we have independently developed the CGM Reporting Management System ("CGMreport," Software Copyright Registration No. 2012SR049264) [21]. On the basis of Visual Basic 6.0, using Access database, the software is able to automatically obtain data from the CGM system and calculate glycemic variability parameters to generate a CGM report according to CGM data.

8.3.2.2 Features of the Software

1. Rapid report preparation and convenient operation: without any settings, the software can directly obtain CGM record from an .mmg file or .csv file and analyze them. The report time is shortened from 10 min to 20 s. The operating interface is user-friendly, and it is easy to master by a CGM operator after simple training. While reducing the workload of CGM operators, the software also helps clinicians gain a timely and accurate understanding of the glycemic information of patients.
2. Report format in accordance with the guidelines: the report is in full compliance with the requirements of the Chinese Clinical Guideline for CGM. In addition to calculating the mean, maximum, and minimum blood glucose values, it presents the PTs spent with various blood glucose levels through the day. The system also provides the normal reference ranges of glycemic parameters (Fig. 8.3). The system is able to directly obtain CGM data from CGM record files and rapidly and comprehensively display the glycemic data of patients.
3. Calculation of multiple glycemic variability parameters: the software can calculate multiple glycemic variability parameters, including MAGE, MODD, SDBG, LAGE, *M*-value, ADRR, LBGI, HBGI, CONGA*n*, LI, *J*-index, MAG, GRADE, and others, which helps physicians to fully grasp the trends of blood glucose fluctuations in patients (Fig. 8.4).
4. CGM graphs: the system for the first time incorporates the normal CGM glucose fluctuations. Also, average multi-day curves are added onto the original CGM glucose curves, allowing more clear observation of the trends in glycemic variability (Fig. 8.5).
5. Convenient searching of CGM data and graphs: the system provides two ways for searching CGM data and graphs, that is, by condition or by graph. The users can quickly find the desired reports by setting the query conditions, and the users can also search CGM graphs to obtain intuitive information regarding glycemic variability.
6. Data export: The obtained CGM data can be exported to Excel files. In the Excel files, a large amount of glycemic data including MBG, SDBG, the highest and lowest glucose values, PTs, and glycemic variability parameters such as MAGE, MODD, CONGA*n*, and ADRR are provided and can be easily used for statistical analysis.

Shanghai 6th People's Hospital

Continuous Glucose Monitoring (CGM) Report

Name: Stone Zhang Sex: Male Age: 46 yr Examination Date: 2015/11/20

Department: Endocrine Ward: 9W Bed: 33 Serial No: 1

Hospitalization No: 1234567 Outpatient No: Diagnosis: Diabetes

Date	Normal Reference (24 hours)	Nov.13	Nov.14	Nov.15	Nov.16
Sensor Glucose measurement times	-	157	288	288	112
Mean sensor glucose (mmol/L)	<6.6	7.7	8.83	8.17	8.38
Standard Deviation (mmol/L)	<1.4	1.78	2.41	1.52	1.71
Maximum (mmol/L)	-	10.44	16.49	12.44	12.77
Minimum (mmol/L)	-	4.22	6.05	6.33	7.05
Duration ≥11.1 mmol/L (hour: minute)	-	0:00 0%	3:55 16%	2:15 9%	1:15 13%
Duration ≥10.0 mmol/L (hour: minute)	-	1:35 12%	6:20 26%	4:05 17%	1:50 20%
Duration ≥7.8 mmol/L (hour: minute)	<4 h (17%)	6:30 50%	11:30 48%	8:55 37%	2:45 29%
Duration ≥7.0 mmol/L (hour: minute)		7:30 57%	17:35 73%	20:15 84%	9:20 100%
Duration ≤3.9 mmol/L (hour: minute)	<3 h (12%)	0:00 0%	0:00 0%	0:00 0%	0:00 0%
Duration ≤2.8 mmol/L (hour: minute)	-	0:00 0%	0:00 0%	0:00 0%	0:00 0%

CGM Reslut: Sensor glucose measurement times are 845, Mean Absolute Difference (MAD) is 10.2%, Mean sensor glucose is 8.34 mmol/L, Standard Deviation is 1.98 mmol/L, Maximum and Minimum of sensor glucose are respectively 16.5 mmol/L, 4.2 mmol/L. The Duration of sensor glucose ≥7.0 mmol/L, ≥7.8 mmol/L, ≥10 mmol/L, and ≥11.1 mmol/L are 54hours(h)40minutes(m)(78%), 29h40m(42%), 13h50m (20%) and 7h25m (11%); The duration of sensor glucose ≤3.9 mmol/L and ≤2.8 mmol/L are 0h00m (0%), and 0h00m (0%).

Reporter: Administrator Auditor: Zhang Report date: 2015/11/23

Fig. 8.3 The CGM report generated by the CGM Reporting Management Software

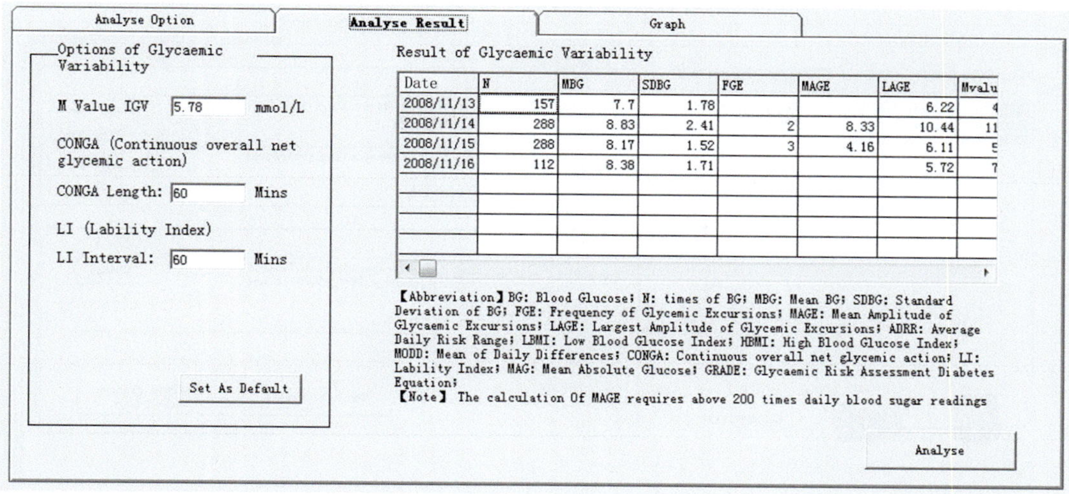

Fig. 8.4 The glycemic variability parameters calculated by CGM Reporting Management Software

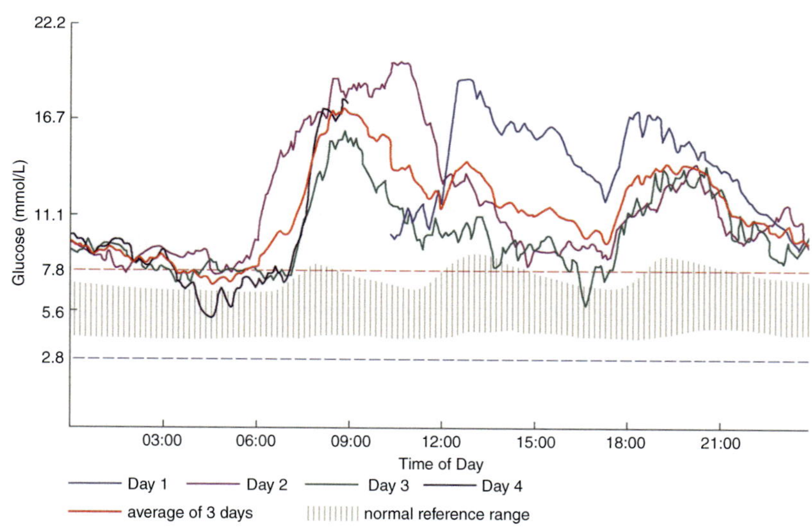

Fig. 8.5 CGM profiles of CGM Reporting Management Software. Notes: The red curve is the average multi-day curve of blood glucose; the shadowed parts show normal reference ranges for CGM parameters

8.3.2.3 Operation of the Software

1. Data acquisition: The Medtronic CGM system is one of the most widely used and mature CGM technologies in China. The CGM Report Management System supports direct analysis of data files for Medtronic CGM systems. The Medtronic CGM system data files can be downloaded via the supporting software "MiniMed Solutions" or "CareLink." For other CGM systems, the data need to be input for analysis according to the required format.

   The system supports two types of file formats, with the suffixes .mmg and .csv. The MMG file is a CGM data file downloaded by "MiniMed Solutions." The CSV file cannot be downloaded directly, and the data must be input manually according to the template. For the Medtronic CGM system, the users can export the data from the CGM system via the "CareLink" software.
2. Data analysis: After data acquisition, start the software "CGM Report Management System." The system comes with a default username "system administrator" and

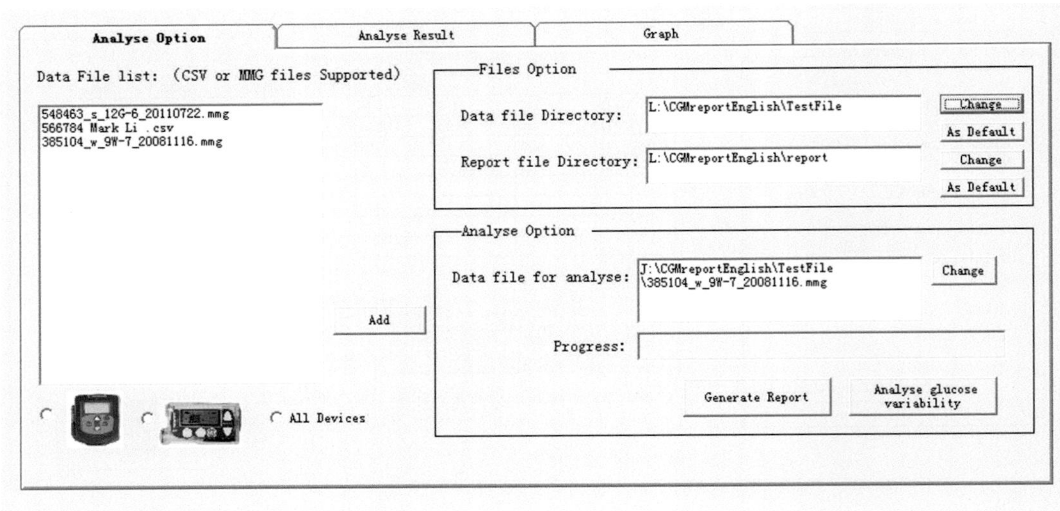

Fig. 8.6 The "Generate Report" interface of the CGM Reporting Management System [21] (Reprint with permission from Chinese Journal of Diabetes Mellitus)

password "6yuannfm." After a successful login into the main interface of the system, click [Generate Report] to enter the subject selection interface. If the subject's information is already in the list, select and double-click the subject; if not, click [New Report], add the subject, and enter the report interface (Fig. 8.6). At the upper part of the interface, the users can input the subject information; the left column shows available CGM data files for analysis. The users can simply select the target CGM data file and click [Generate Report] to generate a CGM report.

In the automatic analysis interface, first input the complete information of the subject, and click [Save] at the top of the menu. Then set the source location of CGM data and the output directory for the CGM report. The source file location is the directory where the CGM file is located, and the CGM data file will be displayed in the list. The CGM report is output to the output directory in Word, and the CGM profiles reflecting glycemic variability are also saved in the same directory. After setting, select the CGM data file to be analyzed (must be a file with the suffix .mmg or .csv) in the list on the left column, and click [Add] to add the data file into the analysis box. Click [Generate Report], and wait for the progress bar to finish, and then the users can view the CGM report and analysis results.

3. Analysis results: The system provides a CGM report in Word format (Fig. 8.3), a CGM graph in JPG format (Fig. 8.5), and up to 15 calculation results of glycemic variability parameters (Fig. 8.4). All results can be exported to the Excel file through the "Data Export" module of the system and then analyzed using statistical software for scientific research.
4. Clinical application of software: At present, the latest version of the system, V3.0, is more powerful and convenient based on the integration of the calculation of glycemic variability parameters and the CGM report, as compared with other software programs, like "EasyGV" and "GlyCulator." Also, the latest version of the system has a powerful glycemic parameter calculation function, and the analysis is more comprehensive and informative in comparison with "CapturAGP," "CareLink," and other software. At present, the system has been utilized nationwide in more than 100 hospitals, facilitating the management of CGM data and the utilization of CGM technology in scientific research and clinical practice. The system is available free of charge for clinicians (if necessary, please send your request via email to CGMreport@163.com).

8.4 Prospects of CGM Reports and Analysis Software

Using software to generate CGM reports and calculate glycemic parameters may standardize CGM reporting, allowing easy interpretation of CGM results and timely understanding of glycemic variability by clinicians, so as to achieve better glycemic control and improve prognosis among patients. However, there are still some problems during utilization of the software. First, there is a variety of blood glucose monitoring systems with various file formats, including FST, MMG, CSV, XLS, and other data types, which increase the difficulty in developing a universal analysis software. The second is unclear definitions of some glycemic variability parameters, which result in inconsistencies in the algorithms among software programs. Different software programs developed by different researchers may yield different calculation results for the same database. The third is the uncertain clinical significance of glycemic variability parameters, and clinical use of these parameters is often not targeted. With the advent of novel computer languages and algorithms, and the development of new pharmaceuticals that target postprandial hyperglycemia such as dipeptidyl peptidase-4 (DPP-4) inhibitors, glucagon-like peptide-1 (GLP-1) receptor agonists, and sodium-dependent glucose transporters 2 (SGLT-2) inhibitors, more glycemic variability parameters will continue to emerge and will require large-sample, long-term, prospective studies to evaluate the effectiveness and clinical significance of various parameters.

In short, data analysis using CGM software can reduce the workload of operators, generate standardized CGM reports, as well as calculate glycemic variability parameters, helping clinicians to understand trends in blood glucose changes. Moreover, CGM and analysis software programs also provide a large amount of glycemic information, contributing to the progression of diabetes-related research.

Statement on Consent for Participation

All the clinical trials carried out by the authors in this book have been reported to the Ethics Committee of Shanghai Jiao Tong University Affiliated Sixth People's Hospital already and were in accordance with the Good Clinical Practice and Standards of China Association for Ethical Studies (approval number: 2007-45).

References

1. Mazze RS, Strock E, Wesley D, Borgman S, Morgan B, Bergenstal R, Cuddihy R. Characterizing glucose exposure for individuals with normal glucose tolerance using continuous glucose monitoring and ambulatory glucose profile analysis. Diabetes Technol Ther. 2008;10:149–59. https://doi.org/10.1089/dia.2007.0293.
2. Bergenstal RM, Ahmann AJ, Bailey T, Beck RW, Bissen J, Buckingham B, Deeb L, Dolin RH, Garg SK, Goland R, Hirsch IB, Klonoff DC, Kruger DF, Matfin G, Mazze RS, Olson BA, Parkin C, Peters A, Powers MA, Rodriguez H, Southerland P, Strock ES, Tamborlane W, Wesley DM. Recommendations for standardizing glucose reporting and analysis to optimize clinical decision making in diabetes: the Ambulatory Glucose Profile (AGP). Diabetes Technol Ther. 2013;15:198–211. https://doi.org/10.1089/dia.2013.0051.
3. Brewer KW, Chase HP, Owen S, Garg SK. Slicing the pie. Correlating HbA–values with average blood glucose values in a pie chart form. Diabetes Care. 1998;21:209–12.
4. Rodbard D. New and improved methods to characterize glycemic variability using continuous glucose monitoring. Diabetes Technol Ther. 2009;11:551–65. https://doi.org/10.1089/dia.2009.0015.
5. Rodbard D. Hypo- and hyperglycemia in relation to the mean, standard deviation, coefficient of variation, and nature of the glucose distribution. Diabetes Technol Ther. 2012;14:868–76. https://doi.org/10.1089/dia.2012.0062.
6. Rodbard D. Interpretation of continuous glucose monitoring data: glycemic variability and quality of glycemic control. Diabetes Technol Ther. 2009;11(Suppl 1):55–67. https://doi.org/10.1089/dia.2008.0132.
7. American Diabetes Association. 6. Glycemic targets. Diabetes Care. 2017;40(Suppl 1):48–56. https://doi.org/10.2337/dc17-S009.
8. International Hypoglycaemia Study Group. Glucose concentrations of less than 3.0 mmol/L (54 mg/dL) should be reported in clinical trials: a joint position statement of the American Diabetes Association and the European Association for the Study of Diabetes. Diabetes Care. 2017;40:155–7. https://doi.org/10.2337/dc16-2215.
9. Chinese Diabetes Society. Chinese clinical guideline for continuous glucose monitoring (2012). Chin J Diabetes Mellitus. 2012;4:582–90. https://doi.org/10.3760/cma.j.issn.1674-5809.2012.10.003.

10. Zhou J, Jia WP. Assessment methods and research progress of glycemic variability. Clin J Endocrinol Metab. 2010;26:261–4. https://doi.org/10.3760/cma.j.issn.1000-6999.2010.03.028.
11. Zhou J, Jia WP. The significance and clinical assessment of glycemic variability. Zhonghua Yi Xue Za Zhi. 2006;86:2154–7. https://doi.org/10.3760/j:issn:0376-2491.2006.30.020.
12. Neylon OM, Baghurst PA, Cameron FJ. The minimum duration of sensor data from which glycemic variability can be consistently assessed. J Diabetes Sci Technol. 2014;8:273–6. https://doi.org/10.1177/1932296813519011.
13. Hill NR, Oliver NS, Choudhary P, Levy JC, Hindmarsh P, Matthews DR. Normal reference range for mean tissue glucose and glycemic variability derived from continuous glucose monitoring for subjects without diabetes in different ethnic groups. Diabetes Technol Ther. 2011;13:921–8. https://doi.org/10.1089/dia.2010.0247.
14. Czerwoniuk D, Fendler W, Walenciak L, Mlynarski W. GlyCulator: a glycemic variability calculation tool for continuous glucose monitoring data. J Diabetes Sci Technol. 2011;5:447–51. https://doi.org/10.1177/193229681100500236.
15. Mo YF, Zhou J, Jia WP. Clinical significance and research progress of parameters for assessing glycemic variability–mean amplitude of glycemic excursion. Clin J Diabetes Mellitus. 2011;3:259–63. https://doi.org/10.3760/cma.j.issn.1674-5809.2011.03.016.
16. Fritzsche G, Kohnert KD, Heinke P, Vogt L, Salzsieder E. The use of a computer program to calculate the mean amplitude of glycemic excursions. Diabetes Technol Ther. 2011;13:319–25. https://doi.org/10.1089/dia.2010.0108.
17. Baghurst PA. Calculating the mean amplitude of glycemic excursion from continuous glucose monitoring data: an automated algorithm. Diabetes Technol Ther. 2011;13:296–302. https://doi.org/10.1089/dia.2010.0090.
18. Sechterberger MK, Luijf YM, Devries JH. Poor agreement of computerized calculators for mean amplitude of glycemic excursions. Diabetes Technol Ther. 2014;16:72–5. https://doi.org/10.1089/dia.2013.0138.
19. Zhou J, Li H, Ran X, Yang W, Li Q, Peng Y, Li Y, Gao X, Luan X, Wang W, Jia W. Establishment of normal reference ranges for glycemic variability in Chinese subjects using continuous glucose monitoring. Med Sci Monit. 2011;17:CR9–13. https://doi.org/10.12659/MSM.881318.
20. Mo Y, Zhou J, Li M, Wang Y, Bao Y, Ma X, Li D, Lu W, Hu C, Li M, Jia W. Glycemic variability is associated with subclinical atherosclerosis in Chinese type 2 diabetic patients. Cardiovasc Diabetol. 2013;12:15. https://doi.org/10.1186/1475-2840-12-15.
21. Zhang L, Zhou J, Lu W, Bao YQ, Jia WP. Establishment and clinical applications of continuous glucose monitoring report and management system. Clin J Diabetes Mellitus. 2012;4:754–5. https://doi.org/10.3760/cma.j.issn.1674-5809.2012.12.012.

9 Clinical Indications for Continuous Glucose Monitoring

W. Jia

As a new type of glucose monitoring technology, continuous glucose monitoring (CGM) is expensive and requires both clinicians and patients to invest considerable time and energy to complete the monitoring process. Moreover, patients must receive education and training to use CGM properly. Therefore, the clinical professionals should understand the indications of CGM and make full use of its advantages, so as to maximize its clinical value. If the investigators use CGM for no specific purpose, even ignoring its indications, or if they fail to apply CGM results in guiding the clinical treatment regimen or improving patients' lifestyle, the benefits will be lost, while patients might suffer from economic and psychological burdens. This chapter focuses on the clinical advantages, application scope, and indications of CGM technology.

9.1 Advantages and Indications of Retrospective CGM

The main advantage of retrospective CGM is its ability to detect occult hyperglycemia and hypoglycemia, especially postprandial hyperglycemia and nocturnal asymptomatic hypoglycemia, which are not easily detected by conventional monitoring methods. For example, (1) CGM can detect glycemic changes relating to factors such as food, exercise, medication, mental factors, and lifestyle; (2) CGM is able to detect postprandial hyperglycemia, nocturnal hypoglycemia, the dawn phenomenon, Somogyi effect, etc.; (3) CGM aids the recommendations for individualized treatment regimens; (4) CGM improves treatment compliance; (5) CGM can be used to analyze the trend and characteristics of blood glucose changes, thus guiding decisions on targeted treatment; and (6) CGM provides visualized method for diabetes education. In short, CGM has unique advantages for the assessment of blood glucose fluctuations and detection of hypoglycemia.

Therefore, according to the *Chinese Clinical Guideline for Continuous Glucose Monitoring (2009)* [1], *Clinical Guideline for Continuous Glucose Monitoring (2012)* [2], and *Clinical Application Guide of Blood Glucose Monitoring in China (Edition 2015)* [3], retrospective CGM is mainly applicable to the following patients or conditions, including:

1. Type 1 diabetes mellitus
2. Type 2 diabetes mellitus that requires intensive insulin therapy including multiple daily injections and continuous subcutaneous insulin infusion therapy
3. Type 2 diabetes mellitus patients who use hypoglycemic treatment under self-monitoring of blood glucose (SMBG) guidance but still encounter one of the following

W. Jia
Department of Endocrinology and Metabolism, Shanghai Clinical Center for Diabetes, Shanghai Diabetes Institute, Shanghai Jiao Tong University Affiliated Sixth People's Hospital, Shanghai, China
e-mail: wpjia@sjtu.edu.cn

W. Jia (ed.), *Continuous Glucose Monitoring*, https://doi.org/10.1007/978-981-10-7074-7_9

situations: severe hypoglycemia or repeated hypoglycemia, asymptomatic hypoglycemia, and nocturnal hypoglycemia; refractory hyperglycemia, especially when fasting; large blood glucose excursions; and diabetic patients who maintain a state of hyperglycemia due to the fear of hypoglycemia
4. Gestational diabetes or diabetes in pregnancy
5. Patients who need diabetes education. CGM facilitates the understanding of blood glucose changes resulting from exercise, diet, stress, and hypoglycemic treatment, thus motivating the patients to establish a healthy lifestyle, improving patients' treatment compliance, and enhancing mutual communication between clinicians and patients. In addition, CGM is also applicable to diabetes patients with gastroparesis or special types of diabetes, in order to understand the characteristics and patterns of blood glucose changes if necessary. The indications of CGM also include other endocrine and metabolic diseases, such as insulinoma. Overall, CGM is primarily recommended to patients with type 1 diabetes and those with type 2 diabetes on intensive insulin therapy or who experience dramatic glycemic variability.

Retrospective CGM can comprehensively reflect the overall glycemic profile, especially for nocturnal and postprandial blood glucose fluctuations that are usually neglected by SMBG, thereby allowing accurate and quantitative assessment of blood glucose fluctuations. Therefore, when appropriate, CGM can also be used as a valuable tool to evaluate the results of clinical studies. For example, we applied CGM to analyze the characteristics of blood glucose fluctuations in patients with polycystic ovary syndrome (PCOS) who had normal glucose tolerance. The results showed that although the blood glucose level had not undergone substantial changes, the pattern of postprandial blood glucose fluctuations was altered, as manifested by a delayed postprandial glucose peak (about 40–50 min after meal) compared to normal, and the postprandial plasma glycemic excursion (PPGE) after breakfast was also increased (Fig. 9.1) [4]. In addition, we utilized CGM to analyze the relationship between mildly elevated alanine transaminase (ALT) and nocturnal mean blood glucose (MBG) in 322 individuals with normal glucose tolerance, including 80 subjects with ALT <13 U/L (group A), 81 with ALT

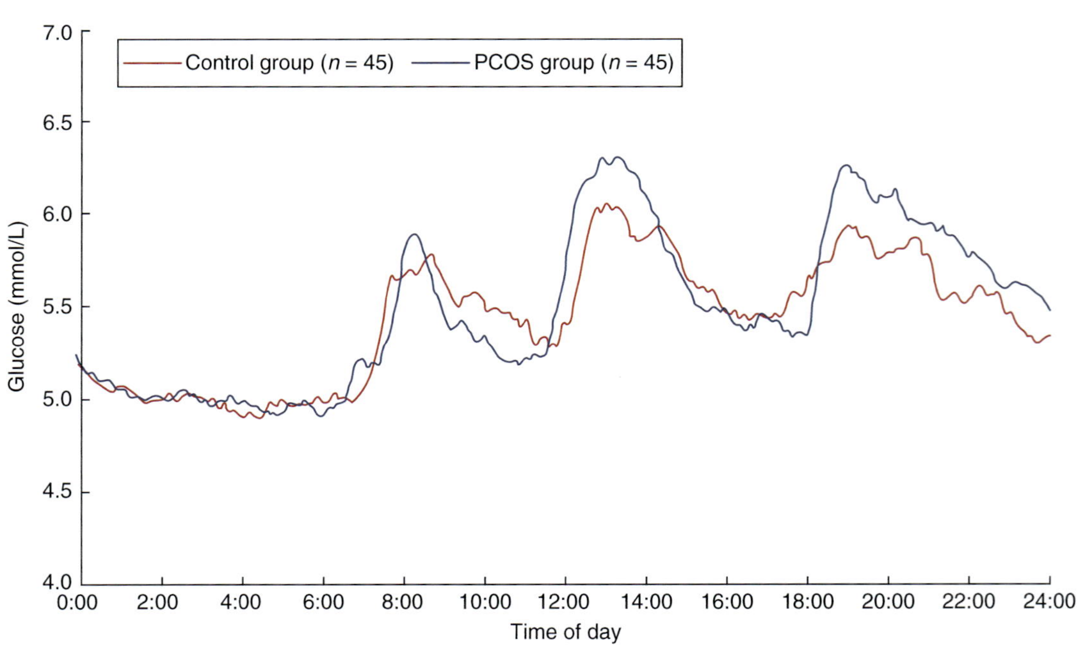

Fig. 9.1 Comparison of CGM profile in 45 female patients with polycystic ovary syndrome (PCOS) who had normal glucose tolerance and 45 age-matched normal females (control group) [4] (Reprint with permission from *Postgraduate Medicine*)

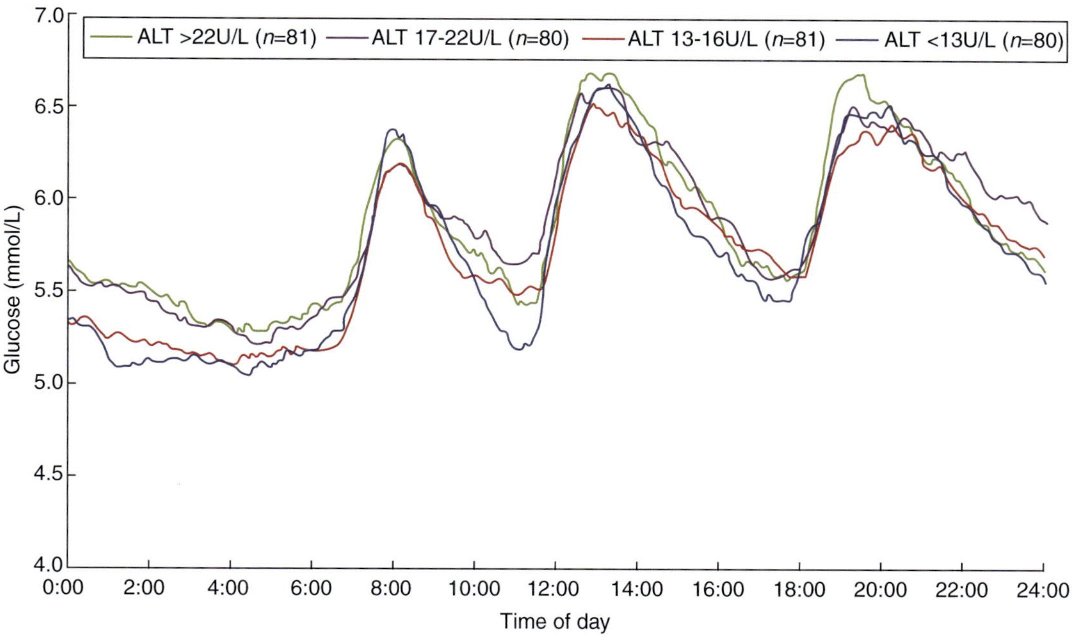

Fig. 9.2 CGM profile of patients with different levels of alanine aminotransferase (ALT) who had normal glucose tolerance [5] (Reprint from *PLoS One*)

13–16 U/L (group B), 80 with ALT 17–22 U/L (group C), and 81 with ALT >22 U/L (group D). After adjustment for age and gender, the nocturnal MBG levels in groups C and D were significantly higher than those in groups A and B ($P < 0.05$). Multiple stepwise regression analysis showed that nocturnal MBG was positively correlated with homeostasis model assessment-insulin resistance (HOMA-IR) and ALT levels and negatively correlated with homeostasis model assessment for β-cell function (HOMA-β). These findings indicated that mildly elevated ALT levels were associated with unfavorable nocturnal glucose profiles in Chinese subjects with normal glucose regulation [5] (Fig. 9.2). Thus, utilization of CGM can clarify the characteristics of nocturnal or postprandial blood glucose. It thereby represents a valuable tool for scientific research, since it is blinded to the patient and thereby eliminates the confounding variable of a patient self-correcting their eating and/or exercise behavior if the studies were real time.

9.2 Advantages and Indications of Real-Time CGM

Retrospective CGM provides a panoramic view of blood glucose fluctuations throughout the day, which can be the basis for guiding safe, effective glycemic control through targeted adjustment of the treatment regimen. The major feature of the real-time CGM system is to provide immediate blood glucose information as well as give hyperglycemic and hypoglycemic alerts, allowing immediate regulation of blood glucose for patients (Table 9.1). Retrospective CGM and real-time CGM have their own advantages and disadvantages in clinical utilization (Table 9.2). Fully understanding the CGM advantages and which populations will benefit most from CGM will make full use of the technology to achieve maximal clinical benefits. With the Medtronic real-time CGM as an example, its clinical features are mainly presented as the following three aspects:

Table 9.1 Comparison of retrospective and real-time CGM [2] (Reprint with permission from *Chinese Journal of Diabetes Mellitus*)

Group	Performance and characteristics	Requirements
Retrospective CGM	• Monitor for 3 consecutive days, retrospective data analysis after download	• Regular and intermittent use, constant outpatient follow-up, and active communication with clinicians
	• Provide accuracy assessment to evaluate the quality of data report	• Monitor blood glucose as required during use
	• "Major events" function, to record glucose-related events	• Record life events related to blood glucose fluctuations
Real-time CGM	• Real-time glucose monitoring and display, including instant blood glucose and trend of blood glucose fluctuations	• Good patient adherence
	• Hyperglycemia/hypoglycemia alerts	• The ability to intervene when there are dramatic glucose fluctuations and manage extreme hyperglycemia or hypoglycemia limits in a timely manner based on real-time glucose data
	• Data storage, data can be reviewed retrospectively after download	• Be willing to monitor blood glucose as required during use; the ability to manage hyperglycemia/hypoglycemia alerts
	• "Major events" function, to record glucose-related events	• Record life events related to blood glucose fluctuations
	• Integration with subcutaneous continuous insulin infusion system	• For patients with real-time CGM-insulin pump integration system, hypoglycemic regimen should be adjusted under the guidance of clinicians when glucose fluctuates significantly or hyperglycemia/hypoglycemia alerts incur

Table 9.2 Advantages and disadvantages of retrospective and real-time CGM systems

	Retrospective CGM	Real-time CGM
Features	• Blind measurement	• Real-time display, hyperglycemia/hypoglycemia alerts
Advantages	• Detect the regularity and trend of blood glucose fluctuations without interference	• Immediate adjustment of treatment regimen
	• Guide targeted treatment	• Early detection of hypoglycemia and severe hyperglycemia
	• Wide scope of application in both clinical practice and scientific research	• Promote alterations in patients' behaviors
Disadvantages	• Lack of timeliness	• Not applicable for diabetes patients with depression or anxiety
		• Requirement for education background

9.2.1 Real-Time Trends of Blood Glucose Fluctuations

This feature benefits most for those patients with frequent blood glucose fluctuations. Real-time CGM is able to display the immediate trend of blood glucose. It gives upward or downward "arrow or arrows" to predict blood glucose changes in the next 30–60 min, for example, an upward "arrow" represents a blood glucose increase between 1.1 and 2.2 mmol/L within the last 20 min; and two upward "arrows" represent a blood glucose rise of more than 2.2 mmol/L within the last 20 min. This function may guide decisions such as to prevent hypoglycemia by additional meal intake or to intensify hypoglycemic measures.

9.2.2 Hyperglycemia and Hypoglycemia Alerts

This feature most benefits those patients who are prone to asymptomatic hypoglycemia or who fail to achieve a glycated hemoglobin A_{1c} (HbA_{1c}) target goal. With the hyperglycemia/hypoglycemia alert feature, the device may give alarms prior to the occurrence of hyperglycemic or hypoglycemic events. Interventions are timely implemented after a recheck of blood glucose by a glucose meter, thus improving the blood glucose fluctuations. For instance, diabetes patients with insulin therapy can work, drive, and exercise as normal individuals when the hypoglycemia alert limits are turned on. Similarly, the hyperglycemia alert limits can help to effectively manage postprandial blood glucose fluctuations.

9.2.3 Adjustment of SMBG Frequency

This feature most benefits those patients who excessively or infrequently use SMBG. For patients with infrequent SMBG, real-time CGM can provide data for guiding diet, exercise, and insulin therapy. For those with frequent SMBG, such as more than 10 measurements daily, real-time CGM helps to properly alleviate the discomfort, inconvenience, and cost.

In 2011, the Endocrine Society published the *Continuous Glucose Monitoring: an Endocrine Society Clinical Practice Guideline*, proposing the indications for real-time CGM [6]. This was updated in November 2016 [7]. In February 2016, the American Association of Clinical Endocrinologists (AACE) together with the American College of Endocrinology published the *Continuous Glucose Monitoring: A Consensus Conference of the American Association of Clinical Endocrinologists and American College of Endocrinology* [8]. With the popularization of real-time CGM technology and its progress in clinical research, the population for which real-time CGM is applicable is under investigation. At present, the indications for real-time CGM include the following:

1. Children and adolescents with type 1 diabetes whose HbA_{1c} <7% (53 mmol/mol). The use of real-time CGM can help to persistently maintain good glycemic control without increasing the risk of hypoglycemia.
2. Children and adolescents with type 1 diabetes who have HbA_{1c} ≥7% (53 mmol/mol) and who are able to use these devices on a nearly daily basis.
3. Adult patients with type 1 diabetes who are able to use these devices on a nearly daily basis.
4. Hospitalized patients with type 2 diabetes on insulin therapy. The use of real-time CGM can reduce blood glucose fluctuations, allowing rapid and stable achievement of glycemic targets, without increasing the risk of hypoglycemia.
5. Perioperative glycemic control in type 2 diabetes patients. The use of real-time CGM can help patients to better control their blood glucose.
6. Non-intensive care unit patients on insulin therapy. The use of real-time CGM facilitates glycemic control and reduces the occurrence of hypoglycemia.

The clinical indications of CGM should be based on accumulated, sufficient data. As the number of cumulative cases utilizing real-time CGM in clinical practice in China is limited, the indications of CGM listed above provide a reference for properly selecting patients for real-time CGM usage. At the same time, it should be emphasized that real-time CGM operators must have good self-awareness and self-management skills for glycemic control, possessing a certain ability to utilize the real-time CGM system, to interpret readings, and to manage hyperglycemia or hypoglycemia alerts.

Statement on Consent for Participation

All the clinical trials carried out by the authors in this book have been reported to the Ethics Committee of Shanghai Jiao Tong University Affiliated Sixth People's Hospital already and were in accordance with the Good Clinical Practice and Standards of China Association for Ethical Studies (approval number: 2007-45).

References

1. Chinese Diabetes Society. Chinese clinical guideline for continuous glucose monitoring (2009). Zhonghua Yi Xue Za Zhi. 2009;89:3388–92. https://doi.org/10.3760/cma.j.issn.0376-2491.2009.48.002.
2. Chinese Diabetes Society. Chinese clinical guideline for continuous glucose monitoring (2012). Chin J Diabetes Mellitus. 2012;4:582–90. https://doi.org/10.3760/cma.j.issn.1674-5809.2012.10.003.
3. Chinese Diabetes Society. Clinical application guide of blood glucose monitoring in China (Edition 2015). Chin J Diabetes Mellitus. 2015;7:603–13. https://doi.org/10.3760/cma.j.issn.1764-5809.2015.10.004.
4. Tao M, Zhou J, Zhu J, Lu W, Jia W. Continuous glucose monitoring reveals abnormal features of postprandial glycemic excursions in women with polycystic ovarian syndrome. Postgrad Med. 2011;123:185–90. https://doi.org/10.3810/pgm.2011.03.2277.
5. Zhou J, Mo Y, Li H, Ran X, Yang W, Li Q, Peng Y, Li Y, Gao X, Luan X, Wang W, Jia W. Alanine aminotransferase is associated with an adverse nocturnal blood glucose profile in individuals with normal glucose regulation. PLoS One. 2013;8:e56072. https://doi.org/10.1371/journal.pone.0056072.
6. Klonoff DC, Buckingham B, Christiansen JS, Montori VM, Tamborlane WV, Vigersky RA, Wolpert H, Endocrine Society. Continuous glucose monitoring: an endocrine society clinical practice guideline. J Clin Endocrinol Metab. 2011;96:2968–79. https://doi.org/10.1210/jc.2010-2756.
7. Peters AL, Ahmann AJ, Battelino T, Evert A, Hirsch IB, Murad MH, Winter WE, Wolpert H. Diabetes technology-continuous subcutaneous insulin infusion therapy and continuous glucose monitoring in adults: an endocrine society clinical practice guideline. J Clin Endocrinol Metab. 2016;101:3922–37.
8. Fonseca VA, Grunberger G, Anhalt H, Bailey TS, Blevins T, Garg SK, Handelsman Y, Hirsch IB, Orzeck EA, Roberts VL, Tamborlane W, Consensus Conference Writing Committee. Continuous glucose monitoring: a consensus conference of the American Association of Clinical Endocrinologists and American College of Endocrinology. Endocr Pract. 2016;22:1008–21. https://doi.org/10.4158/EP161392.CS.

10 Interpretation of the Chinese Clinical Guideline for Continuous Glucose Monitoring

W. Jia

Glucose monitoring is a necessary method for the assessment of glucose metabolism disorders and therapeutic effects. As continuous, dynamic changes occur in blood glucose levels in the body, conventional blood glucose measurements cannot fully reflect the fluctuations in blood glucose throughout the day. Therefore, the achievement of continuous glucose monitoring is pursued by both patients and clinicians. As early as 1967, Updike and Hicks accomplished the first attempt at using continuous glucose monitoring (CGM) in an animal model [1]. Subsequently, CGM technology has become increasingly mature, realizing successful translation from experimental monitoring to clinical application. In 1999, the US Food and Drug Administration (FDA) approved the first retrospective CGM device for clinical use in the USA. In China, after the retrospective CGM device was approved by the China Food and Drug Administration (CFDA) in 2001, CGM has been gradually applied in clinical research and diabetes management.

In December 2009, the Chinese Diabetes Society drafted and published the first *Chinese Clinical Guideline for Continuous Glucose Monitoring (2009)* [2]. In the next 3 years, real-time CGM technology began to be applied in clinical practice, and Chinese scholars published a number of peer-recognized research results that are of certain guidance and reference significance. Thereafter, the guideline was updated in 2012 as the *Chinese Clinical Guideline for Continuous Glucose Monitoring (2012)* [3]. In addition, in order to make CGM guidelines lead clinical practice, the Chinese Diabetes Society published and updated the *Clinical Application Guide of Blood Glucose Monitoring in China (Edition 2011)* [4] and the *Clinical Application Guide of Blood Glucose Monitoring in China (Edition 2015)* [5] in 2011 and 2015, respectively. For the content related to CGM technology, the guidelines were also promptly updated to facilitate the scientific, standardized, and reasonable utilization of CGM technology in China.

Internationally, in October 2010, the American Association of Clinical Endocrinologists (AACE) published an expert consensus on CGM technology in order to clarify the roles of different types of CGM systems and indications for the use of CGM [6], which had been updated in 2016 [7, 8]. Subsequently in 2011, the Endocrine Society together with the Diabetes Technology Society and the European Society of Endocrinology published the *Continuous Glucose Monitoring: An Endocrine Society Clinical Practice Guideline* [9], which had been updated in 2016 as the *Diabetes Technology-Continuous Subcutaneous Insulin Infusion Therapy and Continuous Glucose Monitoring in Adults: An Endocrine Society*

W. Jia
Department of Endocrinology and Metabolism, Shanghai Clinical Center for Diabetes, Shanghai Diabetes Institute, Shanghai Jiao Tong University Affiliated Sixth People's Hospital, Shanghai, China
e-mail: wpjia@sjtu.edu.cn

W. Jia (ed.), *Continuous Glucose Monitoring*, https://doi.org/10.1007/978-981-10-7074-7_10

Clinical Practice Guideline [10]. In this chapter, we will interpret and compare the content and evidence of the above guidelines.

10.1 Classification of CGM Technologies

At present, both Chinese and international guidelines divide CGM technologies into two catalogues: professional CGM technology (retrospective CGM system) and personal CGM technology (real-time CGM system). The two CGM techniques are presented as follows:

1. Professional CGM technology: due to retrospective feature, patients wear the device continuously for 3–7 days, and physicians and patients are unable to view the results during the monitoring period. The retrospective glycemic data are obtained at the end of the monitoring after being downloaded. The glycemic data can be used by clinicians to guide the patient's treatment. This system is usually purchased by hospitals and is mainly applicable for diabetes patients who fail to achieve glycemic target goal or those with recurrent hypoglycemia and/or asymptomatic hypoglycemia as well as pregnant women. The retrospective CGM system has no hyperglycemia/hypoglycemia alert feature, but the operation system is simple. It is generally recommended for regular, intermittent use in patients. A large body of evidence suggests that professional CGM can improve glycemic control in patients with both type 1 and type 2 diabetes.
2. Personal CGM technology: due to the real-time feature, this system provides immediate blood glucose readings as well as glucose alarms and predictive alerts, facilitating the immediate regulation of blood glucose. However, the blood glucose should be rechecked with a glucose meter prior to decision making on treatment adjustment. This system is generally purchased by individual patients for the purpose of achieving better glycemic control by regular use. Real-time CGM operators are required to have good self-awareness and self-management skills of glycemic control, possessing a certain ability to utilize the real-time CGM system, interpret readings, and manage hyperglycemia/hypoglycemia alerts. At present, the existing evidence suggests that patients with type 1 diabetes can achieve better glucose management under the guidance of a real-time CGM system.

10.2 Evidence-Based Medicine of CGM Technology

At present, there are medical evidences confirming the clinical benefits of CGM technology [11]. In adults, the use of real-time CGM systems can significantly reduce glycated hemoglobin A_{1c} (HbA_{1c}) levels without increasing the risk of hypoglycemia in type 1 diabetes patients with $HbA_{1c} \geq 7\%$ (53 mmol/mol); also, the use of real-time CGM systems can reduce the risk of hypoglycemia without increasing the HbA_{1c} level in type 1 diabetes patients with $HbA_{1c} < 7\%$ (53 mmol/mol). In adolescents, the benefits of real-time CGM are related to the frequency of sensor use. HbA_{1c} levels are significantly improved in those patients who use sensors 6–7 day per week. For pregnant women, a retrospective CGM system is able to detect occult hyperglycemia for 94–390 min daily. The use of a retrospective CGM system by women with gestational diabetes helps to achieve better control of blood glucose during pregnancy and to reduce the incidence of macrosomia.

10.3 Indications for CGM Technology in Chinese and International Guidelines

The AACE has recommended specific patient populations for the use of retrospective CGM and real-time CGM [6].

The indicators for retrospective CGM as recommended by the AACE include (1) young adult type 1 diabetes patients who are adjusting their hypoglycemic treatment and (2) young adult type

1 diabetes patients with the following conditions: nocturnal hypoglycemia or the dawn phenomenon, asymptomatic hypoglycemia, or postprandial hyperglycemia. The CGM system should be used on a regular, intermittent basis.

The indicators for real-time CGM as recommended by the AACE include:

1. Type 1 diabetes patients with the following conditions: asymptomatic hypoglycemia or recurrent hypoglycemia, failure to achieve HbA_{1c} target goal or dramatic glucose fluctuation, pregnancy or planning a pregnancy
2. Children or adolescents with HbA_{1c} <7% (53 mmol/mol) who have good self-management skills for glycemic control
3. Young adult type 1 diabetes patients with HbA_{1c} ≥7.0% (53 mmol/mol) who have the ability to use the device daily
4. Young adults who require frequent monitoring of blood glucose and young children (<8 years old), especially with hypoglycemia. For these patients, 2- to 4-week trial use is recommended prior to deciding whether the device should be formally used.

The AACE consensus highlights the patients' selection and benefits of two different types of CGM systems, retrospective CGM and real-time CGM. Although the real-time CGM system represents a step forward, the retrospective CGM still has its unique advantages and clinical scope. It is relatively simpler to operate with higher accuracy over the real-time device; it can truly reflect the blood glucose fluctuations of patients in daily life. Therefore, standardized use of retrospective CGM will bring benefits for inpatients and outpatients with diabetes. It also provides more stable and less interfering glucose information in the field of research.

In China, since the retrospective CGM system had been predominantly utilized before 2009, the CGM guideline (2009 edition) only focused on the indications of retrospective CGM. Moreover, in the USA, patients with type 1 diabetes account for the vast majority of CGM users. Therefore, the AACE consensus specifically elaborates on type 1 diabetes. In contrast, in China, patients with type 2 diabetes account for a large part of CGM users, and numerous research reports are focused on type 2 diabetes. Therefore, in addition to type 1 diabetes, the Chinese CGM guidelines also elaborate on the indications for standardized use of CGM technologies among type 2 diabetes patients in clinical practice. The indications for retrospective CGM recommended by the *Chinese Clinical Guideline for Continuous Glucose Monitoring (2009)* include:

1. Type 1 diabetes mellitus
2. Type 2 diabetes mellitus patients who use hypoglycemic treatment under self-monitoring of blood glucose (SMBG) guidance but still encounter one of the following situations: severe hypoglycemia or repeated hypoglycemia; asymptomatic hypoglycemia and nocturnal hypoglycemia; refractory hyperglycemia, especially when fasting; large blood glucose excursions; diabetic patients who maintain a state of hyperglycemia due to the fear of hypoglycemia
3. Gestational diabetes or diabetes in pregnancy
4. Patients who have a strong willingness to use CGM

Among the abovementioned patients, CGM is primarily recommended to those patients with type 1 diabetes or type 2 diabetes on intensive insulin therapy or patients with dramatic glycemic variability, recurrent hypoglycemia, or asymptomatic hypoglycemia.

As there have been a limited period and number of cumulative cases utilizing real-time CGM in clinical practice in China, the 2012 CGM guideline and 2015 Blood Glucose Monitoring guideline mainly draw on evidences from abroad.

10.4 Support Required in CGM Application

Regular follow-up and proper interpretation of monitoring results by clinicians guarantee the maximized therapeutic benefits of real-time CGM. Therefore, training is critical for real-time CGM users. In other countries, the CGM training is usually provided by manufacturers. The installation of a real-time CGM system and preliminary training generally take 60–90 min.

Compared with the real-time CGM system, the retrospective CGM system is easier to install and requires less training. Before installation, the follow-up schedule for patients needs to be prearranged. After installation, the patients need to be trained for the use of the device (monitoring methods and frequency) and for recording daily events (diet, exercise, medication, etc.). The downloaded glycemic data should be analyzed together with the lifestyle of patients, to guide the adjustment of lifestyle or the hypoglycemic regimen.

In foreign countries, the cost for utilization of retrospective CGM and real-time CGM in type 1 diabetes patients is usually covered by many large-scale healthcare projects, including two parts, data collection (including sensor installation, patient education, glucose calibration with fasting blood glucose concentration from the fingertip, and data download) and data analysis.

10.5 Problems that Need to be Solved in the Development of CGM Technology

10.5.1 Analysis of CGM Data

The use of a CGM system generates considerable data regarding blood glucose levels and relevant glycemic parameters, which can be confusing to some users [12]. Based on studies showing that blood glucose fluctuations may be associated with the occurrence and development of diabetes complications, Chinese and international scholars have developed a number of glycemic parameters for evaluating blood glucose fluctuations based on different statistical ideas, and such information may confuse users who have little idea of how to select the most appropriate information. Therefore, it is necessary to use a systematic method to analyze and interpret these blood glucose data and to establish glucose assessment parameters that are simple but of clinical significance.

10.5.2 Clinical Trials

Although Chinese large-scale clinical trials of CGM with a short period of follow-up have been published and the indications of CGM technology have been preliminarily clarified, there is still a lack of clinical trials that is comparable to the US Diabetes Control and Complications Trial (DCCT) and the UK Prospective Diabetes Study (UKPDS) to validate the long-term efficacy of CGM and to identify the population for maximum benefits. On the other hand, the health economics of CGM technology has been a hot topic of concern. Although there is existing preliminary evidence evaluating the "input/output ratio" of CGM utilization, mature economic modeling and more refined health economic results are required to help healthcare institutions to make rational investment decisions on medical resources, in order to further promote the clinical application of CGM technology.

10.5.3 Development Trend of CGM Technology

The accuracy of CGM technology has always been the focus of attention for the majority of clinicians. Since CGM measures the interstitial glucose concentration, it is different from blood glucose in terms of absolute glucose values and the frequency of changes. The emergence of the real-time CGM system has created even higher requirements for the accuracy of the glucose sensor. Another future development of CGM is to generate a fully closed-loop insulin delivery system as a final goal. Thus, how to establish a CGM algorithm that calculates the physiological insulin infusion dose needed in response to blood glucose changes will become another hot spot in the development of CGM technology. This has already been achieved in part with a hybrid closed-loop system which predictively suspends insulin to prevent hypoglycemia based on sensor glucose levels and trends and changes basal insulin infusion rates accordingly.

In short, with the development of CGM technology and continuous improvement of evidence-based medicine, CGM systems will be used not only as a supplement of SMBG but also as an independent method of glucose monitoring and eventually become the cornerstone of glycemic management in diabetes.

10.6 Interpretation of Clinical Application Guide of Blood Glucose Monitoring in China (Edition 2015)

Comprehensive management of diabetes includes education, diet therapy, exercise therapy, medication, and SMBG. Glucose monitoring is a basic means for assessing the management of diabetes, and it is also an important communication content between clinicians and patients. In 2011, the Chinese Diabetes Society published the *Clinical Application Guide of Blood Glucose Monitoring in China* [4] (hereinafter referred to as "the Guideline") in line with China's national conditions, to promote the standardized management of blood glucose monitoring in diabetes. In recent years, China has made great progress in glucose monitoring in both research and clinical applications. In 2015, the Chinese Diabetes Society once again organized national experts and revised the Guideline [5], increasing new clinical evidence and strengthening the glucose monitoring program, in order to adapt to ever-changing trends and needs.

The new edition of the Guideline (edition 2015) has been updated with regard to four commonly used clinical glucose monitoring methods, including capillary blood glucose monitoring with a glucose meter, continuous monitoring of blood glucose over 3–7 days with CGM, measurement of glycated albumin (GA) reflecting the mean blood glucose (MBG) level over the preceding 2–3 weeks, and HbA_{1c} reflecting MBG over the preceding 2–3 months. The 2015 Guideline for the first time briefly introduces a new glycemic indicator, serum 1,5-anhydroglucitol (1,5-AG), which can accurately and rapidly reflect glycemic control within 1–2 weeks in diabetes patients. We will briefly interpret the 2015 Guideline in this chapter.

10.6.1 Capillary Blood Glucose Monitoring

Capillary blood glucose monitoring is an important part of diabetes management and education. Capillary blood glucose monitoring is divided into point of care testing (POCT) in hospital and SMBG. SMBG is usually performed by patients themselves, and POCT is performed by nurses in hospitals. The 2015 Guideline affirms the role of SMBG in glucose monitoring. It is recommended that all patients should be required to perform SMBG. Moreover, the Guideline adds a new part on POCT, suggesting that all medical and healthcare institutes need to develop specialized standards for POCT management and improve scientific management of POCT. However, it should be noted that the hospital POCT methods can only be used to monitor blood glucose in diabetes patients but not be used as diagnosis method.

With respect to capillary blood glucose monitoring, the frequency of blood glucose monitoring recommended by the 2011 Guideline is not applied consistently in different hospitals at all levels. The 2015 Guideline summarizes the suggestions on SMBG frequency and monitoring time from major academic institutions, such as the International Diabetes Federation (IDF), American Diabetes Association (ADA), and Chinese Diabetes Society, and puts forward the principle of a glucose monitoring program that should be developed in accordance with the patient's condition, treatment goals, and treatment regimen. The 2015 Guideline facilitates implementation of blood glucose monitoring in hospitals of each level based on their own conditions.

Selecting a proper glucose meter and mastering the required operation skill of users are the key factors affecting the accuracy of blood glucose monitoring results. The 2015 Guideline for the first time introduces the International Organization for Standardization (ISO) 15197-2013 Standard for evaluating system accuracy of blood glucose meters, which facilitates hospital blood glucose monitoring management. Moreover, with different bioenzymatic methods, various factors interfere with the accuracy of glucose meters. The 2015 Guideline reviews the interfering factors of glucose meters, providing a reference for clinical selection of appropriate glucose meters and proper interpretation of blood glucose monitoring results. In addition, the technical factors of operators, including improper operation, insufficient blood volume, local extrusion, failure to enter the correct calibration code when changing a new batch of test strips, or improper preservation of test strips, will also affect the accuracy of blood glucose monitoring. The 2015 Guideline puts forward technical requirements for patients regarding SMBG from three aspects, namely, pretest, mid-test, and post-test requirements.

In capillary blood glucose monitoring, blood glucose data management is another important component. With the development of science and technology, mobile medicine, as a new medical mode, is attracting more and more attention in the field of diabetes management. Mobile medicine is currently based on short messages or applications (apps) at a mobile terminal system, such as Android and Apple (IOS). The 2015 Guideline affirms the role of mobile medical care in the comprehensive management of diabetes mellitus. However, there is still a lack of detailed laws and regulations for mobile medical care, which needs further exploration in the management of diabetes.

10.6.2 HbA_{1c}

HbA_{1c} serves as a "gold standard" for clinical evaluation of long-term glycemic control (2–3 months), providing an important basis for guiding treatment decisions. Clinical studies have revealed that the use of HbA_{1c} as the goal to strengthen glycemic control can reduce the risk of microvascular and macrovascular complications of diabetes [13, 14].

Currently, high-performance liquid chromatography (HPLC) is a most commonly used method to detect HbA_{1c}. Standardization of HbA_{1c} assays has yet to be achieved. In 2013, the National Center for Clinical Laboratories of the China Health and Family Planning Commission published the *Guideline for Glycated Hemoglobin Laboratory Assay of China*, which standardizes the analysis of interference factors, selection of methods, procedures, and quality control in HbA_{1c} assays. Our National Center for Clinical Laboratories has approved the primary reference method for HbA_{1c} (IFCC HPLC-LC-MS/MS). The inter-assay coefficient of variation (CV) of HbA_{1c} was reduced from 20–30% in 2000 to 4.6–5.3% in 2012. The 2015 Guideline further emphasizes the importance of HbA_{1c} standardization and the related progress made in the country, especially the promotion of HbA_{1c} standardization in Shanghai, laying a foundation for the future study of HbA_{1c} in the diagnosis of diabetes.

The improvement in HbA_{1c} assay standardization promotes HbA_{1c} research in the screening and diagnosis of diabetes mellitus. Chinese studies reported that the best cut point for HbA_{1c} in the diagnosis of diabetes in Chinese people was 6.2–6.4% (mostly 6.3%) [44–46 mmol/mol (mostly 45 mmol/mol)] [15, 16], which is lower than the diabetes diagnostic criteria [HbA_{1c} ≥6.5% (48 mmol/mol)] published by the ADA and the World Health Organization (WHO). The 2015 Guideline points out that due to an insufficient degree of HbA_{1c} standardization in China, the standardization of HbA_{1c} assays needs to be further strengthened for better implementation of HbA_{1c} assays in the diagnosis of diabetes.

10.6.3 GA

GA is an indicator reflecting short-term glycemic control (2–3 weeks). GA may have an advantage over HbA_{1c} in the evaluation of the curative effect of newly diagnosed diabetes and in short-term hospitalized diabetes patients. The

2015 Guideline adds the latest data on the relationship between GA and diabetes complications and highlights the factors that influence GA measurements. For example, based on research data from the Chinese population, the inverse influence of obesity on GA may be largely attributable to the effects of fat mass and visceral adipose tissue [17].

The 2015 Guideline also points out that compared with HbA_{1c}, there is still a lack of large sample, prospective studies on the relationship between GA and chronic complications of diabetes. Currently, GA is an effective supplement to HbA_{1c} in clinical application.

10.6.4 1,5-AG

1,5-AG is the 1-deoxy form of D-glucose. Its content is significantly reduced in diabetes patients, which can accurately and rapidly reflect blood glucose control within 1–2 weeks. In 2003, the US FDA approved 1,5-AG as a new indicator of short-term glycemic control. The 2015 Guideline for the first time briefly introduces 1,5-AG as a new indicator for glucose monitoring. Despite evidence demonstrating 1,5-AG can be used as an adjunctive indicator to guide the adjustment of treatment regimens for diabetes patients [18], the roles of 1,5-AG in the screening and diagnosis of diabetes require further investigation.

10.6.5 CGM

CGM, as a new type of glucose monitoring technology, is able to provide continuous, comprehensive, and reliable all-day glucose profiles, thereby allowing for an understanding of the trends in blood glucose fluctuations and the detection of occult hyperglycemia and hypoglycemia that cannot be detected by traditional blood glucose monitoring methods. It is an effective supplement to traditional blood glucose monitoring methods. CGM is categorized as a retrospective CGM system or a real-time CGM system. The 2015 Guideline adds a description of real-time CGM, comparing the differences between retrospective and real-time CGM systems. The major feature of the real-time CGM system is to provide immediate blood glucose information as well as give hyperglycemia/hypoglycemia alerts, allowing for stable achievement of the glycemic goal without increasing the risk of hypoglycemia.

10.7 Summary

Glucose monitoring has become an important part of modern comprehensive management of diabetes. It plays an important role in adjustment of clinical treatment regimens, minimizing the risk of complications, patient education, and self-management. The 2015 Guideline adds new contents, including hospital POCT, the frequency of blood glucose monitoring, accuracy requirements for glucose meters, the latest research data on HbA_{1c} and GA, real-time CGM, and others, which help clinicians to standardize practical activities, thus allowing achievement of better glycemic control and diabetes management.

References

1. Updike SJ, Hicks GP. Reagentless substrate analysis with immobilized enzymes. Science. 1967;158:270–2. https://doi.org/10.1126/science.158.3798.270.
2. Chinese Diabetes Society. Chinese clinical guideline for continuous glucose monitoring (2009). Zhonghua Yi Xue Za Zhi. 2009;89:3388–92. https://doi.org/10.3760/cma.j.issn.0376-2491.2009.48.002.
3. Chinese Diabetes Society. Chinese clinical guideline for continuous glucose monitoring (2012). Chin Med J. 2012;125:4167–74. https://doi.org/10.3760/cma.j.issn.0366-6999.2012.23.002.
4. Chinese Diabetes Society. Clinical application guide of blood glucose monitoring in China (Edition 2011). Zhonghua Yi Xue Za Zhi. 2011;91:656–64. https://doi.org/10.3760/cma.j.issn.0376-2491.2011.10.003.
5. Chinese Diabetes Society. Clinical application guide of blood glucose monitoring in China (Edition 2015). Chin J of Diabetes Mellitus. 2015;7:603–13. https://doi.org/10.3760/cma.j.issn.1674-5809.2015.10.004.
6. Blevins TC, Bode BW, Garg SK, Grunberger G, Hirsch IB, Jovanovič L, Nardacci E, Orzeck EA, Roberts VL, Tamborlane WV, AACE Continuous Glucose Monitoring Task Force, Rothermel C.

Statement by the American association of clinical endocrinologists consensus panel on continuous glucose monitoring. Endocr Pract. 2010;16:730–45. https://doi.org/10.4158/EP.16.5.730.

7. Fonseca VA, Grunberger G, Anhalt H, Bailey TS, Blevins T, Garg SK, Handelsman Y, Hirsch IB, Orzeck EA, Roberts VL, Tamborlane W, Consensus Conference Writing Committee. Continuous glucose monitoring: a consensus conference of the American Association of Clinical Endocrinologists and American College of Endocrinology. Endocr Pract. 2016;22:1008–21. https://doi.org/10.4158/EP161392.CS.
8. Bailey TS, Grunberger G, Bode BW, Handelsman Y, Hirsch IB, Jovanovič L, Roberts VL, Rodbard D, Tamborlane WV, Walsh J, American Association of Clinical Endocrinologists (AACE), American College of Endocrinology (ACE). American Association of Clinical Endocrinologists and American College of Endocrinology 2016 outpatient glucose monitoring consensus statement. Endocr Pract. 2016;22:231–61. https://doi.org/10.4158/EP151124.CS.
9. Klonoff DC, Buckingham B, Christiansen JS, Montori VM, Tamborlane WV, Vigersky RA, Wolpert H, Endocrine Society. Continuous glucose monitoring: an endocrine society clinical practice guideline. J Clin Endocrinol Metab. 2011;96:2968–79. https://doi.org/10.1210/jc.2010-2756.
10. Peters AL, Ahmann AJ, Battelino T, Evert A, Hirsch IB, Murad MH, Winter WE, Wolpert H. Diabetes technology-continuous subcutaneous insulin infusion therapy and continuous glucose monitoring in adults: an endocrine society clinical practice guideline. J Clin Endocrinol Metab. 2016;101:3922–37. https://doi.org/10.1210/jc.2016-2534.
11. Vigersky R, Shrivastav M. Role of continuous glucose monitoring for type 2 in diabetes management and research. J Diabetes Complicat. 2017;31:280–7. https://doi.org/10.1016/j.jdiacomp.2016.10.007.
12. Rodbard D. Interpretation of continuous glucose monitoring data: glycemic variability and quality of glycemic control. Diabetes Technol Ther. 2009;11(Suppl 1):55–67. https://doi.org/10.1089/dia.2008.0132.
13. Diabetes Control and Complications Trial Research Group, Nathan DM, Genuth S, Lachin J, Cleary P, Crofford O, Davis M, Rand L, Siebert C. The effect of intensive treatment of diabetes on the development and progression of long-term complications in insulin-dependent diabetes mellitus. N Engl J Med. 1993;329:977–86. https://doi.org/10.1056/NEJM199309303291401.
14. UK Prospective Diabetes Study (UKPDS) Group. Intensive blood-glucose control with sulphonylureas or insulin compared with conventional treatment and risk of complications in patients with type 2 diabetes (UKPDS 33). Lancet. 1998;352:837–53. https://doi.org/10.1016/S0140-6736(98)07019-6
15. Bao Y, Ma X, Li H, Zhou M, Hu C, Wu H, Tang J, Hou X, Xiang K, Jia W. Glycated haemoglobin A1c for diagnosing diabetes in Chinese population: cross sectional epidemiological survey. BMJ. 2010;340:c2249. https://doi.org/10.1136/bmj.c2249.
16. Wu S, Yi F, Zhou C, Zhang M, Zhu Y, Tuniyazi Y, Huang L, Huang X, Wang F, Bi Y, Ning G. HbA1c and the diagnosis of diabetes and prediabetes in a middle-aged and elderly Han population from northwest China (HbA1c). J Diabetes. 2013;5:282–90. https://doi.org/10.1111/1753-0407.12035.
17. Wang F, Ma X, Hao Y, Yang R, Ni J, Xiao Y, Tang J, Bao Y, Jia W. Serum glycated albumin is inversely influenced by fat mass and visceral adipose tissue in Chinese with normal glucose tolerance. PLoS One. 2012;7:e51098. https://doi.org/10.1371/journal.pone.0051098.
18. Liu L, Wan X, Liu J, Huang Z, Cao X, Li Y. Increased 1,5-anhydroglucitol predicts glycemic remission in patients with newly diagnosed type 2 diabetes treated with short-term intensive insulin therapy. Diabetes Technol Ther. 2012;14:756–61. https://doi.org/10.1089/dia.2012.0055.

Continuous Glucose Monitoring and Glycemic Variability

11

J. Zhou and W. Jia

Continuous glucose monitoring (CGM) technology can comprehensively and accurately reflect the characteristics of glycemic variability. Currently, research on glycemic variability using CGM is one of the hot spots (Fig. 11.1). Previously, we have analyzed the glucose profiles of individuals with different glucose tolerances by reviewing retrospective CGM data, and here are some of our findings: (1) despite the influence of various factors, the fasting plasma glucose (FPG) usually fluctuates between 3.9 and 5.6 mmol/L by the regulation of the nervous and endocrine systems and the liver. The blood glucose levels begin to rise about 10 min after meal intake, due to the absorption of carbohydrates in the diet. The peak postprandial blood glucose level and duration time are associated with a variety of factors such as eating time and the amount and content of food intake. Usually, the blood glucose concentration peaks at 1 h after eating and returns to the premeal level after 2–3 h. The intraday and inter-day blood glucose excursions were reported to be approximately 2.0 mmol/L and 0.8 mmol/L [1]. (2) The intraday glycemic variability of patients with impaired glucose tolerance was significantly increased by 50%, as compared with that of those with normal glucose tolerance. However, no significant difference in the inter-day glycemic variability was found [2, 3] (Fig. 11.2). (3) Once the patients were diagnosed as diabetes, the intraday glycemic variability was further increased, accompanied by significantly increased inter-day variability, which are 3- and 2.5-fold increased, respectively, as compared with that in individuals with normal glucose tolerance. However, no significant difference was found in the frequency of intraday glycemic variability [3] (Figs. 11.3 and 11.4). (4) Due to a lack of early-phase insulin secretion, the postprandial glucose concentration excessively rises and lasts for a long time, with predominant hyperglycemia after breakfast [1]. (5) Glycated hemoglobin A_{1c} (HbA_{1c}) represents the overall level of blood glucose but does not reflect the characteristics of glycemic variability. The mean amplitude of glycemic excursion (MAGE) and mean of daily differences (MODD) obtained in CGM glucose profiles can accurately reflect the magnitude of intraday and inter-day glycemic variability of subjects. Both parameters may serve as clinical parameters for assessing whether type 2 diabetes patients achieve the target glycemic control [2].

J. Zhou · W. Jia (✉)
Department of Endocrinology and Metabolism, Shanghai Clinical Center for Diabetes, Shanghai Diabetes Institute, Shanghai Jiao Tong University Affiliated Sixth People's Hospital, Shanghai, China
e-mail: wpjia@sjtu.edu.cn

W. Jia (ed.), *Continuous Glucose Monitoring*, https://doi.org/10.1007/978-981-10-7074-7_11

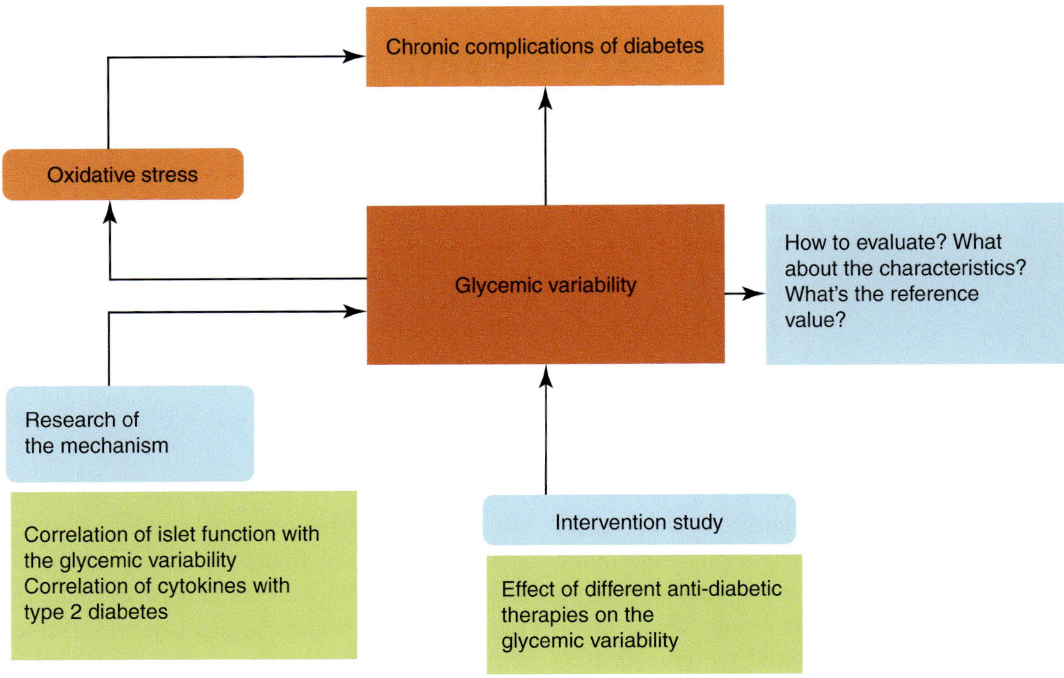

Fig. 11.1 The main content of CGM-based research on glycemic variability

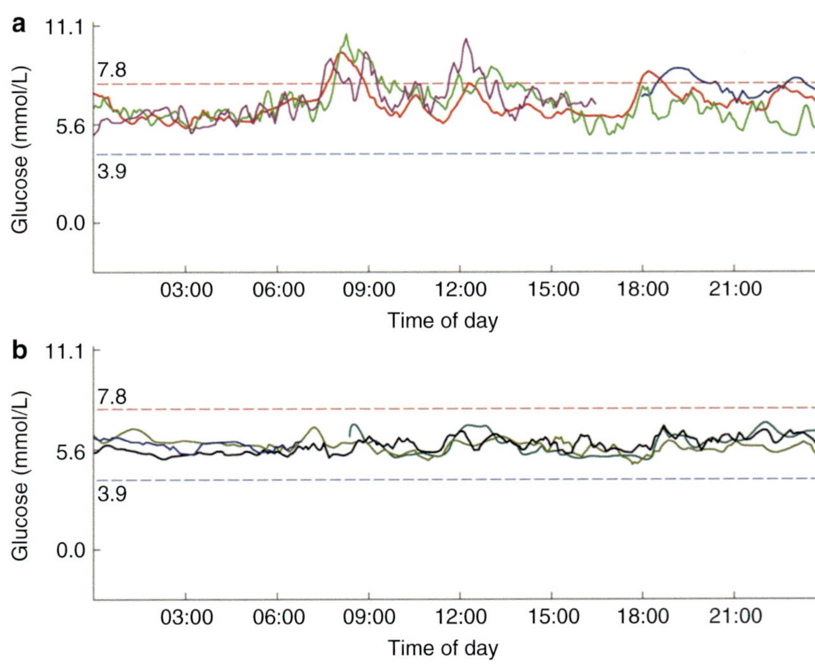

Fig. 11.2 The CGM profiles of one case of impaired glucose tolerance (**a**) and one case of normal glucose tolerance (**b**)

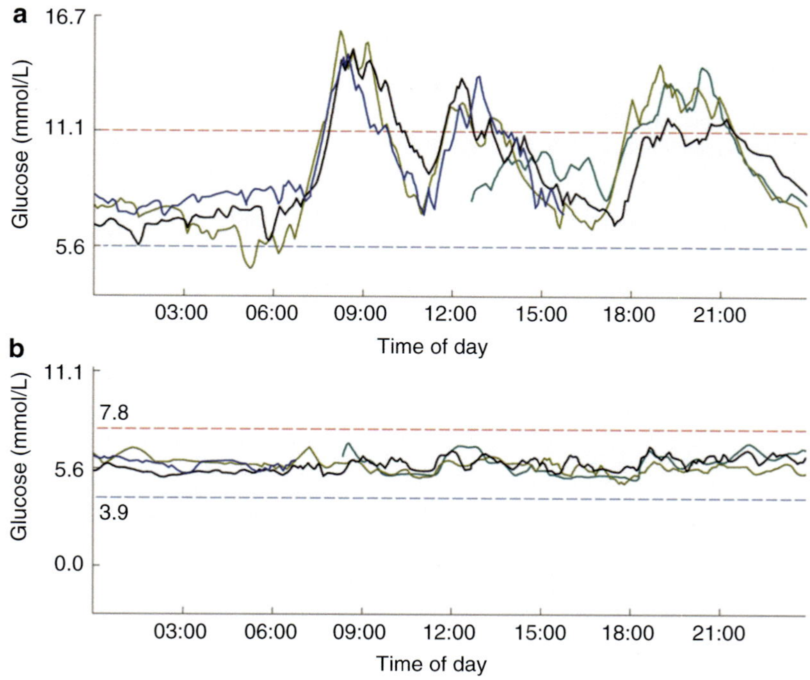

Fig. 11.3 The CGM profiles of one case of type 2 diabetes mellitus (**a**) and one case of normal glucose tolerance (**b**)

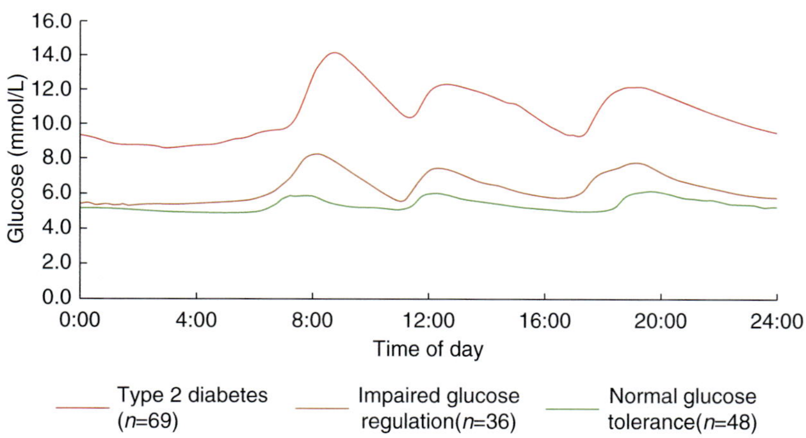

Fig. 11.4 The characteristics of glycemic variability in individuals with different state of glucose tolerance using CGM. Note: The blood glucose levels fluctuate with small amplitudes in healthy individuals. However, individuals with impaired glucose tolerance exhibited increased glycemic variability compared with normal individuals, and the overall glucose level and glycemic variability were significantly increased in type 2 diabetes patients

11.1 Relationship Between Glycemic Variability and Diabetic Microvascular Complications

With advances in CGM technology, further investigation is carried out to explore the relationship between glycemic variability and diabetic microvascular complications. Šoupal et al. [4] found that standard deviation of blood glucose (SDBG) calculated from CGM data was associated with diabetic microangiopathy in 32 type 1 diabetes patients. Similarly, Sartore et al. [5] reported a correlation between SDBG and the development of diabetic retinopathy by analyzing the CGM data from 68 type 1 or type 2 diabetes patients.

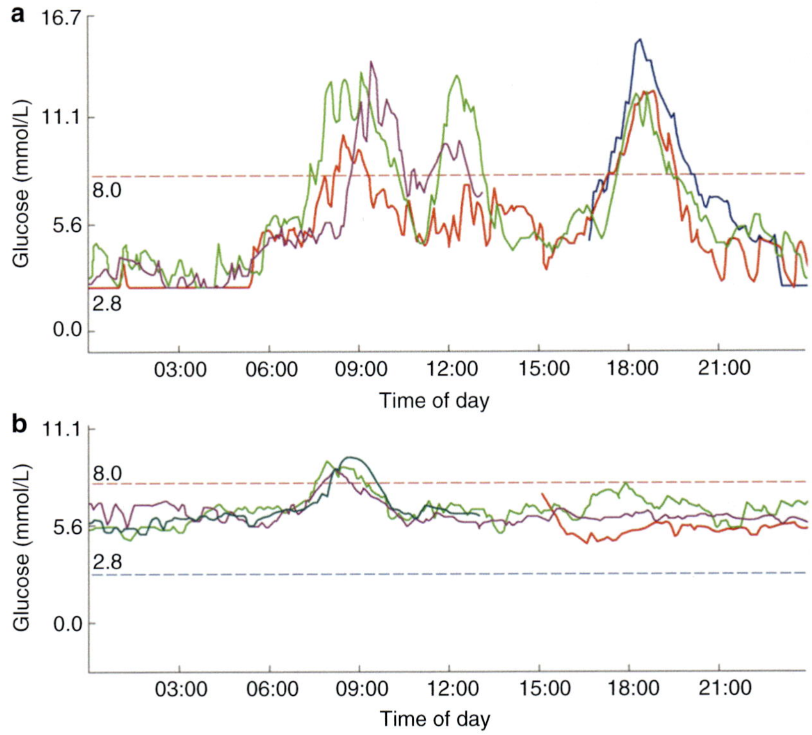

Fig. 11.5 The CGM profiles of two cases of type 2 diabetes with HbA_{1c} <6.5% (48 mmol/mol) [6]. Note: (**a**) HbA_{1c} 6.4% (46 mmol/mol), MAGE 3.0 mmol/L; (**b**) HbA_{1c} 6.2% (44 mmol/mol), MAGE 0.9 mmol/L

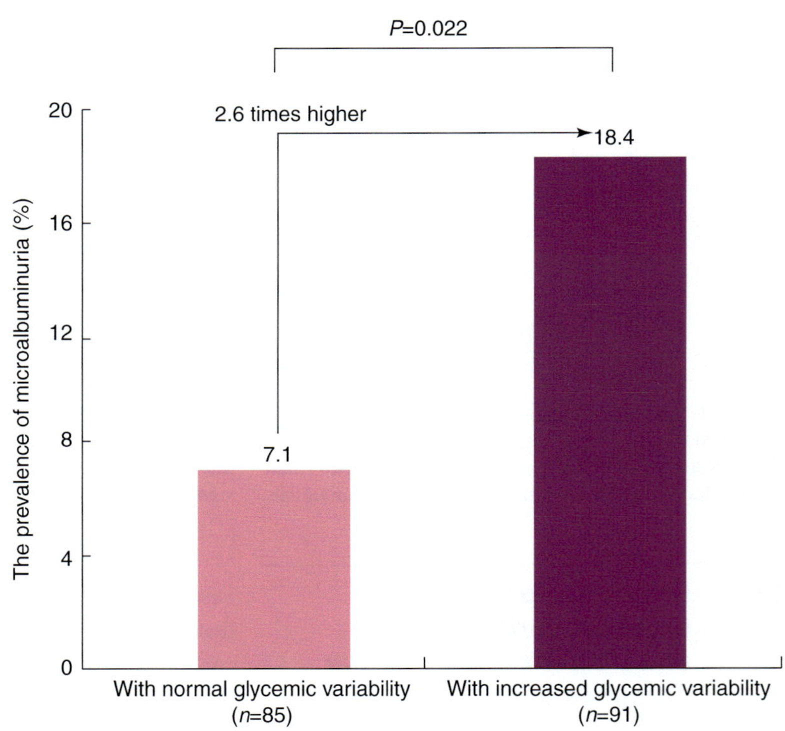

Fig. 11.6 The detection rate of microalbuminuria in type 2 diabetes with HbA_{1c} <6.5% (48 mmol/mol) who had normal or abnormal glycemic variability [6]

We previously investigated the relationship between glycemic variability and microalbuminuria in 176 type 2 diabetes patients with an HbA_{1c} <6.5% (48 mmol/mol) and found that the glycemic variability was very different among these patients (Fig. 11.5). More than half of the patients presented abnormal glycemic variability, which were associated with increased risk of microalbuminuria (Fig. 11.6), indicating that glycemic variability is a risk factor of the occurrence of microalbuminuria in type 2 diabetes [6]. Nevertheless, the Diabetes Control and Complications Trial (DCCT) results show that glycemic variability is not an independent risk factor for complications. Lachin et al. [7] published an article, demonstrating that only the M-value is correlated to microalbuminuria but not retinopathy. At present, however, the correlation between glycemic variability and diabetic microvascular complications still remains undetermined.

11.2 Relationship Between Glycemic Variability and Diabetic Macrovascular Complications

The relationship between glycemic variability and macrovascular complications has also been a hot research topic in recent years. In the study performed by Chen et al. [8], 36 type 2 diabetes patients were classified into two groups according to the levels of carotid intima-media thickness (IMT) as patients with or without atherosclerosis. Compared to controls, the MAGE level calculated from CGM data was gradually increased with the progression of atherosclerosis. Also, the carotid IMT was correlated with age, duration of diabetes, and MAGE by Spearman's correlation analysis. Another study showed that during the DCCT, MBG was a better predictor of the macrovascular complications of type 1 diabetes than HbA_{1c} [9]. These findings suggested that glycemic variability is an important factor contributing to the progression of atherosclerosis in type 2 diabetes patients.

Also, we conducted a cross-sectional study in 216 type 2 diabetes patients to investigate the relationship between glycemic variability and macrovascular complications [10]. Magnetic resonance angiography (MRA) was applied to detect the severity of arterial stenosis, and ultrasonography was used to quantify carotid IMT as an index of subclinical atherosclerosis. Subcutaneous interstitial glucose concentrations of patients were monitored continuously for 3 days using the CGM system. The results revealed that age, increased systolic blood pressure, and increased mean blood glucose (MBG), but not glycemic variability, were independently related to atherosclerotic stenosis. In patients without cervical and/or intracranial lesions evaluated by MRA, SDBG and MAGE were both significantly related to carotid IMT (Figs. 11.7 and 11.8), revealing the intriguing possibility that glycemic variability plays a key role in the subclinical stage of atherosclerosis. Su et al. [11] analyzed the contribution of MAGE, blood glucose, and HbA_{1c} to the major adverse cardiac events in 222 patients with acute myocardial infarction. CGM system was used for 48 consecutive hours after admission. Based on the cutoff reference value of MAGE as 3.9 mmol/L established by our previous study [12], patients were divided into two groups as high MAGE (≥3.9 mmol/L) or low MAGE (<3.9 mmol/L). The results demonstrated that MAGE was independently correlated with the incidence of major adverse cardiac events. Similar findings were obtained by Wang et al. [13]. In another study performed by Su et al. [14], coronary artery angiography was performed in 344 type 2 diabetes with chest pain, and the Gensini score was calculated to assess the severity of coronary artery disease. The results demonstrated that MAGE, calculated from CGM data, was the most distinct independent predictor of coronary artery disease. In addition, in a study of 22 type 1 diabetes patients, MAGE was independently correlated with the change in aortic diastolic pressure during hyperglycemic clamp, suggesting the involvement of daily glucose variability in the progression of macrovascular disease [15]. In 2006, Monnier et al. [16] found that urinary 8-iso prostaglandin $F_{2\alpha}$ excretion rates, an indicator of oxidative stress,

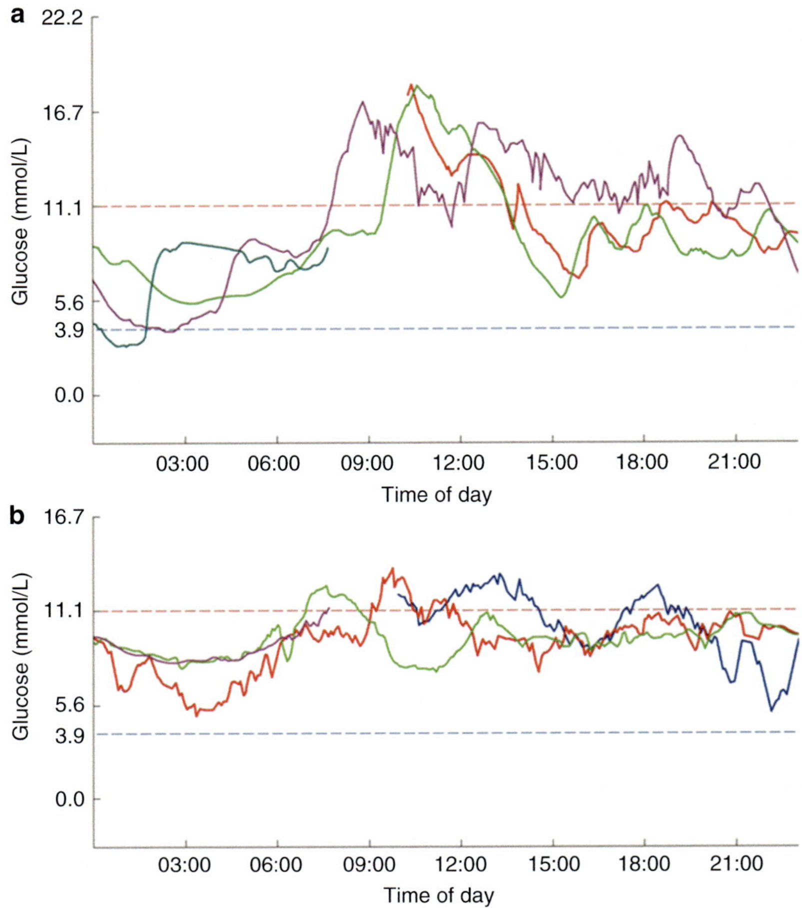

Fig. 11.7 Examples of the CGM profiles and carotid IMT measurements of two cases of type 2 diabetes patients with different glycemic variability. Note: (**a**) carotid IMT 1.0 mm, MAGE 7.99 mmol/L, SDBG 3.43 mmol/L; (**b**) carotid IMT: 0.6 mm, MAGE: 3.06 mmol/L, SDBG 1.42 mmol/L. *carotid IMT* carotid intima-media thickness, *MAGE* mean amplitude of glycemic excursion, *SDBG* standard deviations of blood glucose

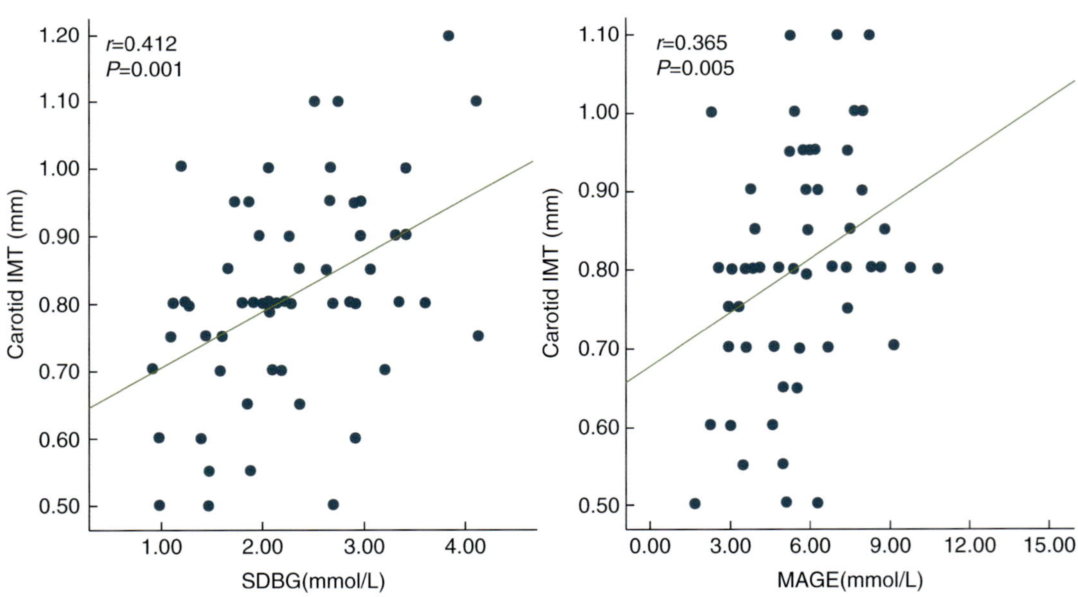

Fig. 11.8 The correlation between glycemic variability and carotid IMT in 63 type 2 diabetes patients without atherosclerotic stenosis as determined by cranial/cervical magnetic resonance angiography [10] (Reprint from Cardiovascular Diabetology). Note: *IMT* intima-media thickness, *SDBG* standard deviations of blood glucose, *MAGE* mean amplitude of glycemic excursion

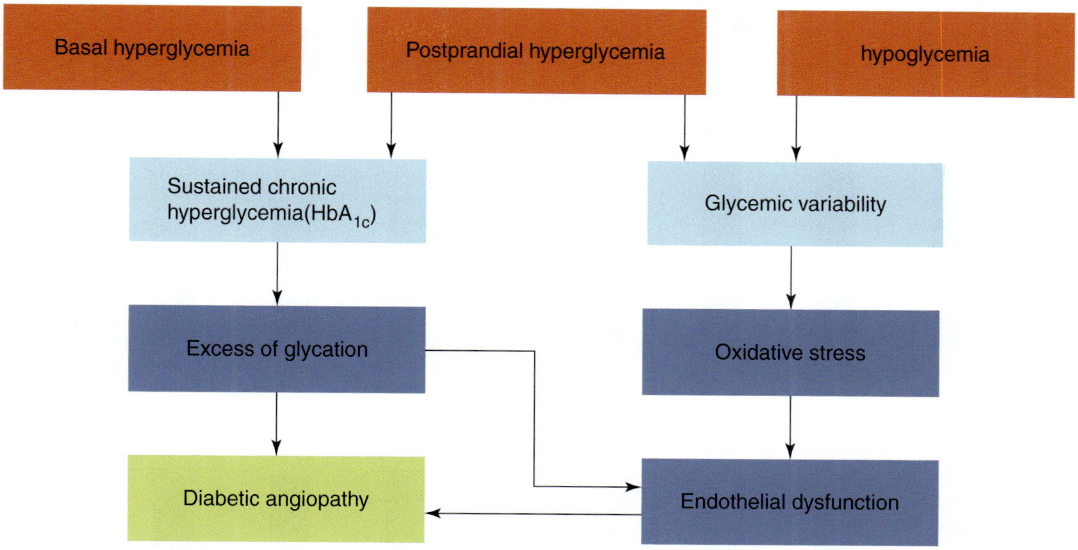

Fig. 11.9 Effect of persistent hyperglycemia (basal hyperglycemia, postprandial hyperglycemia) and glycemic variability (postprandial hyperglycemia and hypoglycemia) on chronic complications of diabetes mellitus

were higher in type 2 diabetes patients than in healthy controls, and it was significantly correlated with MAGE ($r = 0.86$, $P < 0.001$). Thus, they concluded that MAGE is an important parameter reflecting glycemic variability [17], and glycemic variability is involved in macrovascular complications [18]. It is noted that Xu et al. [19] found a significant relationship between MAGE and cardiac autonomic neuropathy in newly diagnosed type 2 diabetes, which demonstrating that glycemic variability is an important risk factor for cardiovascular autonomic neuropathy. Therefore, persistent hyperglycemia (including basal hyperglycemia, postprandial hyperglycemia) and glycemic variability (postprandial hyperglycemia or hypoglycemia) are both involved in macrovascular complications development through different mechanisms (Fig. 11.9).

11.3 Relationship Between Glycemic Variability and Islet Function

Currently, impaired insulin secretion and/or decreased insulin sensitivity are generally accepted as basic pathophysiological characteristics of diabetic patients. Islet β-cell function plays an important role in the progression of diabetes mellitus, and its dynamic changes in "quality" and "quantity" have crucial impact on the regulation of blood glucose and the occurrence of chronic complications. We previously analyzed the relationship between glycemic variability and pathophysiological state in 339 healthy subjects with normal glucose regulation [20]. The results showed that early-phase insulin secretion (expressed as $\Delta I_{30}/\Delta G_{30}$) was significantly different among healthy subjects with different MAGE values, whereas basal insulin secretion and insulin sensitivity were not significantly different (Fig. 11.10). The correlation analysis showed that glycemic variability was negatively correlated with early-phase insulin secretion (Fig. 11.11), indicating that excessive glycemic variability was associated with poor islet function. These data suggested that early changes in islet function could impact glycemic variability. Our previous CGM data from type 2 diabetes patients with HbA_{1c} <6.5% (48 mmol/mol) showed that glucose profiles could greatly differ even among those with HbA_{1c} controlled within the target range. In addition to the duration of diabetes, the postprandial 30-min serum C-peptide level was also an independent factor, which to a certain extent reflects early-phase insulin secretion in type 2 diabetes [6]. These findings were further proven by Kohnert et al. [21], who conducted a study including 59 type 2 diabetes patients (age 64.2 ± 8.6 years

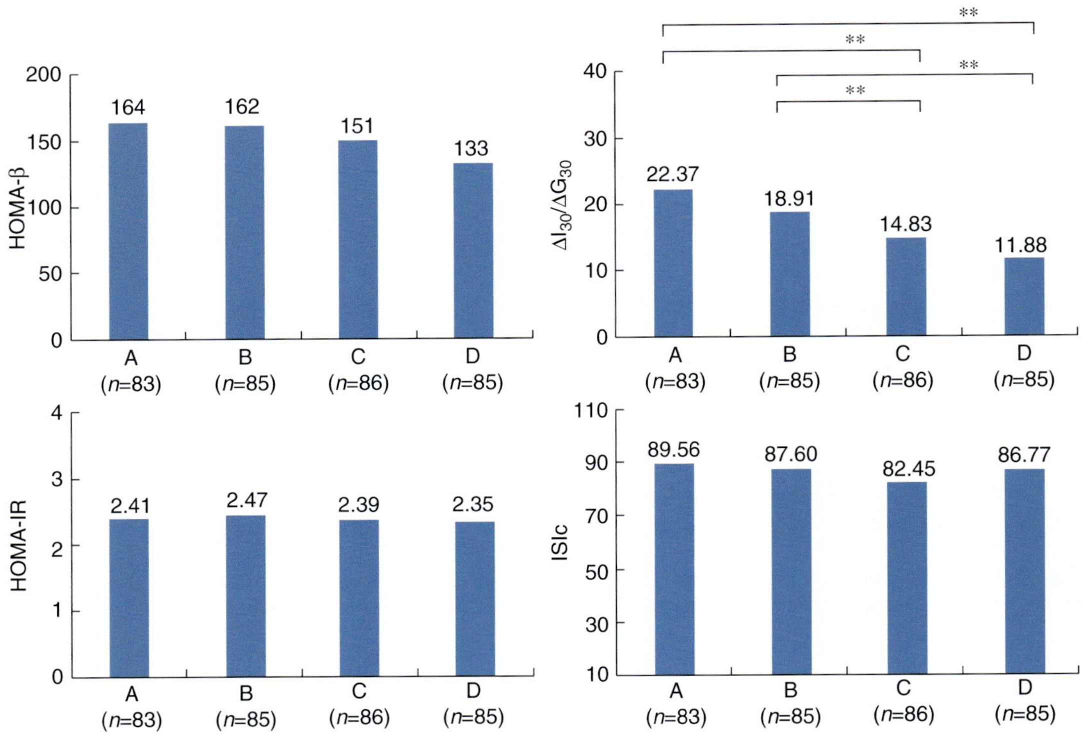

Fig. 11.10 Comparison of insulin secretion function and sensitivity in 339 patients with normal glucose tolerance but different MAGE levels [20] (Reprint with permission from Chinese Journal of Diabetes Mellitus) $^{**}P < 0.01$

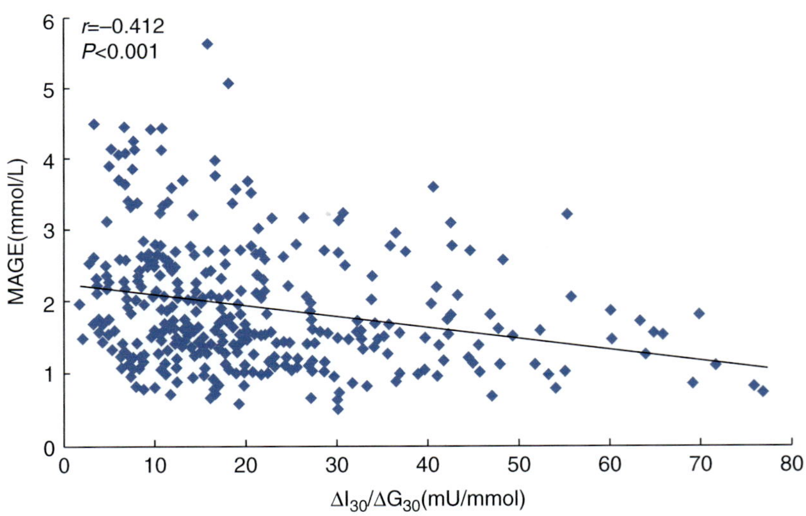

Fig. 11.11 The relationship between MAGE and islet function ($\Delta I_{30}/\Delta G_{30}$) in 339 individuals with normal glucose tolerance [20] (Reprint with permission from Chinese Journal of Diabetes Mellitus)

old; HbA_{1c} 6.5 ± 1.0% (48 ± 11 mmol/mol); body mass index [BMI] 29.8 ± 3.8 kg/m^2) using either oral hypoglycemic agents (n = 34) or diet control alone (n = 25). The glucose profiles obtained from CGM measurements recorded over 3 consecutive days were analyzed. Postprandial β-cell function and basal β-cell function were measured by an insulin secretion model during a mixed-meal test. The insulin sensitivity was assessed by the homeostasis model assessment of insulin resistance

(HOMA-IR). The results showed that MAGE was nonlinearly correlated with postprandial β-cell function ($r = 0.54$, $P < 0.001$) and with basal β-cell function ($r = 0.31$, $P = 0.025$) in oral hypoglycemic agent users but failed to correlate with these parameters in patients treated with diet modification alone. The stepwise multiple regression analysis demonstrated that postprandial β-cell function and treatment with oral hypoglycemic agents were independent contributors to MAGE ($R^2 = 0.50$, $P < 0.01$). This study demonstrated a close relationship between glycemic variability and postprandial β-cell function in type 2 diabetes patients using oral hypoglycemic agents. Therefore, we speculate that compared to other pathophysiological factors such as insulin sensitivity and basal insulin secretion, early-phase islet is more closely associated with glycemic variability. Moreover, improvement in postprandial β-cell function appears to be an important target to reduce glycemic variability, thereby preventing the development and progression of diabetes complications. In addition, we have investigated the relationship between glycemic variability and cytokines. The results showed that the serum osteocalcin concentration increases with a decrease in the glucose concentration, and high initial osteocalcin levels are associated with subsequent improvements in glycemic variability [22].

The above studies show that abnormal glycemic variability may be an important contributor to the development of diabetes-related complications. According to FLAT-SUGAR Trial, compared with basal-bolus insulin, glucagon-like peptide-1 receptor agonist and insulin (GLIPULIN) can reduce glycemic variability, weight, and some cardiometabolic risk markers while maintaining equivalent HbA_{1c} levels [23]. Islet β-cell function and certain cytokines (such as osteocalcin, etc.) can affect blood glucose levels. The data analysis from CGM can accurately and comprehensively reflect glycemic variability. Therefore, it is necessary to carry out further researches in the future, especially prospective, large-scale studies using CGM, to clarify the relationship between glycemic variability and diabetic complications as well as the underlying mechanism, and finally, to provide new strategies for the prevention and treatment of diabetes and complications.

Statement on Consent for Participation
All the clinical trials carried out by the authors in this book have been reported to the Ethics Committee of Shanghai Jiao Tong University Affiliated Sixth People's Hospital already and were in accordance with the Good Clinical Practice and Standards of China Association for Ethical Studies (approval number: 2007-45).

References

1. Zhou J, Jia W, Yu M, Ma X, Bao Y, Lu W. The features of postprandial glucose state in type 2 diabetes mellitus. Zhonghua Yi Xue Za Zhi. 2006;86:970–5. https://doi.org/10.3760/j:issn:0376-2491.2006.14.009.
2. Zhou J, Yu M, Jia WP, Li Q, Li M, Ma XJ, Lu W, Xiang KS. Application of continuous glucose monitoring system in the assessment of within-day and day-to-day blood glucose excursions in type 2 diabetic patients. Chin J Endocrinol Metab. 2006;22:286–8. https://doi.org/10.3760/j:issn:1000-6699.2006.03.028.
3. Zhou J, Jia WP, Yu M, Bao YQ, Ma XJ, Lu W, Hu C, Yu HY, Xiang KS. Characteristics of glycemic stability in subjects with different glucose tolerance: the results of continuous glucose monitoring. Shanghai Med J. 2008;31:10–3.
4. Šoupal J, Škrha J Jr, Fajmon M, Horová E, Mráz M, Škrha J, Prázný M. Glycemic variability is higher in type 1 diabetes patients with microvascular complications irrespective of glycemic control. Diabetes Technol Ther. 2014;16:198–203. https://doi.org/10.1089/dia.2013.0205.
5. Sartore G, Chilelli NC, Burlina S, Lapolla A. Association between glucose variability as assessed by continuous glucose monitoring (CGM) and diabetic retinopathy in type 1 and type 2 diabetes. Acta Diabetol. 2013;50:437–42. https://doi.org/10.1007/s00592-013-0459-9.
6. Zhou J, Jia W, Ma X, Bao YQ, Lu W, Li M, Li Q, Hu C, Xiang KS. Relationship between blood glucose variability and microalbuminuria in type 2 diabetic patients with well-controlled glycosylated hemoglobin. Zhonghua Yi Xue Za Zhi. 2008;88:2977–81. https://doi.org/10.3321/j:issn:0376-2491.2008.42.007.
7. Lachin JM, Bebu I, Bergenstal RM, Pop-Busui R, Service FJ, Zinman B, Nathan DM, DCCT/EDIC Research Group. Association of glycemic variability in type 1 diabetes with progression of microvascular outcomes in the diabetes control and complications trial. Diabetes Care. 2017;40:777–83. https://doi.org/10.2337/dc16-2426.
8. Chen XM, Zhang Y, Shen XP, Huang Q, Ma H, Huang YL, Zhang WQ, Wu HJ. Correlation between glucose fluctuations and carotid intima-media thickness in type 2 diabetes. Diabetes Res Clin Pract. 2010;90:95–9. https://doi.org/10.1016/j.diabres.2010.05.004.

9. Kilpatrick ES, Rigby AS, Atkin SL. Mean blood glucose compared with HbA1c in the prediction of cardiovascular disease in patients with type 1 diabetes. Diabetologia. 2008;51:365–71. https://doi.org/10.1007/s00125-007-0883-x.
10. Mo Y, Zhou J, Li M, Wang Y, Bao Y, Ma X, Li D, Lu W, Hu C, Li M, Jia W. Glycemic variability is associated with subclinical atherosclerosis in Chinese type 2 diabetic patients. Cardiovasc Diabetol. 2013;12:15. https://doi.org/10.1186/1475-2840-12-15.
11. Su G, Mi SH, Tao H, Li Z, Yang HX, Zheng H, Zhou Y, Tian L. Impact of admission glycemic variability, glucose, and glycosylated hemoglobin on major adverse cardiac events after acute myocardial infarction. Diabetes Care. 2013;36:1026–32. https://doi.org/10.2337/dc12-0925.
12. Zhou J, Li H, Ran X, Yang W, Li Q, Peng Y, Li Y, Gao X, Luan X, Wang W, Jia W. Establishment of normal reference ranges for glycemic variability in Chinese subjects using continuous glucose monitoring. Med Sci Monit. 2011;17:CR9–13. https://doi.org/10.12659/MSM.881318.
13. Wang X, Zhao X, Dorje T, Yan H, Qian J, Ge J. Glycemic variability predicts cardiovascular complications in acute myocardial infarction patients with type 2 diabetes mellitus. Int J Cardiol. 2014;172:498–500. https://doi.org/10.1016/j.ijcard.2014.01.015.
14. Su G, Mi S, Tao H, Li Z, Yang H, Zheng H, Zhou Y, Ma C. Association of glycemic variability and the presence and severity of coronary artery disease in patients with type 2 diabetes. Cardiovasc Diabetol. 2011;10:19. https://doi.org/10.1186/1475-2840-10-19.
15. Gordin D, Rönnback M, Forsblom C, Mäkinen V, Saraheimo M, Groop PH. Glucose variability, blood pressure and arterial stiffness in type 1 diabetes. Diabetes Res Clin Pract. 2008;80:e4–7. https://doi.org/10.1016/j.diabres.2008.01.010.
16. Monnier L, Mas E, Ginet C, Michel F, Villon L, Cristol JP, Colette C. Activation of oxidative stress by acute glucose fluctuations compared with sustained chronic hyperglycemia in patients with type 2 diabetes. JAMA. 2006;295:1681–7. https://doi.org/10.1001/jama.295.14.1681.
17. Monnier L, Colette C, Boegner C, Pham TC, Lapinski H, Boniface H. Continuous glucose monitoring in patients with type 2 diabetes: Why? When? Whom? Diabetes Metab. 2007;33:247–52. https://doi.org/10.1016/j.diabet.2006.11.007.
18. Monnier L, Colette C, Owens D. The glycemic triumvirate and diabetic complications: is the whole greater than the sum of its component parts? Diabetes Res Clin Pract. 2012;95:303–11. https://doi.org/10.1016/j.diabres.2011.10.014.
19. Xu W, Zhu Y, Yang X, Deng H, Yan J, Lin S, Yang H, Chen H, Weng J. Glycemic variability is an important risk factor for cardiovascular autonomic neuropathy in newly diagnosed type 2 diabetic patients. Int J Cardiol. 2016;215:263–8. https://doi.org/10.1016/j.ijcard.2016.04.078.
20. Zhou J, Li H, Yang WY, Ran XW, Li Q, Peng YD, Li YB, Gao X, Luan XJ, Wang WQ, Jia W. Relationship between early-phase insulin secretion and blood glucose variability in subject with normal glucose regulation. Chin J Diabetes Mellitus. 2009;1:89–93. https://doi.org/10.3760/cma.j.issn.1674-5809.2009.02.004.
21. Kohnert KD, Augstein P, Zander E, Heinke P, Peterson K, Freyse EJ, Hovorka R, Salzsieder E. Glycemic variability correlates strongly with postprandial beta-cell dysfunction in a segment of type 2 diabetic patients using oral hypoglycemic agents. Diabetes Care. 2009;32:1058–62. https://doi.org/10.2337/dc08-1956.
22. Bao YQ, Zhou M, Zhou J, Lu W, Gao YC, Pan XP, Tang JL, Lu HJ, Jia WP. Relationship between serum osteocalcin and glycaemic variability in type 2 diabetes. Clin Exp Pharmacol Physiol. 2011;38:50–4. https://doi.org/10.1111/j.1440-1681.2010.05463.x.
23. FLAT-SUGAR Trial Investigators. Glucose variability in a 26-week randomized comparison of mealtime treatment with rapid-acting insulin versus glp-1 agonist in participants with type 2 diabetes at high cardiovascular risk. Diabetes Care. 2016;39:973–81. https://doi.org/10.2337/dc15-2782.

12 Continuous Glucose Monitoring and Antidiabetic Therapies

J. Zhou and W. Jia

Continuous glucose monitoring (CGM) reveals an important aspect of blood glucose management, that is, the characteristics of glycemic variability, which facilitates the understanding of the association between glycemic variability and the risk of chronic complications of diabetes. Previous studies have shown that glycemic variability has a significant impact on chronic complications of diabetes. Therefore, in addition to monitoring fasting plasma glucose (FPG), 2-h postprandial plasma glucose (2hPG), glycated hemoglobin A_{1c} (HbA_{1c}), and others, glycemic variability management is also an important component in the adjustment of antidiabetic therapies. Thus, CGM is expected to become an effective means to assess the efficacy of antidiabetic therapies. This chapter describes the clinical trials that used CGM to evaluate antidiabetic therapies as an introduction for future research in this field.

12.1 Evaluation of the Efficacy of Insulin Therapy Using CGM

Previous studies have been carried out to assess the efficacy of insulin therapies via the use of CGM. In our previous study, 48 subjects with normal glucose tolerance and 69 patients with newly diagnosed type 2 diabetes were monitored by using a CGM system. A subset of type 2 diabetes patients ($n = 23$) with HbA_{1c} >8.5% (69 mmol/mol) was monitored a second time after 2–3 weeks of insulin treatment (4 injections daily). The mean amplitude of glycemic excursion (MAGE), the mean of daily differences (MODD), and the incremental areas above preprandial glucose values (AUCpp) were used to assess intraday, inter-day, and postprandial glycemic variability. The results showed that AUCpp after breakfast and dinner were significantly higher than that after lunch in newly diagnosed type 2 diabetes patients. After intensive treatment, significant decreases in MAGE, MODD, and AUCpp were observed (41%, 29%, and 49%, respectively, $P < 0.001$, Fig. 12.1) [1]. Thus, CGM is an effective means to assess glycemic variability and improve glucose management during intensive treatment with insulin.

In the study by Alemzadeh et al. [2], 14 patients with type 1 diabetes were transitioned from flexible multiple daily insulin to continuous subcutaneous insulin infusion (CSII). The results showed that CSII improved glycemic variability as evidenced by MAGE values calculated from CGM data. McNally et al. [3] compared the hypoglycemic efficacy of biphasic insulin aspart 30 (BIAsp 30) versus biphasic human insulin 30 (BHI 30) through CGM. The results showed that compared with BHI 30, BIAsp 30 was associated with similar HbA_{1c} levels but with fewer nocturnal hypoglycemia

J. Zhou · W. Jia (✉)
Department of Endocrinology and Metabolism, Shanghai Clinical Center for Diabetes, Shanghai Diabetes Institute, Shanghai Jiao Tong University Affiliated Sixth People's Hospital, Shanghai, China
e-mail: wpjia@sjtu.edu.cn

W. Jia (ed.), *Continuous Glucose Monitoring*, https://doi.org/10.1007/978-981-10-7074-7_12

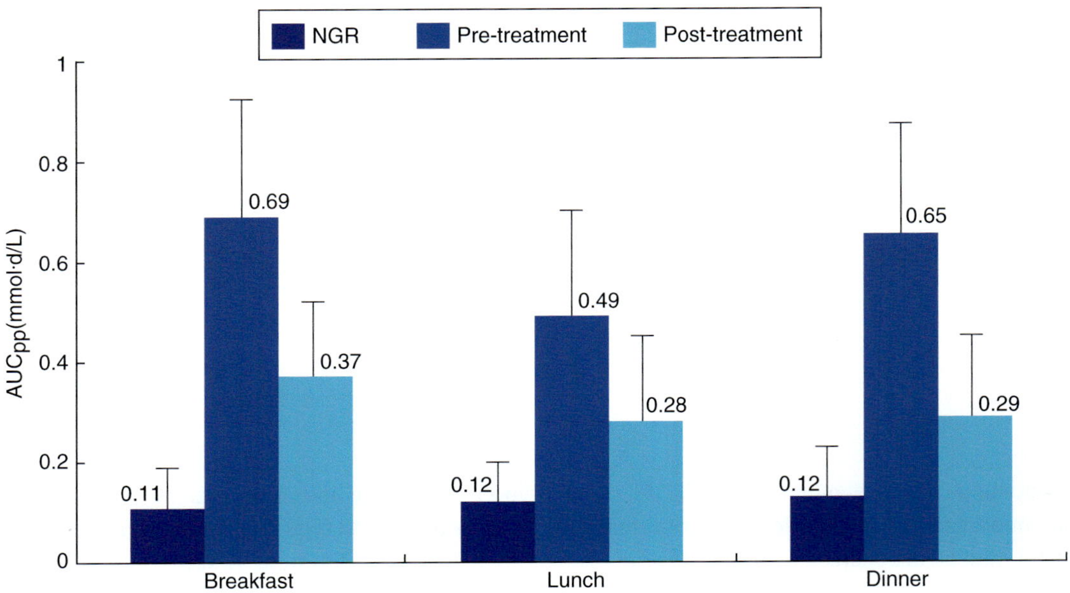

Fig. 12.1 Comparison of incremental areas above preprandial glucose values (AUCpp) in 48 normal individuals and 69 newly diagnosed type 2 diabetes patients [1] (Reprint from *Medical Science Monitor*)

events. The Assessment of Weekly AdministRation of Dulaglutide in Diabetes (AWARD)-4 trial is a phase 3 sub-study of the AWARD clinical program [4], and it was designed by using 24-h CGM to evaluate the effects of glucagon-like peptide-1 (GLP-1) agonist dulaglutide. In the AWARD-4 trial, 884 patients treated with the conventional insulin therapy were randomly divided into three groups: dulaglutide 1.5 mg per week, dulaglutide 0.75 mg per week, and glargine insulin, all in combination with prandial insulin lispro. Of these patients, the CGM system was applied in 144 patients at weeks 0, 13, 26, and 52. The results showed that at week 26, the mean blood glucose (MBG) was decreased in all treatment groups and the intergroup differences were not significantly. The standard deviation of blood glucose (SDBG) was significantly reduced with dulaglutide versus glargine. At week 52, there were no significant differences among groups with regard to overall blood glucose levels, whereas treatment with glargine was associated with a greater risk of hypoglycemia. Tosaka et al. [5] investigated the efficacy of insulin degludec used for basal-bolus insulin regimen after switching from twice-daily basal insulin in 22 Japanese patients with type 1 diabetes mellitus. The frequency of hypoglycemic events, SDBG, and MODD were evaluated by CGM before and 4 weeks after the switch. The results showed that there were no significant differences in HbA_{1c}, the frequency of hypoglycemia, and glycemic variability parameters before and after the switch, suggesting that glycemic control under once-daily insulin degludec injection was comparable to that under twice-daily basal insulin injections in Japanese type 1 diabetes patients. In the study performed by Ma et al. [6], a total of 63 type 2 diabetes were randomized into a liraglutide (GLP-1 agonist) group and neutral protamine Hagedorn (NPH) group, and the patients were followed up for 12 weeks. Through CGM data, FPG, HbA_{1c}, and MBG obtained by CGM were decreased in both groups after 12 weeks of treatment. In the liraglutide group, CGM showed that the frequency of hypoglycemic episodes, MAGE, and SDBG were significantly lower than those in the NPH group. The results revealed that liraglutide achieved improvements in overall glycemic control similar to NPH, whereas liraglutide was superior to NPH with respect to control glycemic variability. Taken together, these results showed that the use of CGM can provide more information, especially in terms of glycemic variability and hypoglycemia, for assessing the efficacy of insulin therapy.

12.2 Evaluation of the Efficacy of Oral Hypoglycemic Agents with CGM

CGM can also provide valuable information on glycemic variability for comparing the efficacy of two oral hypoglycemic agents. According to our previous study, the glycemic excursion was higher at breakfast or dinner than that at lunch in newly diagnosed type 2 diabetic patients [1] (Fig. 12.1). We thus designed the corresponding interventional study. A total of 40 newly diagnosed type 2 diabetes patients whose HbA_{1c} levels ranged from 7.0 to 9.8% (53–84 mmol/mol) were randomized to either glipizide controlled-release tablets monotherapy (5 mg, QD) or combination therapy of glipizide tablets (5 mg, QD) plus acarbose (50 mg, BID) for 8 weeks. CGM was used at the beginning and end of the study (Fig. 12.2). The results showed that HbA_{1c}, 24-h MBG, MAGE, and AUCpp were significantly improved in both groups. Also, glycemic variability parameters including MAGE, MODD, and AUCpp were significantly improved in the combination therapy group than in the monotherapy group, but no difference in HbA_{1c} improvement or glycated albumin (GA) improvement was found between two groups [7]. These findings suggested that glipizide tablets alone or in combination with acarbose can improve overall blood glucose levels and intraday glycemic variability, and combination therapy was more effective at reducing inter-day glycemic variability than monotherapy in newly diagnosed type 2 diabetic patients.

Based on the results of this study, we conducted a multicenter clinical study to further compare the efficacy of non-sulfonylurea insulin secretagogues (nateglinide) and acarbose on postprandial glycemic excursions in Chinese subjects

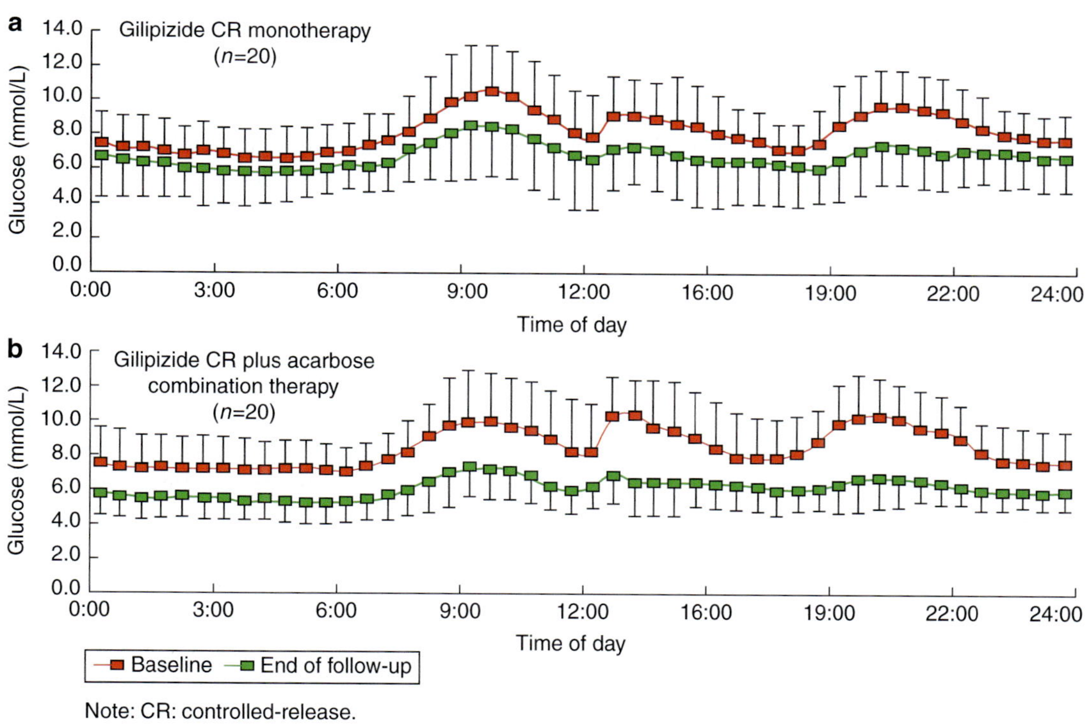

Fig. 12.2 The CGM profiles of newly diagnosed type 2 diabetes patients treated with glipizide controlled-release tablet monotherapy (**a**) or combination therapy of glipizide controlled-release tablets plus acarbose (**b**) [7] (Reprint with permission from *Clinical Experimental Pharmacology and Physiology*). Note: CR, controlled-release

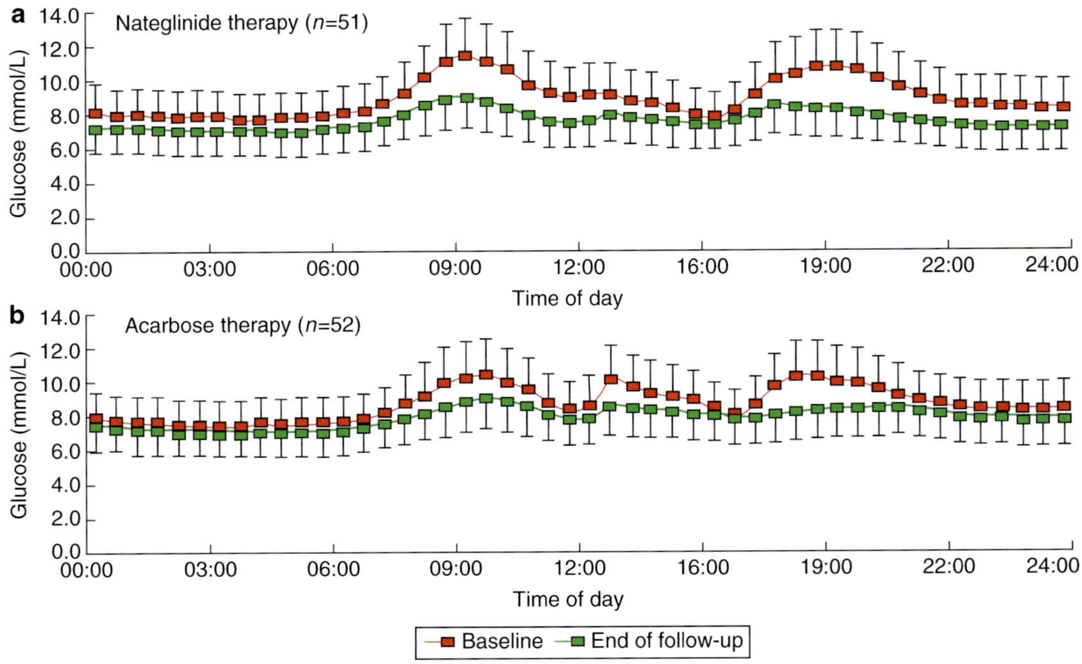

Fig. 12.3 The CGM glucose profiles before and after treatment with nateglinide (**a**) or acarbose (**b**) of type 2 diabetes patients who have not been previously treated with hypoglycemic agents [8] (Reprint with permission from *Diabetes Technology & Therapeutics*)

with type 2 diabetes. A total of 103 patients with type 2 diabetes who have not been previously treated with hypoglycemic agents [HbA_{1c} ranging from 6.5 to 9.0% (48–75 mmol/mol)] were included in the study. Patients were randomized to receive nateglinide (120 mg, TID) or acarbose (50 mg, TID) for 2 weeks. AUCpp, MAGE, SDBG, MODD, and 24-h MBG were calculated using the CGM system (Fig. 12.3), and GA and serum insulin levels were measured as well. The results showed that AUCpp, 24-h MBG, and GA levels were significantly decreased in both treatment groups, but no significant intergroup differences were found (Fig. 12.4). Moreover, the nateglinide-treated group had significantly increased insulin levels at 30 min and 120 min after a standard meal compared with the baseline level, whereas the acarbose-treated group had decreased insulin levels at both time points. Thus, nateglinide and acarbose were comparably effective at reducing postprandial glycemic excursions in Chinese patients with type 2 diabetes as their initial therapy, possibly through different pathophysiological mechanisms [8].

A similar study was conducted by Abrahamian et al. [9] in 18 type 2 diabetes patients (7 treated with modified diet only and 11 with metformin monotherapy). The patients were given nateglinide, 120 mg orally TID before meals. Glycemic parameters, including 24-h MBG, FPG, and 2hPG obtained from CGM data, were significantly decreased. Nishimura et al. [10] conducted a randomized, double-blind clinical study to determine the efficacy of luseogliflozin (a selective inhibitor of sodium glucose cotransporter 2 [SGLT-2]) in combination with a low-carbohydrate diet on 24-h glucose variability assessed by CGM in 18 type 2 diabetes patients. The results revealed that luseogliflozin could significantly improve glycemic variability. Marfella et al. [11] used CGM to assess the effects of the dipeptidyl peptidase-4 (DPP-4) inhibitors

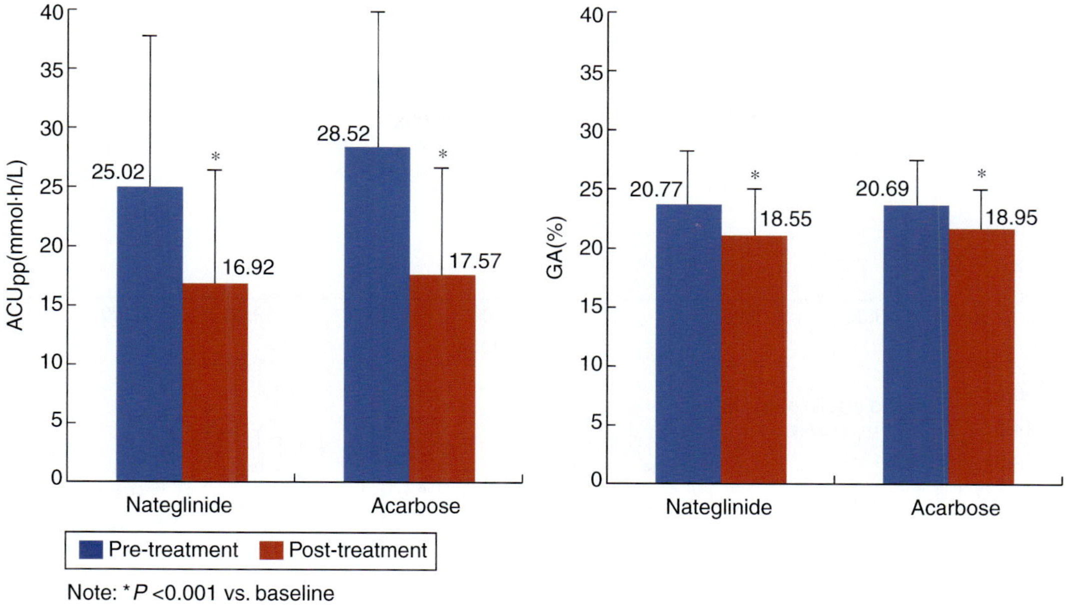

Fig. 12.4 Comparison of AUCpp and GA before and after treatment with nateglinide ($n = 51$) or acarbose ($n = 52$) [8] (Reprint with permission from *Diabetes Technology & Therapeutics*). Note: $*P < 0.001$ vs. baseline

sitagliptin and vildagliptin on glycemic variability. A total of 38 patients with type 2 diabetes mellitus were treated with metformin plus sitagliptin 100 mg daily or vildagliptin 50 mg BID over a period of 3 months. The results showed a larger decrease in MAGE in the vildagliptin group as compared with the sitagliptin group. The above studies suggest that CGM, as an effective means for assessing glycemic variability, plays an important role in assessments of the efficacy of oral hypoglycemic agents.

12.3 Evaluation of the Efficacy of Combined Oral Hypoglycemic Agents and Insulin with CGM

We conducted a multicenter, randomized, open-label, parallel clinical trial to compare the efficacy of combination therapy of basal insulin and oral hypoglycemic agents versus twice-daily premixed insulin monotherapy in Chinese type 2 diabetes patients by using CGM. The study enrolled 105 type 2 diabetes patients in whom blood glucose was insufficiently controlled by oral antidiabetic agents [FPG $\geq$7.0 mmol/L and 7.5% (58 mmol/mol) < HbA_{1c} $\leq$10% (86 mmol/mol)] from eight hospitals in China, and they were randomized at a ratio of 1:1 with the treatment group for combination therapy (once-daily insulin glargine plus gliclazide modified-release) or monotherapy (twice-daily premixed insulin) for 12 weeks. The results showed that the combination therapy could more stably decrease 24-h MBG, but there was no difference in the reduction of MAGE between the two groups [12] (Fig. 12.5).

In a similar study conducted by Wan et al. [13], 60 newly diagnosed type 2 diabetes were randomized into two groups and treated with CSII alone or with CSII plus sitagliptin. The latter group achieved a significant improvement in MAGE and SDBG through the analysis of CGM glucose profiles. A 26-week, randomized controlled clinical study included 102 participants on metformin and basal insulin [14]. The patients continued metformin and basal insulin and were randomized to

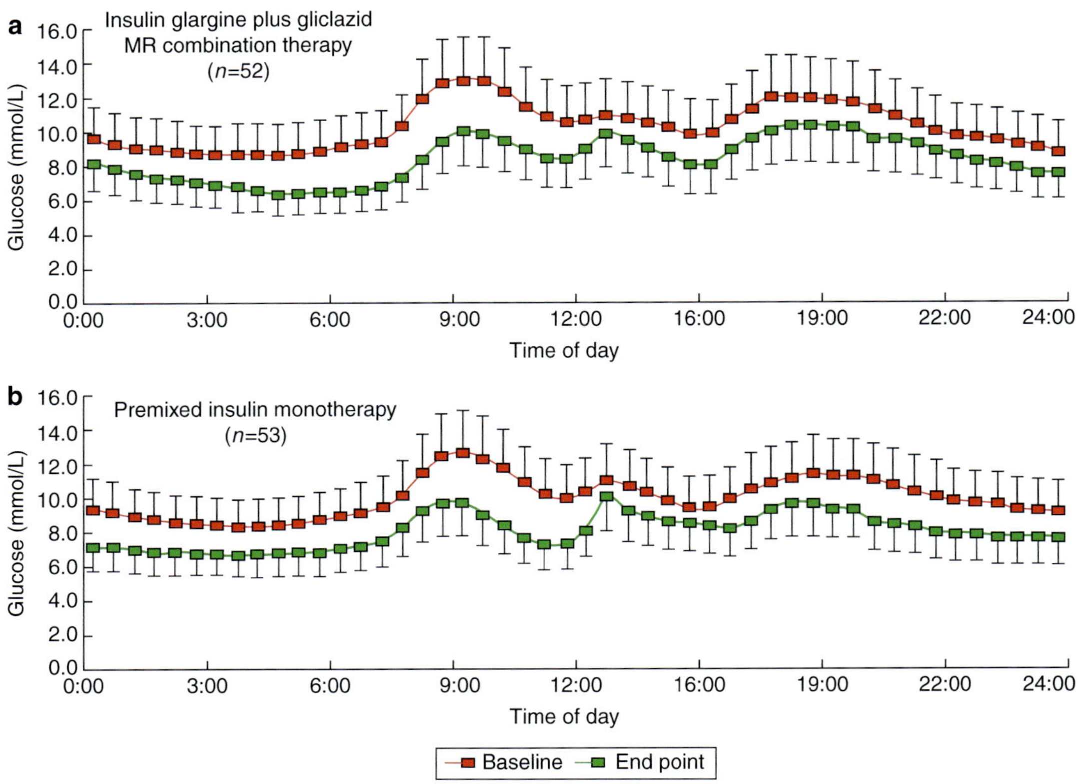

Fig. 12.5 The CGM glucose profiles after combination therapy with gliclazide modified-release tablets and basal insulin (**a**) or premixed insulin (**b**) of type 2 diabetes patients whose blood glucose was insufficiently controlled by oral hypoglycemic agents [12] (Reprint with permission from *Diabetes/Metabolism Research and Reviews*)

additional administration of exenatide twice daily or rapid-acting insulin analogs before meals. The primary endpoint of the study was the comparison of coefficient of variation (CV) calculated from CGM profiles after 26 weeks of treatment. The results revealed that exenatide significantly reduced CV while maintaining equivalent HbA_{1c} levels versus insulin therapy. Tanaka et al. [15] conducted a study in 26 type 2 diabetes patients who were treated with insulin therapy with or without additional administration of the DPP-4 inhibitor teneligliptin. CGM measurements were performed for 7 consecutive days. On days 1–3, patients received insulin with or without other antidiabetic drugs, and on days 4–7, teneligliptin 20 mg once daily was added to ongoing therapy. The results showed that addition of teneligliptin to insulin therapy led to significant improvements in 24-h MBG, MAGE, and postprandial 2-h area under the curve (AUC).

All clinical trials and studies illustrated above have suggested that CGM plays an important role in the evaluation of diabetes mellitus (Tables 12.1 and 12.2). With further advances in our understanding of glycemic variability, CGM will become an effective tool for assessing hypoglycemic efficacy, providing a basis for developing more optimized and effective antidiabetic therapies.

Table 12.1 Clinical trials evaluating hypoglycemic drugs by retrospective review of CGM data and conducted by Shanghai Clinical Center for Diabetes [16] (Reprint from *Journal of Diabetes Investigation*)

Year	Reference	Subjects	Inclusion criteria	Treatment duration	Intervention	Endpoint events
2008	Zhou et al. [1]	23 newly diagnosed type 2 diabetes mellitus	HbA_{1c} >8.5% (69 mmol/mol)	2–3 weeks	Daily multiple injections of insulin	MAGE, MODD, and AUCpp were significantly reduced after treatment
2010	Bao et al. [7]	40 newly diagnosed type 2 diabetes mellitus	HbA_{1c} 7.0–9.8% (53–84 mmol/mol)	8 weeks	Glipizide controlled-release tablets monotherapy vs. combination therapy of glipizide controlled-release tablets plus acarbose	The improvements in MBG, MAGE, MODD, and AUCpp were more significant in the combination therapy group than in the monotherapy group
2013	Zhou et al. [8]	103 type 2 diabetes patients who have not been previously treated with hypoglycemic agents	HbA_{1c} 6.5–9.0% (48–75 mmol/mol)	2 weeks	Nateglinide vs. acarbose	No significant differences in AUCpp, MAGE, SDBG, MODD, and 24-h MBG between the two groups
2015	Zhou et al. [12]	105 type 2 diabetes patients whose glucose was insufficiently controlled by oral hypoglycemic agents	HbA_{1c} 7.5–10% (58–86 mmol/mol)	12 weeks	Gliclazide modified-release tablets combined with basal insulin vs. premixed insulin	Both treatments could significantly improve the 24-h MBG, but no significant improvements in MAGE, SDBG, and MODD were found

Note: *MBG* mean blood glucose, *AUCpp* incremental areas above preprandial glucose values, *MAGE* mean amplitude of glycemic excursion, *MODD* mean of daily differences, *SDBG* standard deviations of blood glucose

Table 12.2 Clinical trials evaluating the effect of antidiabetic therapies by CGM

Year	Reference	Country	Patient type	N	Intervention	Primary endpoint
2012	Sakamoto et al. [17]	Japan	T2DM adults	20	DPPi	Glycemic variability
2015	Mianowska et al. [18]	Poland	Young children with T1DM	3	Insulin	Glycemic variability
2014	Ebrahim et al. [19]	Canada	Adolescent with exercise-induced hyperglycemia	1	None	Phenotype characterization
2014	Mohan et al. [20]	India	Overweight adults without diabetes	15	Diet	Glycemic variability
2014	Yates et al. [21]	Australia	Kidney transplant recipients	22	Steroid	Glycemic variability
2015	Didangelos et al. [22]	Greece	T2DM adults	14	Insulin	Glycemic variability
2013	Ando et al. [23]	Japan	T2DM adults	30	None	Glycemic variability

Statement on Consent for Participation

All the clinical trials carried out by the authors in this book have been reported to the Ethics Committee of Shanghai Jiao Tong University Affiliated Sixth People's Hospital already and were in accordance with the Good Clinical Practice and Standards of China Association for Ethical Studies (approval number: 2007-45).

References

1. Zhou J, Jia W, Bao Y, Ma X, Lu W, Li H, Hu C, Xiang K. Glycemic variability and its responses to intensive insulin treatment in newly diagnosed type 2 diabetes. Med Sci Monit. 2008;14:CR552–8.
2. Alemzadeh R, Palma-Sisto P, Holzum M, Parton E, Kicher J. Continuous subcutaneous insulin infusion attenuated glycemic instability in preschool children with type 1 diabetes mellitus. Diabetes Technol Ther. 2007;9:339–47. https://doi.org/10.1089/dia.2006.0038.
3. McNally PG, Dean JD, Morris AD, Wilkinson PD, Compion G, Heller SR. Using continuous glucose monitoring to measure the frequency of low glucose values when using biphasic insulin aspart 30 compared with biphasic human insulin 30: a double-blind crossover study in individuals with type 2 diabetes. Diabetes Care. 2007;30:1044–8. https://doi.org/10.2337/dc06-1328.
4. Jendle J, Testa MA, Martin S, Jiang H, Milicevic Z. Continuous glucose monitoring in patients with type 2 diabetes treated with glucagon-like peptide-1 receptor agonist dulaglutide in combination with prandial insulin lispro: an AWARD-4 substudy. Diabetes Obes Metab. 2016;18:999–1005. https://doi.org/10.1111/dom.12705.
5. Tosaka Y, Kanazawa A, Ikeda F, Iida M, Sato J, Matsumoto K, Uchida T, Tamura Y, Ogihara T, Mita T, Shimizu T, Goto H, Ohmura C, Fujitani Y, Watada H. Switching from twice-daily basal insulin injections to once-daily insulin degludec injection for basal-bolus insulin regimen in japanese patients with type 1 diabetes: a pilot study. Int J Endocrinol. 2015;2015:176261. https://doi.org/10.1155/2015/176261.
6. Ma Z, Chen R, Liu Y, Yu P, Chen L. Effect of liraglutide vs. NPH in combination with metformin on blood glucose fluctuations assessed using continuous glucose monitoring in patients with newly diagnosed type 2 diabetes. Int J Clin Pharmacol Ther. 2015;53:933–9. https://doi.org/10.5414/CP202415.
7. Bao YQ, Zhou J, Zhou M, Cheng YJ, Lu W, Pan XP, Tang JL, Lu HJ, Jia WP. Glipizide controlled-release tablets, with or without acarbose, improve glycaemic variability in newly diagnosed type 2 diabetes. Clin Exp Pharmacol Physiol. 2010;37:564–8. https://doi.org/10.1111/j.1440-1681.2010.05361.x.
8. Zhou J, Li H, Zhang X, Peng Y, Mo Y, Bao Y, Jia W. Nateglinide and acarbose are comparably effective reducers of postprandial glycemic excursions in chinese antihyperglycemic agent-naive subjects with type 2 diabetes. Diabetes Technol Ther. 2013;15:481–8. https://doi.org/10.1089/dia.2013.0046.
9. Abrahamian H, Francesconi M, Loiskandl A, Dzien A, Prager R, Weitgasser R. Evaluation of a new insulinotropic agent by using an innovative technology: efficacy and safety of nateglinide determined by continuous glucose monitoring. Diabetes Technol Ther. 2004;6:31–7. https://doi.org/10.1089/152091504322783387.
10. Nishimura R, Omiya H, Sugio K, Ubukata M, Sakai S, Samukawa Y. Sodium-glucose cotransporter 2 inhibitor luseogliflozin improves glycaemic control, assessed by continuous glucose monitoring, even on a low-carbohydrate diet. Diabetes Obes Metab. 2016;18:702–6. https://doi.org/10.1111/dom.12611.
11. Marfella R, Barbieri M, Grella R, Rizzo MR, Nicoletti GF, Paolisso G. Effects of vildagliptin twice daily vs. sitagliptin once daily on 24-hour acute glucose fluctuations. J Diabetes Complicat. 2010;24:79–83. https://doi.org/10.1016/j.jdiacomp.2009.01.004.
12. Zhou J, Zheng F, Guo X, Yang H, Zhang M, Tian H, Guo L, Li Q, Mo Y, Jia W. Glargine insulin/gliclazide MR combination therapy is more effective than premixed insulin monotherapy in Chinese patients with type 2 diabetes inadequately controlled on oral antidiabetic drugs. Diabetes Metab Res Rev. 2015;31:725–33. https://doi.org/10.1002/dmrr.2661.
13. Wan H, Zhao D, Shen J, Lu L, Zhang T, Chen Z. Comparison of the effects of continuous subcutaneous insulin infusion and add-on therapy with sitagliptin in patients with newly diagnosed type 2 diabetes mellitus. J Diabetes Res. 2016;2016:9849328. https://doi.org/10.1155/2016/9849328.
14. FLAT-SUGAR Trial Investigators. Glucose variability in a 26-week randomized comparison of mealtime treatment with rapid-acting insulin versus glp-1 agonist in participants with type 2 diabetes at high cardiovascular risk. Diabetes Care. 2016;39:973–81. https://doi.org/10.2337/dc15-2782.
15. Tanaka S, Suzuki K, Aoki C, Niitani M, Kato K, Tomotsune T, Aso Y. Add-on treatment with teneligliptin ameliorates glucose fluctuations and improves glycemic control index in Japanese patients with type 2 diabetes on insulin therapy. Diabetes Technol Ther. 2014;16:840–5. https://doi.org/10.1089/dia.2014.0095.
16. Jia W. Continuous glucose monitoring in China: then, now and in the future. J Diabetes Investig. 2017;8:3–5. https://doi.org/10.1111/jdi.12521.
17. Sakamoto M, Nishimura R, Irako T, Tsujino D, Ando K, Utsunomiya K. Comparison of vildagliptin twice daily vs. sitagliptin once daily using continuous glucose monitoring (CGM): crossover pilot study (J-VICTORIA study). Cardiovasc Diabetol. 2012;11:92. https://doi.org/10.1186/1475-2840-11-92.

18. Mianowska B, Fendler W, Tomasik B, Młynarski W, Szadkowska A. Effect of insulin dilution on lowering glycemic variability in pump-treated young children with inadequately controlled type 1 diabetes. Diabetes Technol Ther. 2015;17:605–10. https://doi.org/10.1089/dia.2014.0392.
19. Ebrahim MS, Lawson ML, Geraghty MT. A novel heterozygous mutation in the glucokinase gene conferring exercise-induced symptomatic hyperglycaemia responsive to sulfonylurea. Diabetes Metab. 2014;40:310–3. https://doi.org/10.1016/j.diabet.2013.12.012.
20. Mohan V, Spiegelman D, Sudha V, Gayathri R, Hong B, Praseena K, Anjana RM, Wedick NM, Arumugam K, Malik V, Ramachandran S, Bai MR, Henry JK, Hu FB, Willett W, Krishnaswamy K. Effect of brown rice, white rice, and brown rice with legumes on blood glucose and insulin responses in overweight Asian Indians: a randomized controlled trial. Diabetes Technol Ther. 2014;16:317–25. https://doi.org/10.1089/dia.2013.0259.
21. Yates CJ, Fourlanos S, Colman PG, Cohney SJ. Divided dosing reduces prednisolone-induced hyperglycaemia and glycaemic variability: a randomized trial after kidney transplantation. Nephrol Dial Transplant. 2014;29:698–705. https://doi.org/10.1093/ndt/gft377.
22. Didangelos T, Margaritidis C, Iliadis F, Hitoglou A, Makedou K, Savopoulos C, Hatzitolios A. Premix insulin analogs preserve good glycemic control in patients with type 2 diabetes previously treated with premix human insulin: a CGM study. In: Diabetes, vol. 64. Alexandria, VA: American Diabetes Association; 2015. p. A245.
23. Ando K, Nishimura R, Tsujino D, Seo C, Utsunomiya K. 24-hour glycemic variations in drug-naïve patients with type 2 diabetes: a continuous glucose monitoring (CGM)-based study. PLoS One. 2013;8:e71102. https://doi.org/10.1371/journal.pone.0071102.

13 Using Continuous Glucose Monitoring for Patients with Hypoglycemia

X. J. Ma and J. Zhou

Hypoglycemia remains to be a clinical challenge in diabetes management. In 2013, the American Diabetes Association (ADA) and the Endocrine Society recommended that hypoglycemia is diagnosed as blood glucose concentration of ≤3.9 mmol/L [1]. Hypoglycemia in diabetic patients can be classified into five categories as follows:

1. Severe hypoglycemia. Severe hypoglycemia is an event typically presenting with impairment of consciousness and neurological symptoms. The neurological recovery following the return of plasma glucose to normal is considered sufficient evidence that the event was induced by a low plasma glucose concentration.
2. Documented symptomatic hypoglycemia. Documented symptomatic hypoglycemia is an event during which typical symptoms of hypoglycemia are accompanied by a measured plasma glucose concentration of ≤3.9 mmol/L.
3. Asymptomatic hypoglycemia. Asymptomatic hypoglycemia is an event not accompanied by typical symptoms of hypoglycemia but with a blood glucose of ≤3.9 mmol/L.
4. Probable symptomatic hypoglycemia. Probable symptomatic hypoglycemia is an event when patients present with hypoglycemic symptoms but without blood glucose measurements.
5. Pseudo-hypoglycemia. Pseudo-hypoglycemia is an event when patients present with typical hypoglycemia symptoms but with blood glucose of >3.9 mmol/L.

In 2017, the ADA published updated criteria for the diagnosis and treatment of hypoglycemia [2]. The International Hypoglycemia Study group proposed the following classification: (1) Level 1 (glucose alert value), a glucose value of 3.9 mmol/L or less, which is sufficiently low for treatment with fast-acting carbohydrate and dose adjustment of glucose-lowering therapy; (2) Level 2 (clinically significant hypoglycemia), a glucose level of 3.0 mmol/L or less, which is sufficiently low to indicate serious, clinically important hypoglycemia; and (3) Level 3 (severe hypoglycemia), hypoglycemia associated with severe cognitive impairment requiring external assistance for recovery.

The Diabetes Control and Complications Trial (DCCT) study showed that intensive glycemic treatment can reduce the risk of long-term complications but also increase the incidence of hypoglycemia [3]. Hypoglycemia leads to hypoglycemic symptoms, cognitive dysfunction, and corresponding regulation of counterregulatory hormones [4]. Hypoglycemia is closely related to cognitive impairment among juvenile, middle-aged, and elderly diabetic patients, regardless of

X. J. Ma · J. Zhou (✉)
Department of Endocrinology and Metabolism, Shanghai Clinical Center for Diabetes, Shanghai Diabetes Institute, Shanghai Jiao Tong University Affiliated Sixth People's Hospital, Shanghai, China
e-mail: zhoujian@sjtu.edu.cn

W. Jia (ed.), *Continuous Glucose Monitoring*, https://doi.org/10.1007/978-981-10-7074-7_13

patients' age. In addition, hypoglycemia can also lead to behavioral abnormalities, such as psychosensorial symptoms [5], fear of hypoglycemia [6, 7], depressive symptoms [8], impaired exercise capacity [9], motor function deficit [10], and some other disorders. All these are major challenges for the achievement of target glycemic control.

Moreover, hypoglycemia can cause fatal outcomes such as dead-in-bed syndrome. Tanenberg et al. [11] reported a case of sudden death due to hypoglycemia confirmed by continuous glucose monitoring (CGM): a 23-year-old type 1 diabetic patient treated with insulin pump suffered from sudden death during sleep. The CGM showed that the patient had a linear drop in blood glucose at midnight after injection of insulin, and his blood glucose was <1.7 mmol/L (31 mg/dL) at death. This is the first case with CGM-based evidence showing that hypoglycemia caused dead-in-bed syndrome. Dead-in-bed syndrome refers to unexpected sudden death of young people with type 1 diabetes. The mechanism is complicated and may be associated with recurrent episodes of severe hypoglycemia. Repeated hypoglycemia can cause hemorrhage of brain tissues at the early stage, followed by cellular swelling and focal tissue necrosis caused by sodium and potassium ions transferring into cells, and ultimately leads to neuronal necrosis and brain death. Additionally, severe hypoglycemia can also induce cardiac electrophysiological disorder that results in sudden death [12].

CGM can provide continuous, comprehensive, and reliable blood glucose information and facilitate early detection and evaluation of hypoglycemia, providing guidance for the treatment for hypoglycemia.

13.1 Clinical Application of Retrospective CGM in Diabetic Hypoglycemia

Retrospective CGM can be used for early monitoring of hypoglycemia incidents and describing the characteristics of hypoglycemia in diabetic patients. Here we present two examples: Fig. 13.1 is a CGM profile showing a hypoglycemia episode before lunch of a type 1 diabetes patient

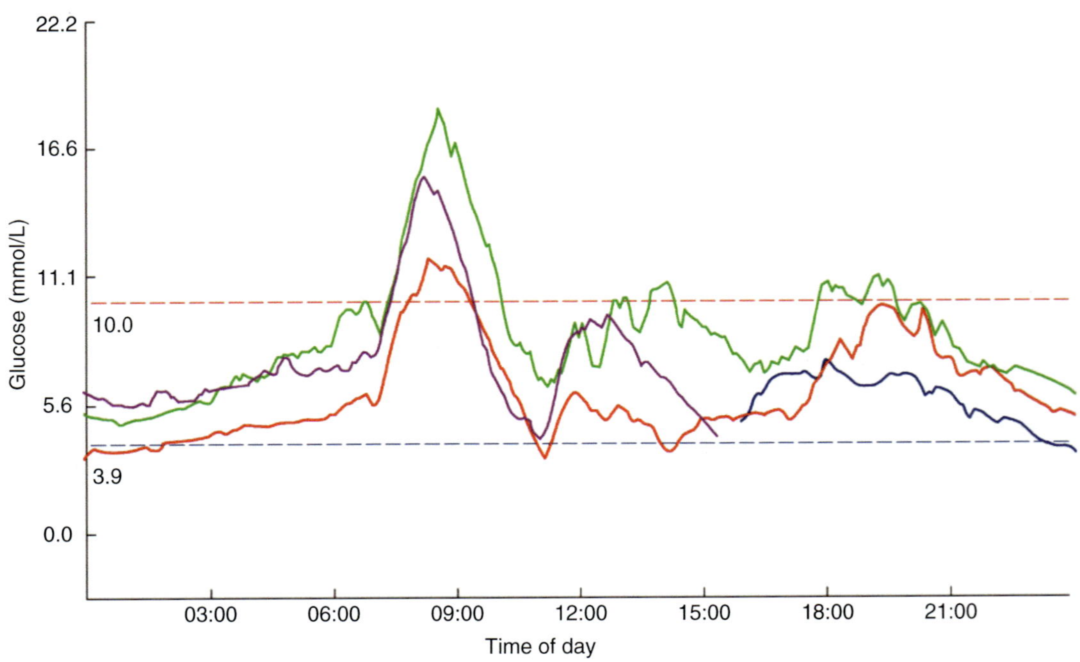

Fig. 13.1 The CGM profiles of one type 1 diabetes patient treated with subcutaneous premixed insulin 30R BID daily

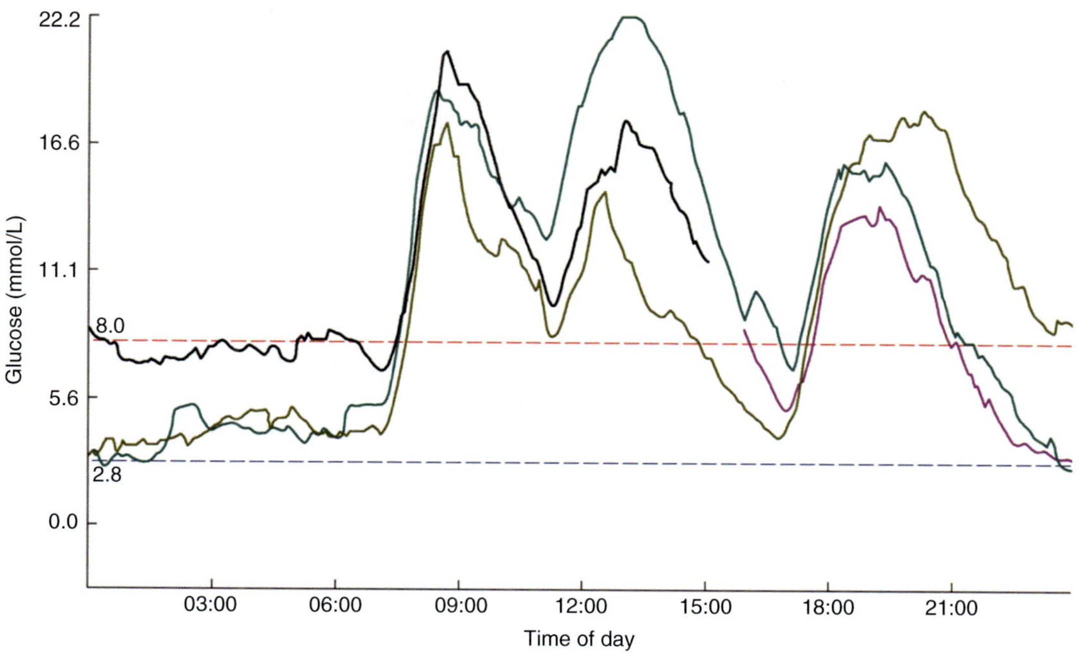

Fig. 13.2 The CGM profiles of one type 1 diabetes patient treated with subcutaneous short-acting insulin TID daily

treated with subcutaneous premixed insulin 30R (BID, 20 U before breakfast and 16 U before dinner). Figure 13.2 is a CGM profile showing hypoglycemia episodes before dinner and during nighttime of a type 1 diabetic patient treated with subcutaneous short-acting insulin (TID, 5 U, 3 U, and 3 U before meals).

Previously, we reviewed the CGM data of 61 hospitalized, elderly patients with type 2 diabetes who were treated with insulin pump for a short period of time. Patients were divided into hypoglycemic group and non-hypoglycemic group, according to the incidence of hypoglycemic events from the CGM results on the third and fourth days. The results showed that about 1/3 of patients experienced hypoglycemia during initial use with an insulin pump, and CGM achieved a significantly higher rate of hypoglycemia detection than self-monitoring of blood glucose (SMBG) [13]. In addition, Maia et al. [14] analyzed retrospective CGM data of 17 children with type 1 diabetes and found that 56.2% of patients had asymptomatic hypoglycemia, with sensitivity of 63.3% and specificity of 96.6% for the detection of hypoglycemia by CGM. Therefore, retrospective CGM has more advantages in early detection of hypoglycemia in adult type 2 diabetes patients as well as asymptomatic hypoglycemia in children with type 1 diabetes with low sensitivity but high specificity compared to SMBG.

Moreover, application of retrospective CGM can provide information for adjusting treatment of diabetic patients and facilitate understanding of glucose fluctuations patterns. In 2010, we reviewed the CGM data from 257 adult type 2 diabetes patients treated with insulin pump and analyzed the relationship between bedtime blood glucose and the presence of nocturnal hypoglycemic events. Patients were divided into a hypoglycemic group and a non-hypoglycemic group according to the occurrence of nocturnal hypoglycemia. The study showed large glycemic variability when insulin pump was initiated and an increased risk of nocturnal hypoglycemia when bedtime blood glucose was <5.9 mmol/L [15]. Similarly, Wentholt et al. [16] applied retrospective CGM in type 1 diabetes who were treated with an insulin pump (n = 24) and subcutaneous insulin injections (n = 33). The results demonstrated that CGM enabled more precise detection of nocturnal hypoglycemia frequency and duration in type 1 diabetic patients, and the frequency and duration of nocturnal hypoglycemia were closely associated with bedtime glucose concentration. It is feasible to apply CGM at the early stage of intensive insulin therapy in adult diabetic patients so that the dose of insulin or diet can be adjusted timely, thus achieving safe and effective therapy regimen by preventing hypoglycemia, especially nocturnal hypoglycemia.

13.2 Clinical Application of Real-Time CGM in Diabetic Hypoglycemia

Real-time CGM provides glucose values that allow for early detection of hypoglycemia and immediate therapeutic adjustments, thus promoting patients' behavior improvement and significantly reducing the duration of hypoglycemia. Pettus et al. [17] surveyed 222 type 1 diabetes patients who used real-time CGM and found that when the CGM device showed two arrows down ("↓↓" glucose decreasing >0.11 mmol/L per min), 42% of the respondents would reduce their insulin dosage to prevent hypoglycemia. With a glucose value of 6.7 mmol/L and a falling glucose trend, 70% of respondents would intake carbohydrates to avoid hypoglycemia. Additional studies are needed to determine insulin adjustments based on glucose trend data.

In the study conducted by Peyser et al. [18], CGM values were compared with Yellow Springs Instrument (YSI) analyzer measurements in 51 diabetes patients. The results showed that when the CGM hypoglycemic alert value was set at 4.4 mmol/L, the device could provide warnings for 95% of asymptomatic hypoglycemia episodes about 10 min in advance. Therefore, real-time CGM plays an important role in early detection of hypoglycemia, especially asymptomatic hypoglycemia, thus preventing the onset of cognitive impairment via a timely warning of hypoglycemia. Battelino et al. [19] conducted a clinical study in 120 type 1 diabetic patients on intensive therapy who were randomly assigned to a control group with both SMBG and retrospective CGM performed every other week for 5 days or to a group with real-time CGM. The primary outcome was the time spent in hypoglycemia over a period of 26 weeks. The results showed that the use of real-time CGM was associated with significantly less time spent with hypoglycemia for children and adults with type 1 diabetes on intensive therapy compared to SMBG.

In addition, studies have suggested that age is an important factor that involved in the hypoglycemia improvement when using CGM among type 1 diabetes patients. In the study conducted by the Juvenile Diabetes Research Foundation (JDRF) CGM Study Group [20], 322 adults and children with type 1 diabetes were randomly assigned to a group with CGM or to a control group with SMBG according to age. The results showed that compared to SMBG, CGM was associated with better glycemic control without increasing risk of asymptomatic hypoglycemia among patients aged 25 years old or older, but not in patients aged 8–14 years old and 15–24 years old. This may be related to more frequent use of CGM and better ability to manage hypoglycemia in adult type 1 diabetes patients.

As mentioned above, CGM is useful in monitoring hypoglycemia incidents and enables practitioners to analyze glucose characteristics and to guide the individualized treatment. A practical example described below illustrates the utilization of CGM in the management of severe hypoglycemia in patients with type 1 diabetes [21].

Example case: A 16-year-old female patient was diagnosed with type 1 diabetes 3 years ago. Twelve days prior to admission, she experienced hypoglycemic coma, with a glycated hemoglobin A_{1c} (HbA_{1c}) of 13.9% (128 mmol/mol). The patient was treated with subcutaneous short-acting insulin (10 U, 4 U, and 6 U at 30 min before meals) and subcutaneous intermediate-acting insulin (1 U at 10:00 p.m.). The patient had a body mass index (BMI) of 22.96 kg/m^2 and a waist circumference of 93 cm. Results of complete blood count tests, liver and kidney function, electrolytes, and blood lipids were all within the normal reference ranges. The patient had a strong positive urine glucose (++++) and glycated albumin (GA) of 35.2% (reference range 11.0–17.0%). Fasting and postprandial 2-h serum C peptide levels were 0.66 ng/ml and 1.47 ng/ml, respectively (reference range, fasting state, 0.82–2.50 ng/ml). The glutamic acid decarboxylase antibody (GAD-Ab) was positive, and islet cell antibody and insulin autoantibody (IAA) were negative.

After admission, the patient was equipped with a retrospective CGM system for 72-h blood glucose monitoring, and hypoglycemic regimens were adjusted based on the CGM results.

1. On the day of admission, the patient was given a subcutaneous short-acting insulin injection (8 U, 12 U at 30 min before lunch and dinner) and subcutaneous Humulin N (8 U at 10:00 p.m.). The CGM showed large glycemic fluctuations. The percentage of time (PT) spent with glucose <2.8 mmol/L was 4% (20 min), and the PT spent with glucose >7.8 mmol/L was 67% (320 min). The blood glucose levels gradually dropped from 7:23 p.m., until reaching 2.8 mmol/L at 11:38 p.m., lasted until 01:03 a.m. on the next day (Fig. 13.3a).
2. On the second day, the hypoglycemic regimen was adjusted to subcutaneous Humulin R

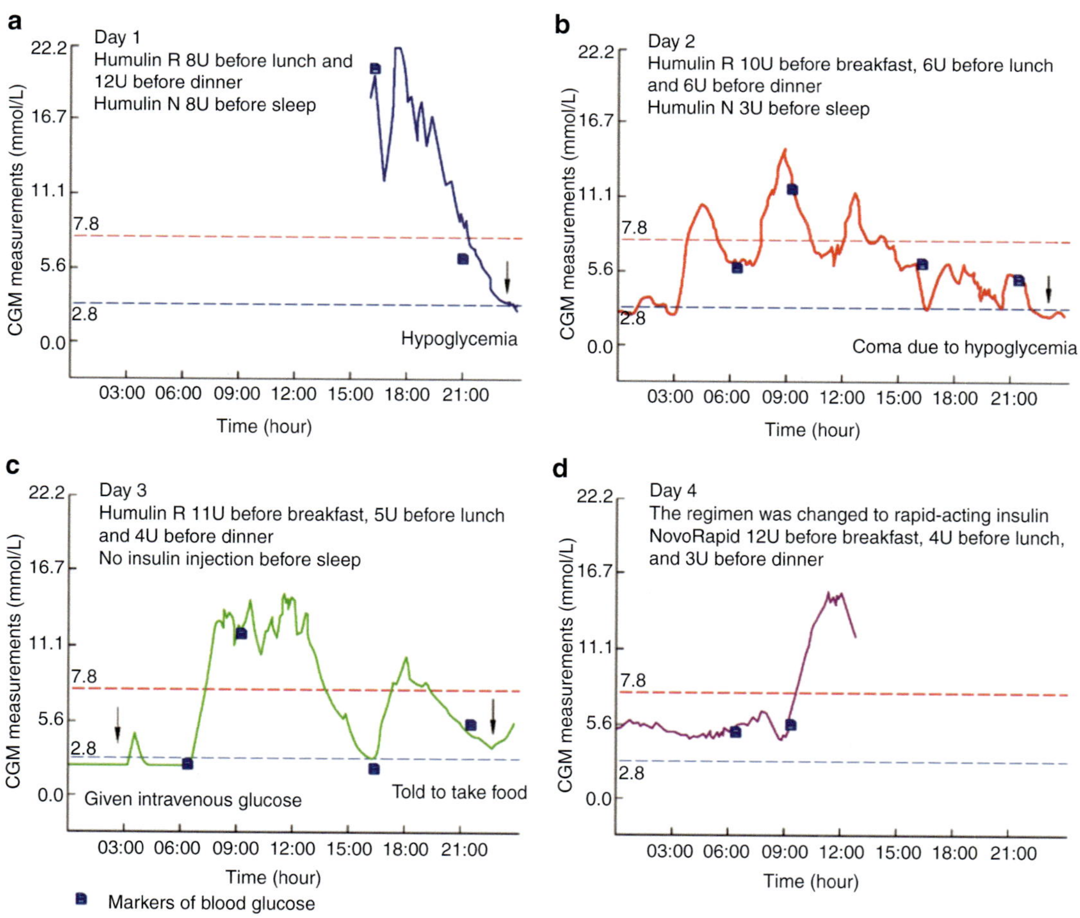

Fig. 13.3 The CGM profiles of one type 1 diabetes patient with concomitant secondary adrenocortical insufficiency and resultant recurrent, severe hypoglycemia [21] (Reprint with permission from Shanghai Medical Journal)

(10 U, 6 U, and 6 U before meals) and subcutaneous intermediate-acting insulin (3 U at 10:00 p.m.). The patient continued to experience recurrent hypoglycemic episodes during the dinner-to-bedtime period, and the PT spent with glucose <2.8 mmol/L was 16% (230 min; Fig. 13.3b).

3. On the third day, the patient was found unconscious at 3:00 a.m., with a blood glucose level of 1.6 mmol/L, and was diagnosed with hypoglycemic coma. She recovered after intravenous infusion of glucose. Her blood pressure was 96/74 mmHg, and her heart rate was 91 beats/min at that time. CGM showed that the hypoglycemia (blood glucose < 2.8 mmol/L) lasted up to 310 min (from Day 2 at 10:08 p.m. to Day 3 at 3:18 a.m.). Thus, the bedtime insulin was discontinued from Day 3. In addition, the patient also experienced a 25-min asymptomatic hypoglycemic event before dinner. The PT spent with glucose <2.8 mmol/L was 26% (380 min; Fig. 13.3c).
4. On the fourth day, the hypoglycemic regimen was adjusted to subcutaneous rapid-acting insulin NovoRapid (12 U, 4 U, and 3 U at 5 min before meals). No hypoglycemia occurred on that day (Fig. 13.3d).
5. The patient had no hypoglycemic event until the seventh day when she experienced nocturnal hypoglycemia again, with blood glucose of 2.6 mmol/L at 3:00 a.m. Thus, the insulin was discontinued and changed to metformin 250 mg with dinner. Subsequently, the patient underwent relevant examinations to further clarify the causes of the hypoglycemia. No abnormalities were detected in the adrenal gland computed tomography (CT) scan or pituitary magnetic resonance imaging (MRI) examination. Repeated measures of sex hormones, growth hormone, cortisol, and adrenocorticotropic hormone (cortisol and adrenocorticotropic hormone (ACTH), at 8:00 a.m., 4:00 p.m., and 12:00 a.m.) and 24-h urinary cortisol were tested. The last menstrual period of the patient was February 16, 2011. The sex hormone tests showed that the follicle-stimulating hormone concentration was 3.34 IU/L (reference range, 5.0–20.9 IU/L); the luteinizing hormone concentration was 4.1 IU/L (reference range, 18.1–90.2 IU/L); the progesterone concentration was 0.1 μg/L (reference range, 1.2–15.9 μg/L); the testosterone level was 1.28 μg/L (reference range, 0.1–1.1 μg/L); the dehydroepiandrosterone concentration was 172.5 μg/dL (reference range, 8.6–169.8 μg/dL); and the growth hormone levels were within normal ranges. The cortisol levels were 0.68 μg/dL and 0.69 μg/dL in the early mornings on March 2, 2011, and March 6, 2011, when hypoglycemic events occurred, and the corresponding ACTH were 4.23 ng/L and 6.22 ng/L (reference range, 7.20–63.30 ng/L), respectively. The cortisol levels were 10.23 μg/dL and 13.53 μg/dL at 8:00 a.m. on March 2, 2011, and March 6, 2011, respectively (reference range, 4.30–22.4 μg/dL), and the corresponding ACTH concentrations were 17.29 ng/L and 43.65 ng/L, respectively (reference range, 7.20–63.30 ng/L). The cortisol level was 2.92 μg/dL at 4:00 p.m. (reference range, 3.09–16.70 μg/dL), and the corresponding ACTH was 14.82 ng/L (reference range, 7.20–63.30 ng/L). The 24-h urinary cortisol was 202.24 μg and 190.60 μg (reference range, 28.5–214.0 μg per 24 h), respectively. Taking these results together, the patient was considered to have recurrent, persistent nocturnal hypoglycemia concomitant with secondary adrenocortical insufficiency (Fig. 13.4). Since the patient had insufficient secretion of cortisol and ACTH in response to hypoglycemia, the patient was treated with prednisone 2.5 mg at bedtime on the 11th day. There has been no recurrence of hypoglycemia since then.
6. Summary: The CGM data revealed recurrent, persistent episodes of severe hypoglycemia that were difficult to detect by other blood glucose monitoring methods and were likely to cause unpredictable serious outcomes for the patient. In this case, the hypoglycemic regimen was adjusted based on the CGM data, and the concomitant disease that exacerbated hypoglycemia was diagnosed.

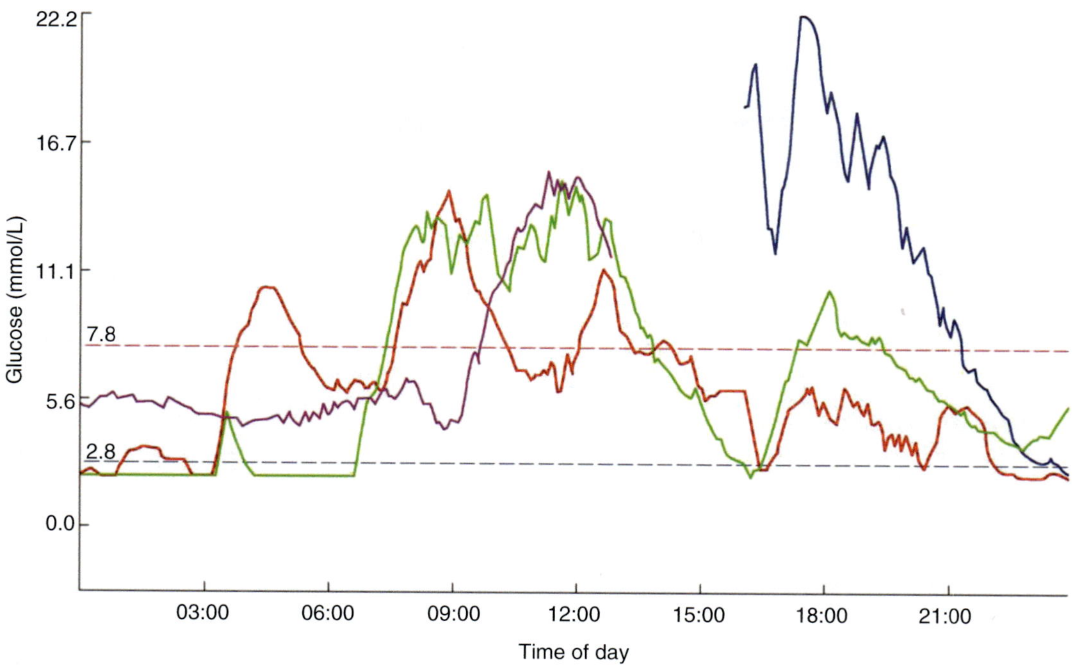

Fig. 13.4 The CGM profiles of one type 1 diabetic patient with concomitant secondary adrenocortical insufficiency and recurrent, severe hypoglycemia [21]

Statement on Consent for Participation

All the clinical trials carried out by the authors in this book have been reported to the Ethics Committee of Shanghai Jiao Tong University Affiliated Sixth People's Hospital already and were in accordance with the Good Clinical Practice and Standards of China Association for Ethical Studies (approval number: 2007-45).

References

1. Seaquist ER, Anderson J, Childs B, Cryer P, Dagogo-Jack S, Fish L, Heller SR, Rodriguez H, Rosenzweig J, Vigersky R. Hypoglycemia and diabetes: a report of a workgroup of the American Diabetes Association and the Endocrine Society. Diabetes Care. 2013;36:1384–95. https://doi.org/10.2337/dc12-2480.
2. American Diabetes Association. 6. Glycemic targets. Diabetes Care. 2017;40(Suppl 1):48–56. https://doi.org/10.2337/dc17-S009.
3. The Diabetes Control and Complications (DCCT) Research Group. Effect of intensive therapy on the development and progression of dibetic nephropathy in the Diabetes Control and Complications Trial. Kidney Int. 1995;47:1703–20.
4. Warren RE, Frier BM. Hypoglycaemia and cognitive function. Diabetes Obes Metab. 2005;7:493–503. https://doi.org/10.1111/j.1463-1326.2004.00421.x.
5. Law JR, Yeşiltepe-Mutlu G, Helms S, Meyer E, Özsu E, Çizmecioğlu F, Lin FC, Hatun Ş, Calikoglu AS. Adolescents with Type 1 diabetes mellitus experience psychosensorial symptoms during hypoglycaemia. Diabet Med. 2014;31:1245–51. https://doi.org/10.1111/dme.12533.
6. Hendrieckx C, Halliday JA, Bowden JP, Colman PG, Cohen N, Jenkins A, Speight J. Severe hypoglycaemia and its association with psychological well-being in Australian adults with type 1 diabetes attending specialist tertiary clinics. Diabetes Res Clin Pract. 2014;103:430–6. https://doi.org/10.1016/j.diabres.2013.12.005.
7. Nefs G, Bevelander S, Hendrieckx C, Bot M, Ruige J, Speight J, Pouwer F. Fear of hypoglycaemia in adults with Type 1 diabetes: results from Diabetes MILES - The Netherlands. Diabet Med. 2015;32:1289–96. https://doi.org/10.1111/dme.12739.
8. Kikuchi Y, Iwase M, Fujii H, Ohkuma T, Kaizu S, Ide H, Jodai T, Idewaki Y, Nakamura U, Kitazono T. Association of severe hypoglycemia with depressive symptoms in patients with type 2 diabetes: the Fukuoka Diabetes Registry. BMJ Open Diabetes Res Care. 2015;3:e000063. https://doi.org/10.1136/bmjdrc-2014-000063.
9. Kelly D, Hamilton JK, Riddell MC. Blood glucose levels and performance in a sports cAMP for adolescents with type 1 diabetes mellitus: a field

study. Int J Pediatr. 2010;2010:216167. https://doi.org/10.1155/2010/216167.
10. Sherin A, Peeyush KT, Naijil G, Chinthu R, Paulose CS. Hypoglycemia induced behavioural deficit and decreased GABA receptor, CREB expression in the cerebellum of streptozoticin induced diabetic rats. Brain Res Bull. 2010;83:360–6. https://doi.org/10.1016/j.brainresbull.2010.09.004.
11. Tanenberg RJ, Newton CA, Drake AJ. Confirmation of hypoglycemia in the "dead-in-bed syndrome", as captured by a retrospective glucose monitoring system. Endocr Pract. 2010;16:244–8. https://doi.org/10.4158/EP09260.CR.
12. Mo YF, Zhou J, Jia WP. Research progress of dead-in-bed syndrome in type 1 diabetes. Chin J Endocrinol Metab. 2011;27:1032–5. https://doi.org/10.3760/cma.j.issn.1000-6699.2011.12.018.
13. Li M, Zhou J, Bao YQ, Lu W, Jia WP, Xiang KS. Evaluating the feature of hypoglycemia detected by continuous glucose monitoring system during temporary continuous subcutaneous insulin infusion in type 2 diabetes patients. Zhonghua Yi Xue Za Zhi. 2008;88:1679–82. https://doi.org/10.3321/j.issn:0376-2491.2008.24.008.
14. Maia FF, Araújo LR. Efficacy of continuous glucose monitoring system to detect unrecognized hypoglycemia in children and adolescents with type 1 diabetes. Arq Bras Endocrinol Metabol. 2005;49:569–74.
15. Li M, Zhou J, Bao YQ, Lu W, Jia WP. Prediction of nocturnal hypoglycaemia with bedtime glucose level during continuous subcutaneous insulin infusion in type 2 diabetics. Zhonghua Yi Xue Za Zhi. 2010;90:2962–6. https://doi.org/10.3760/cma.j.issn.0376-2491.2010.42.005.
16. Wentholt IM, Maran A, Masurel N, Heine RJ, Hoekstra JB, DeVries JH. Nocturnal hypoglycaemia in Type 1 diabetic patients, assessed with continuous glucose monitoring: frequency, duration and associations. Diabet Med. 2007;24:527–32. https://doi.org/10.1111/j.1464-5491.2007.02107.x.
17. Pettus J, Price DA, Edelman SV. How patients with type 1 diabetes translate continuous glucose monitoring data into diabetes management decisions. Endocr Pract. 2015;21:613–20. https://doi.org/10.4158/EP14520.OR.
18. Peyser TA, Nakamura K, Price D, Bohnett LC, Hirsch IB, Balo A. Hypoglycemic accuracy and improved low glucose alerts of the latest Dexcom G4 Platinum continuous glucose monitoring system. Diabetes Technol Ther. 2015;17:548–54. https://doi.org/10.1089/dia.2014.0415.
19. Battelino T, Phillip M, Bratina N, Nimri R, Oskarsson P, Bolinder J. Effect of continuous glucose monitoring on hypoglycemia in type 1 diabetes. Diabetes Care. 2011;34:795–800. https://doi.org/10.2337/dc10-1989.
20. Juvenile Diabetes Research Foundation Continuous Glucose Monitoring Study Group, Tamborlane WV, Beck RW, Bode BW, Buckingham B, Chase HP, Clemons R, Fiallo-Scharer R, Fox LA, Gilliam LK, Hirsch IB, Huang ES, Kollman C, Kowalski AJ, Laffel L, Lawrence JM, Lee J, Mauras N, O'Grady M, Ruedy KJ, Tansey M, Tsalikian E, Weinzimer S, Wilson DM, Wolpert H, Wysocki T, Xing D. Continuous glucose monitoring and intensive treatment of type 1 diabetes. N Engl J Med. 2008;359:1464–76. https://doi.org/10.1056/NEJMoa0805017.
21. Mo YF, Zhou J, Bao YQ, Gao F, Lu W, Jia WP. A case of repeated severe hypoglycemia caused by type 1 diabetes complicated with secondary adrenal insufficiency. Shanghai Med J. 2013;36:474–6.

Using Continuous Glucose Monitoring for Patients with Fasting Hyperglycemia

14

J. Zhou

The dawn phenomenon and Somogyi effect are two important causes of fasting hyperglycemia. With the application of continuous glucose monitoring (CGM) technology, it is possible to explore the mechanisms and clinical features of the dawn phenomenon and Somogyi effect, which greatly improves the accurate understanding and management of the two phenomena and facilitates stable control of overall blood glucose level in patients with diabetes mellitus.

14.1 Definitions and Epidemiological Characteristics of the Dawn Phenomenon and Somogyi Effect

14.1.1 Definition

The concept of the dawn phenomenon was first put forward by Schmidt et al. [1] in 1981, when the authors observed an abnormal rise in glucose concentration at early morning and after breakfast in patients with type 1 diabetes and called it the "dawn phenomenon." In 1984, Bolli et al. [2] also reported this phenomenon in type 2 diabetes patients. Since then, the dawn phenomenon has gradually attracted the attention of researchers. The characteristics and definitions of the dawn phenomenon have been further elaborated. The current definition of the dawn phenomenon is the need for more insulin dosage to prevent a spontaneous rise in blood glucose levels in the predawn and dawn in patients with good glycemic control at nighttime without hypoglycemic events. In recent years, the utilization of CGM clinically has been shown to facilitate the detection of the dawn phenomenon and promote an in-depth understanding of the dawn phenomenon as well. At present, the scope of the dawn phenomenon includes hyperglycemia from early morning to before breakfast, and an abnormally high postprandial glucose excursion after breakfast is commonly referred to as the extended dawn phenomenon [3–5].

Somogyi effect is a rebound hyperglycemia episode following a nocturnal hypoglycemia episode as a result of excessive insulin during the nighttime. In 1959, the scientist Somogyi first proposed the concept that "hypoglycemia induced by excessive insulin dose can lead to rebound hyperglycemia" in his paper and put forward the hypothesis that "this rebound hyperglycemia is due to the regulation by hypothalamus-pituitary-adrenal axis" [6]. Subsequent studies have confirmed the existence of Somogyi effect [7–9], but at the same time, many scholars still have a skeptical attitude toward this phenomenon [10, 11]. Although both the dawn phenomenon and Somogyi effect are manifested as hyperglycemia

J. Zhou
Department of Endocrinology and Metabolism, Shanghai Clinical Center for Diabetes, Shanghai Diabetes Institute, Shanghai Jiao Tong University Affiliated Sixth People's Hospital, Shanghai, China
e-mail: zhoujian@sjtu.edu.cn

W. Jia (ed.), *Continuous Glucose Monitoring*, https://doi.org/10.1007/978-981-10-7074-7_14

Table 14.1 Comparison of the dawn phenomenon and the Somogyi effect [4] (Reprinted from Endokrynologia Polska)

Features	The dawn phenomenon	The Somogyi effect
Definition	Recurring early morning hyperglycemia	Early morning hyperglycemia due to treatment with excessive amount of exogenous insulin
Cause	Decrease of insulin secretion between 03:00 a.m. and 05:00 a.m. and increase of insulin-antagonistic hormones	Nocturnal hypoglycemia due to excessive dose of insulin and hyperglycemia the next early morning due to increase of insulin-antagonistic hormones
Occurrence	Type 1 diabetes Type 2 diabetes with no insulin therapy	Type 1 diabetes Type 2 diabetes with insulin therapy
Incidence	Type 1 diabetic children—27.4%; Type 1 diabetic adults—24.1%; Type 2 diabetic adults—3%; Type 1 diabetes generally—54%; Type 2 diabetes generally—55%	Type 1 and 2 diabetic patients—12.6–67.0%; Type 1 diabetic patients—18%
Diagnosis	Measurement of the plasma glucose concentration between 03:00 a.m. and 05:00 a.m. for next several nights CGM Confirmative result: high/normal plasma glucose level	Measurement of the plasma glucose concentration between 03:00 a.m. and 05:00 a.m. for next several nights CGM Confirmative result: low plasma glucose level
Prevention/treatment	Increase evening physical activity Increase protein-to-carbohydrate ratio in the last meal of the day Eat breakfast as usual even though the dawn phenomenon is presented Individual diet modification only if $HbA_{1c} < 7.0\%$ (53 mmol/mol) Antidiabetic oral agent therapy only if $HbA_{1c} < 7.0\%$ (53 mmol/mol) Long-acting insulin analogs like glargine insulin Use an insulin pump	Modify insulin dosage More protein than carbohydrates in the last meal of the day Go to bed with higher level of plasma glucose than usual Long-acting insulin analogs like glargine insulin Use an insulin pump

in early morning, they differ completely from their pathogenesis to treatment. Thus, it is important to accurately identify and distinguish them (Table 14.1).

14.1.2 Epidemiological Characteristics

The exact incidences of the two phenomena are not yet clear. The incidence of Somogyi effect varies widely among studies, as previous studies have reported an incidence of approximately 12.6% in diabetic patients [12], but some scholars believe that this percentage is likely much higher up to 67% [13]. Another report suggests an incidence of Somogyi effect is about 18% in type 1 diabetes [4].

The reported incidence for the dawn phenomenon ranges from 3 to 55%, with estimated incidences of 24.1% and 27.4% in adults and children with type 1 diabetes, respectively [12, 14]. Another study showed an overall incidence of the dawn phenomenon as high as 55% in type 1 diabetes patients and as high as 54% in type 2 diabetes [15]. Generally, the common understanding on the incidence of both phenomena includes (1) the dawn phenomenon is more common than Somogyi effect; (2) compared with adult diabetes, children with type 1 diabetes are more susceptible to the dawn phenomenon [4].

14.2 Pathogenesis of the Dawn Phenomenon and Somogyi Effect

14.2.1 Pathogenesis of the Dawn Phenomenon

The pathophysiological mechanisms of the dawn phenomenon are complex and not yet clear. It is believed that the dawn phenomenon is the result of decline in β-cell function, followed by increased endogenous glucose production and sustained insulin resistance in the early morning. In the early morning, the increase in insulin-antagonistic hormones such as growth hormone leads to impairment of the signal transduction of insulin system and enhanced lipolysis and further exaggerates insulin resistance and promotes endogenous glucose production (hepatic glycogenolysis, gluconeogenesis, etc.). With a weakened effect of insulin on peripheral tissues, especially at 08:00 a.m. when insulin sensitivity is the lowest through a day [16], together the above factors eventually trigger a dawn phenomenon. The mechanisms may involve the following aspects:

14.2.1.1 Growth Hormone

The role of growth hormone in the pathogenesis of insulin resistance has been widely studied [17]. Growth hormone is considered as the primary factor contributing to the dawn phenomenon in type 1 diabetes, and in type 2 diabetes, and it is the cause only secondary to insulin resistance contributing to the dawn phenomenon. In healthy individuals, growth hormone appears to be secreted in large amounts during slow-wave sleep and peaks from 12:00 a.m. to 2:00 a.m. However, it is known that growth hormone administration leads to substantial impairment of both hepatic and peripheral insulin sensitivity after a latency period of approximately 4 h in a healthy individual (from 04:00 a.m. to 06:00 a.m.) [15]. In 2013, Shih et al. [18] found an elevated blood glucose concentration, increased free fatty acid concentration, and decreased metabolic clearance rate of insulin (reflecting insulin sensitivity) at 16 h after treatment with exogenous growth hormone in 15 type 2 diabetes patients, and this effect was weakened by the growth hormone antagonist octreotide. It is currently considered that growth hormone may lead to insulin resistance through the following pathways:

1. Impairment of the signal transduction system: growth hormone and insulin mediate intracellular glucose and lipid metabolism through a critical, common signal transduction pathway, that is, the insulin receptor substrate 1 (IRS-1)-phosphatidylinositol 3-kinase (PI-3 K) signaling pathway. Activation of the IRS-1/PI-3 K pathway activates their downstream protein kinase B to initiate a cascade of phosphorylation reactions that lead to cellular events such as activation of glycogen synthase and promotion of glucose transporter 4 (GLUT4) expression [19].
2. Enhanced lipolysis: in fasting state, growth hormone stimulates lipid oxidation and decomposition and then leads to intracellular accumulation of lipid metabolites, which competitively inhibit glucose uptake and glycogen synthesis.
3. Insulin-like growth factor (IGF) and insulin-like growth factor-binding protein (IGFBP): in 2010, Yagasaki et al. [20] found that IGFBP-1 also plays an important role in the occurrence of the dawn phenomenon. The authors divided 48 patients with type 1 diabetes into three treatment groups. The plasma glucose, IGFBP-1, and free IGF-1 levels of the patients were measured. The results showed that the serum IGFBP-1 levels were markedly increased at breakfast, and free IGF-1 levels were inversely decreased ($P < 0.05$) in patients with poor glycemic control who experienced the dawn phenomenon. In contrast, for those with good glycemic control, the serum IGFBP-1 levels remained stable in the morning. Therefore, the increase in circulating IGFBP-1 in the morning due to the waning of insulin action could be another mechanism behind the dawn phenomenon. The increase of IGBP-1 leads to reduced free IGF-1 levels and increases the growth hormone levels and may finally cause decreased insulin sensitivity and the dawn phenomenon.

14.2.1.2 Circadian Rhythm of Insulin Sensitivity

The dawn phenomenon is related to the circadian rhythm of insulin sensitivity in diabetic patients, with the lowest insulin sensitivity typically occurring at eight o'clock in the morning [4, 21, 22]. Endogenous glucose production also changes with circadian rhythmicity, reaching a peak in the early morning and dropping to a valley after noon.

Diabetic patients have peak endogenous glucose 30–50% greater than that of the healthy individuals, resulting in elevated blood glucose levels [23].

14.2.1.3 Fibroblast Growth Factor 21 (FGF-21)

In 2011, Chen et al. [24] found that growth hormone-induced lipolysis was enhanced in FGF-21 knockout mice. FGF-21 interacts with growth hormone through the hypothalamus-pituitary-adrenal axis to regulate lipolysis and promote fasting gluconeogenesis. In the human body, circulating FGF-21 levels begin to rise at midnight, reach a peak in the early morning, and then decline to basal concentrations early in the afternoon. The circulating FGF-21 levels display a circadian rhythm and resemble the oscillation of free fatty acids [25]. In conclusion, FGF-21 plays a regulatory role in growth hormone-induced dawn phenomenon.

14.2.1.4 Others

1. The effects of other insulin-antagonistic hormones such as glucagon, catecholamine, and cortisol might be involved. Carroll et al. [15] found an elevation of insulin-antagonistic hormones such as glucagon, catecholamine, and cortisol between 12:00 a.m. and 08:00 a.m., with the increases in glucagon and cortisol being the most dramatic [4].
2. Dietary factors include dinner intake (amount and time) of previous day or snacking at bedtime.
3. Treatment: inadequate use of oral hypoglycemic agents or insulin in the prevention of nocturnal hypoglycemia of previous day.

14.2.2 Pathogenesis of Somogyi Effect

The pathogenesis of Somogyi effect is mainly related to the body's negative feedback mechanisms. During a hypoglycemic event, the central nervous system is stimulated to send signals to mobilize the body to produce a series of responses against hypoglycemia, mainly through the following two pathways: (1) a direct hyperglycemic effect and (2) stimulation of the secretion of hyperglycemic hormone to antagonize the action of insulin and promote the ability of sympathetic nerve and adrenaline on the mobilization of stored energy. Hypoglycemia and the resultant excitation of the sympathetic system and increase in the plasma catecholamine levels can all inhibit the secretion of insulin, resulting in low insulinemia. Moreover, excitation of the sympathetic system and an increased plasma catecholamine level can promote the secretion of glucagon, thus increasing glycogen decomposition and gluconeogenesis. In hypoglycemic events, an inadequate supply of glucose can cause excitation of the sympathetic system with increased secretion of adrenocortical hormones, promoting the elevation of the cortisol level. Growth hormone secretion is also increased, which can inhibit the utilization of glucose in muscle tissue and directly promote the decomposition of lipid in adipose tissues.

14.3 Utilization of CGM for the Dawn Phenomenon and Somogyi Effect

14.3.1 Utilization of CGM for Distinguishing the Dawn Phenomenon and Somogyi Effect

Previously, the distinction between the dawn phenomenon and Somogyi effect was made mainly based on multiple blood glucose measurements at 03:00 a.m. to 05:00 a.m., especially in type 1 diabetes patients [12]. If the glucose levels were consistently low during this period, the Somogyi effect was probably the cause; if it was normal or elevated, the dawn phenomenon was more likely the reason. The dawn phenomenon is quantified by the absolute increase in glucose from nocturnal nadir to pre-breakfast value [∂ glucose (∂G)], which is commonly defined as a rise in plasma glucose levels $\partial G > 0.56$ mmol/L (10 mg/dL) between 05:00 a.m. and 09:00 a.m. (every half hour), occurring after a growth hormone surge of ≥ 5 μg/L. In recent years, blood glucose excursion after breakfast, which is regarded as an extended dawn phenomenon, has also attracted more attention. The abnormal increase in blood glucose concentration after breakfast is considered as an obstacle to achieving stable glycemic control throughout the day. In 2002, Monnier et al. [21] measured the levels of blood glucose and insulin at four time points, namely, pre-breakfast (08:00 a.m.), at the postprandial state (11:00 a.m., 02:00 p.m.), and at the postabsorptive state (05:00 p.m.), and found that the blood glucose level at 11:00 a.m. was significantly higher than those at other time points. However, a certain cutoff point for identifying Somogyi effect has not yet been identified. Cryer, an American researcher, believed that the nocturnal glucose nadir relating to the Somogyi effect is probably between 3.8 mmol/L (which may cause the secretion of insulin-antagonistic hormones such as growth hormone, glucagon, epinephrine, and cortisol) and 3.0 mmol/L (which may cause hypoglycemic symptoms) [26].

In recent years, the application of CGM technology has allowed for visual observation of the circadian changes in blood glucose concentrations and for differentiation of the dawn phenomenon and Somogyi effect (Fig. 14.1). CGM techniques can be used to identify nocturnal hypoglycemia and the Somogyi effects that cannot be detected by glucose concentrations measured in venous blood samples [27, 28]. Schaepelynck-Bélicar et al. [28] observed the CGM data of 12 patients with poorly controlled type 1 diabetes. Prolonged overnight hyperglycemia was observed in five patients, the dawn phenomenon in four patients, and nighttime hypoglycemia in four patients. These data revealed that CGM enables the analysis of various glucose patterns from nighttime to early morning in these patients.

The ∂G value can be easily and accurately obtained by CGM for quantifying the dawn phenomenon. If nocturnal glucose readings at any time points are greater than that before breakfast, $\partial G = 0$, the dawn phenomenon is excluded. Currently, the dawn phenomenon is quantified by an absolute increase $\partial G > 0.56$ mmol/L (10 mg/dL) or by an absolute increase $\partial G > 1.11$ mmol/L (20 mg/dL) or a relative increase ($\partial G\%$) >6.9% [3]. In 2013, Monnier et al. [5] found that $\partial G > 1.11$ mmol/L (20 mg/dL) was the best cutoff value for quantifying in the application of CGM. The median of ∂G value and the median of inter-day difference from nocturnal glucose nadir to pre-breakfast glucose value among the 248 participants were 0.89 mmol/L and 0.83 mmol/L, respectively.

14.3.2 Utilization of CGM for Evaluation of the Dawn Phenomenon and Somogyi Effect

CGM technology improves the detection of asymptomatic nocturnal hypoglycemia and the Somogyi effect through whole-day glucose profiles. However, there are some doubts about the existence of Somogyi effect. Guillod et al. [29] and Høi-Hansen et al. [30] suggested that nocturnal hypoglycemia is a common phenomenon in type 1 diabetes patients based on an analysis of CGM data and that nocturnal hypoglycemia is not directly related to fasting hyperglycemia. On the contrary, nocturnal hypoglycemia is more likely to trigger morning hypoglycemia. Choudhary et al. [31] analyzed the CGM data of 89 patients with type 1 diabetes. They found that 94% of patients with fasting fingertip blood glucose <5 mmol/L had nocturnal hypoglycemia (defined as glucose <3.5 mmol/L), and only two subjects experienced a rebound elevation in fasting plasma glucose (FPG) after nocturnal hypoglycemia.

The existence and influence of the dawn phenomenon are well known. CGM technology promotes a better understanding of the characteristics of the extended dawn phenomenon. In 2005, Colette et al. [32] applied CGM in 14 type 2 diabetes on short-term calorie-restricted diet. They found that the daytime glucose peaked at 120 ± 24 min after breakfast, and there was no significant difference before and after calorie-restricted dieting. The study also found that, during periods of poor insulin sensitivity, a calorie-restricted diet failed to improve the

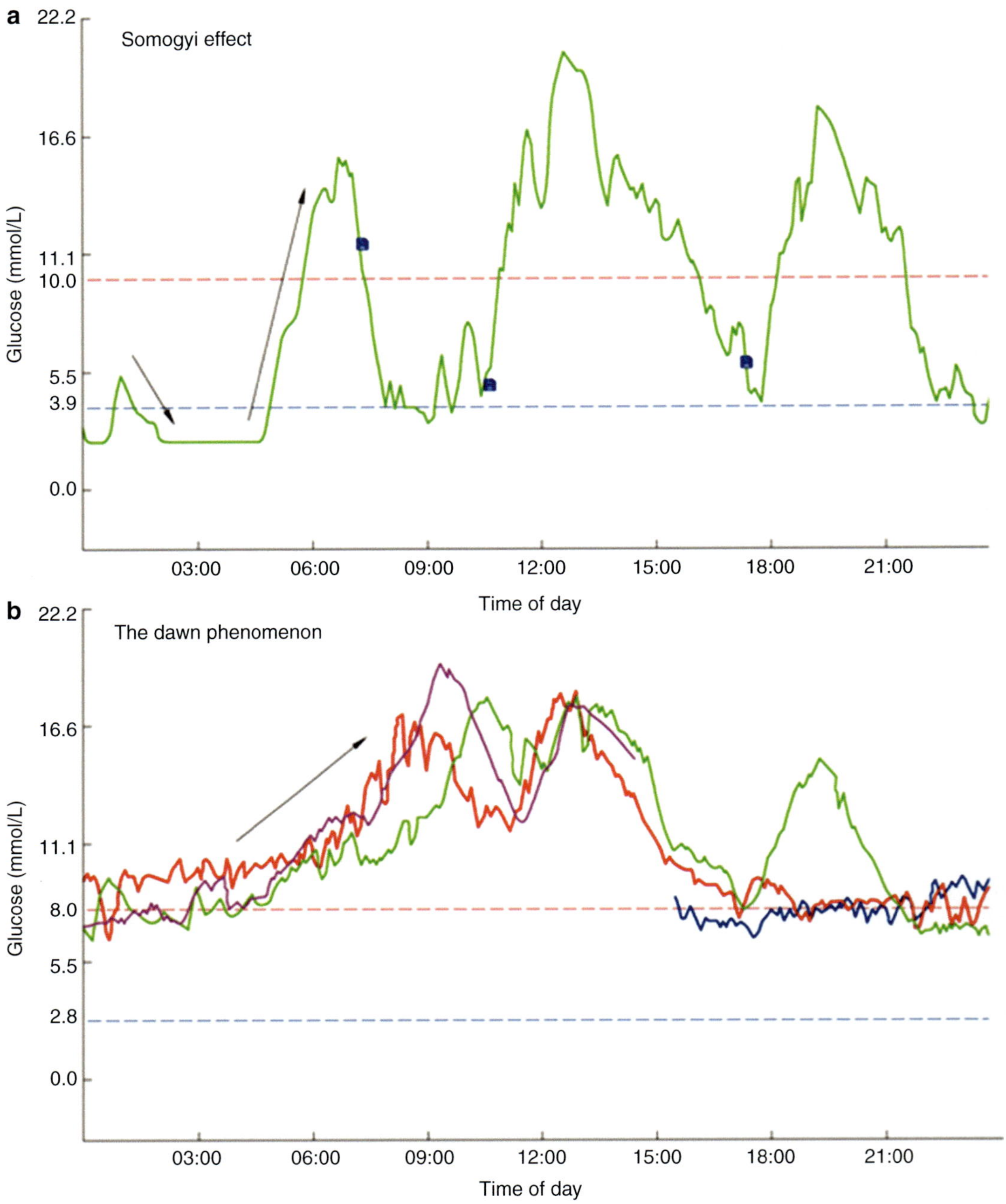

Fig. 14.1 CGM profiles showing the Somogyi effect (**a**) and dawn phenomenon (**b**)

postprandial blood glucose fluctuations, and post-breakfast was considered as the period least sensitive to caloric restriction therapy. In our previous study, 69 newly diagnosed type 2 diabetes patients and 48 normal subjects were monitored using the CGM system. The results showed that among normal subjects, the area under the curve (AUC), glucose peak value, and glucose peak time were not significantly different after meals. In type 2 diabetes, postprandial glucose fluctuations were most prominent following breakfast and less evident during lunch and dinner. The

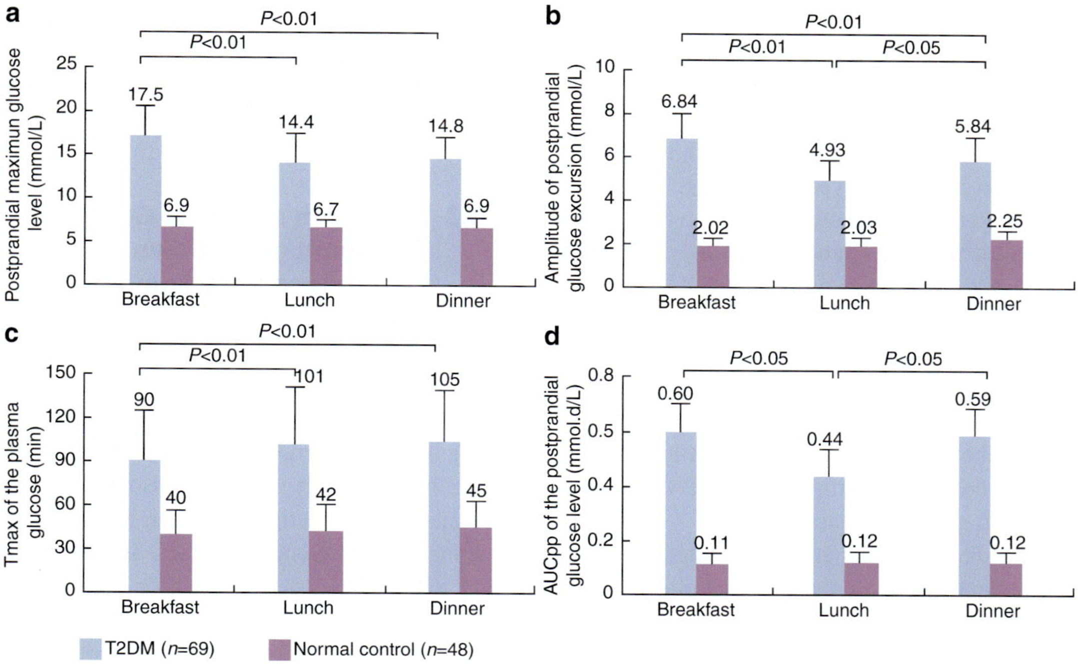

Fig. 14.2 The characteristics of postprandial glucose fluctuation of type 2 diabetes patients [33, 34] (Reprinted from Medical Science Monitor and reprinted with permission from National Medical Journal of China)

peak intraday glucose values occurred at 90 ± 37 min after breakfast, with a significantly shorter peak time than those after lunch and dinner. In addition, the peak blood glucose value after breakfast was significantly higher than those after lunch and dinner [33] (Fig. 14.2).

In 2013, Monnier et al. [5] applied CGM in 248 non-insulin-treated patients with type 2 diabetes and found that the median magnitude of the dawn glucose increase was 0.89 mmol/L and the postprandial glucose after breakfast was higher than those after lunch and dinner, emphasizing that the abnormal hyperglycemia caused by the dawn phenomenon also influences postprandial glucose after breakfast to a great extent (also called "extended dawn phenomenon").

The magnitude of the dawn phenomenon is affected by the course of diabetes, glycemic control, and insulin sensitivity. In the study conducted by Perriello et al. [27], 114 type 1 diabetes patients were given insulin infusion, and the increased magnitude of the dawn phenomenon was associated with a short duration of diabetes, poor glycemic control, increased hepatic glucose production, and reduced peripheral glucose utilization. In addition, seven patients with poor glycemic control were selected. After 5–9 months of intensive insulin therapy, glycated hemoglobin A_{1c} (HbA_{1c}) decreased from 12.4% (112 mmol/mol) to 7.9% (63 mmol/mol) after treatment, and the magnitude of the dawn phenomenon was also decreased (evaluated by % increase between morning and nocturnal insulin requirements, 24% before treatment and 18% after treatment, $P < 0.05$). For another six poorly controlled patients without intensive insulin therapy, HbA_{1c} remained unchanged, so did the magnitude of the dawn phenomenon, during an observation period of 6–8 months. For five cases with intensive insulin therapy, the HbA_{1c} increased from 7.9% (63 mmol/mol) to 9.1% (76 mmol/mol) by 2 weeks after discontinuation of intensive treatment, and the magnitude of the dawn was also increased. These findings fully explain an intricate link between glycemic control and the magnitude of the dawn phenomenon. A similar conclusion was reached in a study of patients with type 2 diabetes. A comparison was made between morning glucose levels in seven patients with poorly controlled diabetes [HbA_{1c} 11.2% (99 mmol/mol), five type 2 and two type 1 diabetes] and levels in seven patients with well-controlled diabetes [HbA_{1c} 7.6% (60 mmol/mol), five type 2 and two type 1 diabetes]. The mean plasma glucose concentrations in the two groups increased from 6.1 mmol/L and 4.4 mmol/L at 03:00 a.m. to 12.2 mmol/L and 5.7 mmol/L at 08:00 a.m., respectively. Patients with poorly controlled diabetes exhibited a significant dawn increment in glucose levels as compared with patients with well-controlled diabetes, irrespective of the type of diabetes, suggesting that the magnitude of the dawn glucose rise was associated with glycemic control [35].

The dawn phenomenon and extended dawn phenomenon have a greater impact on blood glucose level than Somogyi effect. In the study performed by Monnier et al. [5], diabetic patients were divided into two groups based on the presence/absence of a dawn phenomenon (defined as $\partial G > 1.11$ mmol/L). This study was the first to investigate the impact of the magnitude of the dawn phenomenon and extended dawn phenomenon on HbA_{1c} and 24-h mean glucose in type 2 diabetes. The comparison between paired subsets of subjects for the nocturnal glucose nadir showed that the change caused by the dawn phenomenon was 0.67 mmol/L (12 mg/dL) in the mean glucose concentration and 0.4% (4 mmol/mol) in HbA_{1c}, which could not be eliminated by antidiabetic agents. These findings were consistent with the relationship previously established by the A1c-Derived Average Glucose study (an increment of 1.6 mmol/L in mean glucose concentration corresponds to a 1% increment in HbA_{1c}) [36]. As another study illustrated, the deterioration of glucose homeostasis in individuals with type 2 diabetes progresses from postprandial to fasting hyperglycemia, and the dawn phenomenon state and extended dawn phenomenon are intermediate steps during the progression [37]. The morning glucose levels (pre-breakfast to 3 h after breakfast) have been found to differ significantly (7.5 mmol/L and 9.3 mmol/L, $P < 0.01$) between subjects with HbA_{1c} 6.5–6.9% (48–52 mmol/mol) and 7.0–7.9% (53–63 mmol/mol), suggesting that the elimination of the dawn phenomenon facilitates achievement of target glycemic control [$HbA_{1c} < 7.0\%$ (53 mmol/mol)] for patients with $HbA_{1c} < 8.0\%$ (64 mmol/mol).

14.3.3 Utilization of CGM to Guide Treatment of the Dawn Phenomenon and Somogyi Effect

Application of CGM in diabetes can facilitate an improvement in glycemic control not only by preventing the dawn phenomenon and the occurrence of nocturnal hypoglycemia but also via timely adjustment of the treatment regimen for the dawn phenomenon and Somogyi effect. In the study conducted by Schaepelynck-Bélicar et al. [28], insulin treatment was adjusted based on CGM measurements in 12 adolescents with poorly controlled type 1 diabetes. The incidence of the dawn phenomenon reduced from four episodes in two patients to one episode in one patient. The mean HbA_{1c} decreased from 10.3 ± 2.1% (89 ± 23 mmol/mol) to 8.8 ± 1.1% (73 ± 12 mmol/mol). For Somogyi effect, it is important to prevent or reduce nocturnal hypoglycemia. CGM has been reported to reduce the risk of nocturnal hypoglycemia in 75% of patients [29]. CGM provides accurate data for the formulation of hypoglycemic regimen and significantly improves glycemic management. Through 24-h continuous monitoring, the CGM directly reflects the glycemic characteristics of each patient and facilitates the personalized selection of rational targeted therapies.

14.4 Principles for the Treatment of the Somogyi Effect and Dawn Phenomenon

Since the Somogyi effect is mainly due to the use of excess insulin, adjustment of insulin dose and type is first considered, e.g., replacing the neutral protamine Hagedorn (NPH) with long-acting insulin analogs (glargine or detemir insulin, etc.) [38, 39]. As an intermediate-acting insulin, NPH starts working 30–60 min after injection, peaks

4–5 h after injection, and lasts 10–16 h. The onset of action of insulin glargine is a little later than insulin NPH (1–2 h after injection), but its duration of action is 24 h. Insulin glargine or detemir acts relatively constant with no pronounced peak, which significantly reduces the risk of hypoglycemia and improves the dawn phenomenon and Somogyi effect. An insulin pump is also an effective measure to reduce the risk of nocturnal hypoglycemia. Somogyi effect may be prevented by increasing the protein-to-carbohydrate ratio in the last meal of the day, and a patient should go to bed with a reasonably high level of plasma glucose.

The essential rule for the treatment of the dawn phenomenon is to restore the normal balance of hormone in the body. Another therapeutic option is the selection of suitable hypoglycemic agents to control the morning hyperglycemia. Although some oral antidiabetic agents can improve the dawn phenomenon to varying degrees, effective control of the dawn phenomenon depends on an increase in insulin requirements at dawn. Thus, basal insulin is an optimal choice. The specific treatments are introduced as follows:

14.4.1 Basic Treatment

When $HbA_{1c} < 7.0\%$ (53 mmol/mol), the dawn phenomenon is generally manageable with diet and exercise therapy or combined with oral hypoglycemic agents. The dawn phenomenon may be prevented by increasing evening physical activity, increasing the protein-to-carbohydrate ratio in the last meal of the day, and eating breakfast as usual. These measures help to decrease the secretion of insulin-antagonistic hormones. In some cases, the mild dawn phenomenon can be controlled by the basic treatment combined with oral hypoglycemic agents [40].

14.4.2 Oral Hypoglycemic Agents

Low-dose metformin is usually used to treat the dawn phenomenon. However, it is currently believed that none of the oral hypoglycemic agents, either alone or in combination, can fully manage the dawn phenomenon. Especially, sulfonylureas are not recommended due to their potential side effect of nocturnal hypoglycemia [5].

Other medications that control the dawn phenomenon include cyproheptadine, which acts on the anterior pituitary gland to inhibit the secretion of growth hormone and adrenocorticotropic hormone (ACTH) through potent inhibitory effects against histamine and 5-hydroxytryptamine [41]. Suppression of cortisol secretion using metyrapone may also decrease the magnitude of the dawn phenomenon. In addition, administration of somatostatin can reduce FPG levels in type 1 and type 2 diabetes and resultantly decreases the magnitude of the dawn phenomenon in type 1 diabetes. However, some patients are not sensitive to this treatment. This is because somatostatin inhibits the secretion of not only glucagon and growth hormone but also insulin as well. Given that long-term inhibition of nocturnal growth hormone secretion may handicap the physical growth and development of diabetic children and adolescents, it should be used with caution clinically. The novel growth hormone antagonist pegvisomant overcomes the undesirable side effect of decreased glucose tolerance in conventional growth hormone inhibitors and provides a new direction for the treatment of the dawn phenomenon.

14.4.3 Insulin Therapy

Insulin should be first considered for the control of the dawn phenomenon, especially for those with $HbA_{1c} > 7.0\%$ (53 mmol/mol). The latest study confirms that even in patients with $HbA_{1c} < 7.0\%$ (53 mmol/mol), basal insulin therapy can reduce nocturnal hyperglycemia and the dawn phenomenon, facilitating achievement of HbA_{1c} under 7.0% (53 mmol/mol) [42, 43]. At present, the following insulin regimens are commonly used for the control of the dawn phenomenon.

14.4.3.1 Long-Acting Insulin Analog at Bedtime

Compared with NPH, long-acting insulin analogs have the advantages of no significant absorption peak, lower risk of nocturnal hypoglycemia, and longer duration of action. Pistrosch et al. [44] found that 36-week treatment with long-acting insulin analog at bedtime resulted in a more pronounced reduction in FPG as compared with oral administration with metformin at bedtime (Δ: 3.1 ± 2.5 mmol/L vs. 1.4 ± 1.5 mmol/L; $P < 0.001$). Both insulin glargine and detemir are basal insulin analogs. Patients treated with insulin glargine and detemir of the same dose achieve similar glycemic control with similar all-day blood glucose spectrum. Therefore, insulin glargine and detemir are capable of regulating the blood glucose level in similar ways [45, 46]. However, there is a lower glucose variability and less weight gain with insulin detemir versus insulin glargine [47, 48]. Tone et al. [39] found that insulin detemir versus glargine could reduce the frequency of hypoglycemia in type 1 diabetes, but not type 2 diabetic patients.

Moreover, some of the emerging drugs also provide new possibilities for the control of the dawn phenomenon. Insulin degludec (IDeg) is a new basal insulin that is ultralong-acting, which improves glycemic control to a similar degree to insulin glargine but confers lower risks of overall and nocturnal hypoglycemia [49]. In fact, the day-to-day variability in the glucose-lowering effect of IDeg is less than that for glargine, so the effect of IDeg is more predictable. The safe, predictable, and flexible profile of IDeg may be an advantage in the management of fasting hyperglycemia and nocturnal hypoglycemia [50]. Furthermore, the previous study reported that basal insulin regime changing from Lantus to Toujeo resulted in fewer hypoglycemic episodes and glucose fluctuations [51].

14.4.3.2 Insulin Pump

The insulin pump has a unique advantage in controlling nighttime and dawn blood glucose fluctuations, precisely modeling insulin secretion patterns of β-cells by adjustment of pump settings (basal rate, bolus dose). In the study conducted by Yagasaki et al. [20], the use of the insulin pump led to improved glycemic control from 03:00 a.m. to 07:00 a.m. and increased circulating IGFBP-1, showing the suppression of the dawn phenomenon. Papargyri et al. [52] reported their experience with the use of continuous subcutaneous insulin infusion (CSII) in 112 type 1 diabetes patients followed up for 7 years. They found that HbA_{1c} was reduced by 0.7–0.9% (8–10 mmol/mol) in the first 3 years, and 21% of patients had asymptomatic nocturnal hypoglycemia. The frequency of hypoglycemia decreased with the prolongation of treatment time, confirming the safety of insulin pump therapy. However, Bouchonville et al. [53] put forward the notion that the dawn phenomenon occurs unpredictably; therefore, programming of the insulin pump for an early morning increase in insulin delivery is ineffective for both the frequency and magnitude of the dawn phenomenon and may cause an increased risk of hypoglycemia. This defect can be avoided when applying an insulin pump with a threshold-suspend function and closed-loop insulin delivery system.

The latest study using CGM compared the efficacy of three insulin regimens, NPH (0.22 ± 0.03 U/kg), CSII (infusion of basal insulin as rapid-acting analog at single rate 0.7 ± 0.1 U/h), or long-acting insulin analogs (0.25 ± 0.02 U/kg). The results showed that bedtime NPH resulted in a magnitude of dawn phenomenon of 3.06 mmol/L, whereas CSII at single rate partly prevented the dawn phenomenon with magnitude of 0.94 mmol/L and long-acting insulin glargine eliminated the dawn phenomenon ($\partial G = 0$) [42]. Additionally, eight diabetic patients with HbA_{1c} of 6.89 ± 0.05% (52 ± 1 mmol/mol) were treated with evening dose of insulin glargine (0.25 ± 0.02 U/kg) as add-on to metformin. After 6 months of treatment, the dawn phenomenon was basically eliminated with a decrease in the magnitude of 1.00 mmol/L; the removal of the dawn phenomenon resulted in a decrease in HbA_{1c} to 6.5 ± 0.1% (mean decrease of 0.39%) (48 ± 1 mmol/mol), which validated the estimated contribution of the dawn phenomenon to the 0.4% (4 mmol/mol) increase in HbA_{1c} calculated by Monnier et al. [5].

Overall, the use of long-acting insulin at a reasonable time is the most convenient and practical measure for the control of the dawn phenomenon and Somogyi effect: at 06:00 a.m. to 09:00 a.m. for reducing the risk of nocturnal hypoglycemia and improving the Somogyi effect and at 06:00 p.m. to 09:00 p.m. for preventing the dawn phenomenon.

Recently, the US Food and Drug Administration (FDA) has approved the MiniMed 670G (Medtronic), a hybrid closed-loop insulin delivery system for use in patients ≥14 years old with type 1 diabetes [54]. The system uses an algorithm to automatically adjust basal insulin doses based on readings from a CGM. The new device appears to have the potential to keep blood glucose levels more stable and to improve the control of the dawn phenomenon.

14.5 Summary and Outlook

The dawn phenomenon and Somogyi effect have negative effects on the overall glycemic control of patients that cannot be ignored. The extensive application of CGM not only promotes an in-depth understanding of the dawn phenomenon and Somogyi effect but also facilitates clinical identification of the two phenomena and thus improves morning glycemic control. In the future, it is necessary to further investigate their pathophysiological mechanisms, for example, the role of novel cytokines involved in particular so as to find potential targets for intervention. Also, large-scale, multicenter studies utilizing CGM technology are needed to determine the criteria for identifying the dawn phenomenon and Somogyi effect and hence further improve clinical diagnosis and treatment of these conditions.

Statement on Consent for Participation

All the clinical trials carried out by the authors in this book have been reported to the Ethics Committee of Shanghai Jiao Tong University Affiliated Sixth People's Hospital already and were in accordance with the Good Clinical Practice and Standards of China Association for Ethical Studies (approval number: 2007-45).

References

1. Schmidt MI, Hadji-Georgopoulos A, Rendell M, Margolis S, Kowarski A. The dawn phenomenon, an early morning glucose rise: implications for diabetic intraday blood glucose variation. Diabetes Care. 1981;4:579–85.
2. Bolli GB, Gerich JE. The "dawn phenomenon"--a common occurrence in both non-insulin-dependent and insulin-dependent diabetes mellitus. N Engl J Med. 1984;310:746–50. https://doi.org/10.1056/NEJM198403223101203.
3. Monnier L, Colette C, Sardinoux M, Baptista G, Regnier-Zerbib A, Owens D. Frequency and severity of the dawn phenomenon in type 2 diabetes: relationship to age. Diabetes Care. 2012;35:2597–9. https://doi.org/10.2337/dc12-0385.
4. Rybicka M, Krysiak R, Okopień B. The dawn phenomenon and the Somogyi effect - two phenomena of morning hyperglycaemia. Endokrynol Pol. 2011;62:276–84.
5. Monnier L, Colette C, Dejager S, Owens D. Magnitude of the dawn phenomenon and its impact on the overall glucose exposure in type 2 diabetes: is this of concern? Diabetes Care. 2013;36:4057–62. https://doi.org/10.2337/dc12-2127.
6. Somogyi M. Exacerbation of diabetes by excess insulin action. Am J Med. 1959;26:169–91.
7. Perriello G, De Feo P, Torlone E, Calcinaro F, Ventura MM, Basta G, Santeusanio F, Brunetti P, Gerich JE, Bolli GB. The effect of asymptomatic nocturnal hypoglycemia on glycemic control in diabetes mellitus. N Engl J Med. 1988;319:1233–9. https://doi.org/10.1056/NEJM198811103191901.
8. Bolli GB, Gottesman IS, Campbell PJ, Haymond MW, Cryer PE, Gerich JE. Glucose counterregulation and waning of insulin in the Somogyi phenomenon (posthypoglycemic hyperglycemia). N Engl J Med. 1984;311:1214–9. https://doi.org/10.1056/NEJM198411083111904.
9. Matyka KA, Crowne EC, Havel PJ, Macdonald IA, Matthews D, Dunger DB. Counterregulation during spontaneous nocturnal hypoglycemia in prepubertal children with type 1 diabetes. Diabetes Care. 1999;22:1144–50.
10. Tordjman KM, Havlin CE, Levandoski LA, White NH, Santiago JV, Cryer PE. Failure of nocturnal hypoglycemia to cause fasting hyperglycemia in patients with insulin-dependent diabetes mellitus. N Engl J Med. 1987;317:1552–9. https://doi.org/10.1056/NEJM198712173172502.
11. Havlin CE, Cryer PE. Nocturnal hypoglycemia does not commonly result in major morning hyperglycemia in patients with diabetes mellitus. Diabetes Care. 1987;10:141–7.
12. Mozersky RP, Bahl VK, Patel H, Patel N, Palushock S, Yamakawa H, Mook W, Basuray R, Velez-Giraldo JR. Fasting hyperglycemia in type I diabetes mellitus. J Am Osteopath Assoc. 1993;93:769–74.

13. Cohen M, Zimmet PZ. Home blood-glucose monitoring: a new approach to the management of diabetes mellitus. Med J Aust. 1980;2:713–6.
14. Kapellen TM, Heidtmann B, Bachmann J, Ziegler R, Grabert M, Holl RW. Indications for insulin pump therapy in different age groups: an analysis of 1,567 children and adolescents. Diabet Med. 2007;24:836–42. https://doi.org/10.1111/j.1464-5491.2007.02224.x.
15. Carroll MF, Hardy KJ, Burge MR, Schade DS. Frequency of the dawn phenomenon in type 2 diabetes: implications for diabetes therapy. Diabetes Technol Ther. 2002;4:595–605. https://doi.org/10.1089/152091502320798213.
16. Ando H, Ushijima K, Shimba S, Fujimura A. Daily fasting blood glucose rhythm male mice: a role of the circadian clock in the liver. Endocrinology. 2016;157:463–9. https://doi.org/10.1210/en.2015-1376.
17. Campbell PJ, Bolli GB, Cryer PE, Gerich JE. Pathogenesis of the dawn phenomenon in patients with insulin-dependent diabetes mellitus. Accelerated glucose production and impaired glucose utilization due to nocturnal surges in growth hormone secretion. N Engl J Med. 1985;312:1473–9. https://doi.org/10.1056/NEJM198506063122302.
18. Shih KC, Hsieh SH, Kwok CF, Hwu CM, Hsieh PS, Ho LT. Effect of growth hormone on dawn phenomenon in patients with type 2 diabetes. Growth Factors. 2013;31:66–73. https://doi.org/10.3109/08977194.2013.772996.
19. Møller N, Jørgensen JO. Effects of growth hormone on glucose, lipid, and protein metabolism in human subjects. Endocr Rev. 2009;30:152–77. https://doi.org/10.1210/er.2008-0027.
20. Yagasaki H, Kobayashi K, Saitou T, Nagamine K, Mitsui Y, Mochizuki M, Kobayashi K, Cho H, Ohyama K, Amemiya S, Nakazawa S. Nocturnal blood glucose and IGFBP-1 changes in type 1 diabetes: Differences in the dawn phenomenon between insulin regimens. Exp Clin Endocrinol Diabetes. 2010;118:195–9. https://doi.org/10.1055/s-0029-1239518.
21. Monnier L, Colette C, Rabasa-Lhoret R, Lapinski H, Caubel C, Avignon A, Boniface H. Morning hyperglycemic excursions: a constant failure in the metabolic control of non-insulin-using patients with type 2 diabetes. Diabetes Care. 2002;25:737–41.
22. Boden G, Chen X, Urbain JL. Evidence for a circadian rhythm of insulin sensitivity in patients with NIDDM caused by cyclic changes in hepatic glucose production. Diabetes. 1996;45:1044–50.
23. Radziuk J, Pye S. Diurnal rhythm in endogenous glucose production is a major contributor to fasting hyperglycaemia in type 2 diabetes. Suprachiasmatic deficit or limit cycle behaviour? Diabetologia. 2006;49:1619–28. https://doi.org/10.1007/s00125-006-0273-9.
24. Chen W, Hoo RL, Konishi M, Itoh N, Lee PC, Ye HY, Lam KS, Xu A. Growth hormone induces hepatic production of fibroblast growth factor 21 through a mechanism dependent on lipolysis in adipocytes. J Biol Chem. 2011;286:34559–66. https://doi.org/10.1074/jbc.M111.285965.
25. Yu H, Xia F, Lam KS, Wang Y, Bao Y, Zhang J, Gu Y, Zhou P, Lu J, Jia W, Xu A. Circadian rhythm of circulating fibroblast growth factor 21 is related to diurnal changes in fatty acids in humans. Clin Chem. 2011;57:691–700. https://doi.org/10.1373/clinchem.2010.155184.
26. Cryer PE. Hierarchy of physiological responses to hypoglycemia: relevance to clinical hypoglycemia in type I (insulin dependent) diabetes mellitus. Horm Metab Res. 1997;29:92–6. https://doi.org/10.1055/s-2007-978997.
27. Perriello G, De Feo P, Torlone E, Fanelli C, Santeusanio F, Brunetti P, Bolli GB. The dawn phenomenon in type 1 (insulin-dependent) diabetes mellitus: magnitude, frequency, variability, and dependency on glucose counterregulation and insulin sensitivity. Diabetologia. 1991;34:21–8.
28. Schaepelynck-Bélicar P, Vague P, Simonin G, Lassmann-Vague V. Improved metabolic control in diabetic adolescents using the continuous glucose monitoring system (CGMS). Diabetes Metab. 2003;29:608–12.
29. Guillod L, Comte-Perret S, Monbaron D, Gaillard RC, Ruiz J. Nocturnal hypoglycaemias in type 1 diabetic patients: what can we learn with continuous glucose monitoring? Diabete Metab. 2007;33:360. https://doi.org/10.1016/j.diabet.2007.03.007.
30. Høi-Hansen T, Pedersen-Bjergaard U, Thorsteinsson B. The Somogyi phenomenon revisited using continuous glucose monitoring in daily life. Diabetologia. 2005;48:2437–8. https://doi.org/10.1007/s00125-005-1946-5.
31. Choudhary P, Davies C, Emery CJ, Heller SR. Do high fasting glucose levels suggest nocturnal hypoglycaemia? The Somogyi effect-more fiction than fact? Diabet Med. 2013;30:914–7. https://doi.org/10.1111/dme.12175.
32. Colette C, Ginet C, Boegner C, Benichou M, Pham TC, Cristol JP, Monnier L. Dichotomous responses of inter and postprandial hyperglycaemia to short-term calorie restriction in patients with type 2 diabetes. Eur J Clin Investig. 2005;35:259–64. https://doi.org/10.1111/j.1365-2362.2005.01482.x.
33. Zhou J, Jia W, Bao Y, Ma X, Lu W, Li H, Hu C, Xiang K. Glycemic variability and its responses to intensive insulin treatment in newly diagnosed type 2 diabetes. Med Sci Monit. 2008;14:CR552–8. https://doi.org/10.3760/j:issn:0376-2491.2006.14.009.
34. Zhou J, Jia WP, Yu M, Ma XJ, Bao YQ, Lu W. The features of postprandialglucose state in type 2 diabetes mellitus. Zhonghua Yi Xue Za Zhi. 2006;86:970–5.
35. Atiea JA, Luzio S, Owens DR. The dawn phenomenon and diabetes control in treated NIDDM and IDDM patients. Diabetes Res Clin Pract. 1992;16:183–90.
36. Nathan DM, Kuenen J, Borg R, Zheng H, Schoenfeld D, Heine RJ, A1c-Derived Average Glucose Study Group. Translating the A1C assay into estimated aver-

age glucose values. Diabetes Care. 2008;31:1473–8. https://doi.org/10.2337/dc08-0545.
37. Monnier L, Colette C, Dunseath GJ, Owens DR. The loss of postprandial glycemic control precedes stepwise deterioration of fasting with worsening diabetes. Diabetes Care. 2007;30:263–9. https://doi.org/10.2337/dc06-1612.
38. Matyka K, Ford-Adams M, Dunger DB. Hypoglycaemia and counterregulation during childhood. Horm Res. 2002;57(Suppl 1):85–90.
39. Tone A, Iseda I, Higuchi C, Tsukamoto K, Katayama A, Matsushita Y, Hida K, Wada J, Shikata K. Comparison of insulin detemir and insulin glargine on glycemic variability in patients with type 1 and type 2 diabetes. Exp Clin Endocrinol Diabetes. 2010;118:320–4. https://doi.org/10.1055/s-0029-1243230.
40. Sheehan JP. Fasting hyperglycemia: etiology, diagnosis, and treatment. Diabetes Technol Ther. 2004;6:525–33. https://doi.org/10.1089/152091504170591O.
41. Hanew K, Sugawara A, Shimizu Y, Sato S, Sasaki A, Tazawa S, Ishii K, Saitoh T, Saso S, Yoshinaga K. The combination therapy with bromocriptine and cyproheptadine in patients with acromegaly. Endocrinol Jpn. 1989;36:429–38.
42. Porcellati F, Lucidi P, Bolli GB, Fanelli CG. Thirty years of research on the dawn phenomenon: lessons to optimize blood glucose control in diabetes. Diabetes Care. 2013;36:3860–2. https://doi.org/10.2337/dc13-2088.
43. ORIGIN Trial Investigators, Gerstein HC, Bosch J, Dagenais GR, Díaz R, Jung H, Maggioni AP, Pogue J, Probstfield J, Ramachandran A, Riddle MC, Rydén LE, Yusuf S. Basal insulin and cardiovascular and other outcomes in dysglycemia. N Engl J Med. 2012;367:319–28. https://doi.org/10.1056/NEJMoa1203858.
44. Pistrosch F, Köhler C, Schaper F, Landgraf W, Forst T, Hanefeld M. Effects of insulin glargine versus metformin on glycemic variability, microvascular and beta-cell function in early type 2 diabetes. Acta Diabetol. 2013;50:587–95. https://doi.org/10.1007/s00592-012-0451-9.
45. King AB. Once-daily insulin detemir is comparable to once-daily insulin glargine in providing glycaemic control over 24 h in patients with type 2 diabetes: a double-blind, randomized, crossover study. Diabetes Obes Metab. 2009;11:69–71. https://doi.org/10.1111/j.1463-1326.2008.01014.x.
46. King AB. No higher dose requirements with insulin detemir than glargine in type 2 diabetes: a crossover, double-blind, and randomized study using continuous glucose monitoring. J Diabetes Sci Technol. 2010;4:151–4. https://doi.org/10.1177/193229681000400119.
47. Heise T, Nosek L, Rønn BB, Endahl L, Heinemann L, Kapitza C, Draeger E. Lower within-subject variability of insulin detemir in comparison to NPH insulin and insulin glargine in people with type 1 diabetes. Diabetes. 2004;53:1614–20.
48. Swinnen SG, Simon AC, Holleman F, Hoekstra JB, Devries JH. Insulin detemir versus insulin glargine for type 2 diabetes mellitus. Cochrane Database Syst Rev. 2011:CD006383. https://doi.org/10.1002/14651858.CD006383.pub2.
49. Hollander P, King AB, Del Prato S, Sreenan S, Balci MK, Muñoz-Torres M, Rosenstock J, Hansen CT, Niemeyer M, Garber AJ. Insulin degludec improves long-term glycaemic control similarly to insulin glargine but with fewer hypoglycaemic episodes in patients with advanced type 2 diabetes on basal-bolus insulin therapy. Diabetes Obes Metab. 2015;17:202–6. https://doi.org/10.1111/dom.12411.
50. Simioni N, Filippi A, Scardapane M, Nicolucci A, Rossi MC, Frison V. Efficacy and safety of insulin degludec for hyperglycemia management in noncritical hospitalized patients with diabetes: an observational study. Diabetes Ther. 2017;8:941–6. https://doi.org/10.1007/s13300-017-0271-6.
51. Shields A, Sankaranarayanan S. Basal insulin regime change from Lantus to Toujeo resulted in fewer hypoglycaemic episodes in a 28-year-old man with diabetes mellitus. BMJ Case Rep. 2016;2016:bcr2016215831. https://doi.org/10.1136/bcr-2016-215831.
52. Papargyri P, Ojeda Rodríguez S, Corrales Hernández JJ, Mories Álvarez MT, Recio Córdova JM, Delgado Gómez M, Sánchez Marcos AI, Iglesias López RA, Herrero Ruiz A, Beaulieu Oriol M, Miralles García JM. An observational 7-year study of continuous subcutaneous insulin infusion for the treatment of type 1 diabetes mellitus. Endocrinol Nutr. 2014;61:141–6. https://doi.org/10.1016/j.endonu.2013.09.003.
53. Bouchonville MF, Jaghab JJ, Duran-Valdez E, Schrader RM, Schade DS. The effectiveness and risks of programming an insulin pump to counteract the dawn phenomenon in type 1 diabetes. Endocr Pract. 2014;20:1290–6. https://doi.org/10.4158/EP144198.OR.
54. Garg SK, Weinzimer SA, Tamborlane WV, Buckingham BA, Bode BW, Bailey TS, Brazg RL, Ilany J, Slover RH, Anderson SM, Bergenstal RM, Grosman B, Roy A, Cordero TL, Shin J, Lee SW, Kaufman FR. Glucose outcomes with the in-home use of a hybrid closed-loop insulin delivery system in adolescents and adults with type 1 diabetes. Diabetes Technol Ther. 2017;19:155–63. https://doi.org/10.1089/dia.2016.0421.

Using Continuous Glucose Monitoring for Patients with Fulminant Type 1 Diabetes

15

J. Zhou

Fulminant type 1 diabetes was first reported by Imagawa et al. [1] in 2000 and is characterized by a sudden onset of severe metabolic disorders, markedly elevated blood glucose with normal or slightly elevated glycated hemoglobin A_{1c} (HbA_{1c}), and almost complete, irreversible loss of islet function. Fulminant type 1 diabetes can be classified as one subtype of idiopathic type 1 diabetes (type 1B), with an acute onset of ketosis or ketoacidosis. The associated serious complications such as rhabdomyolysis, acute renal failure, and cerebral edema have been reported [2–4], and the outcomes could be fatal if without timely diagnose and treatment. Therefore, fulminant type 1 diabetes, as an acute and critical disease of the endocrine and metabolic system, requires special attention by all clinicians. In addition, due to almost complete, irreversible damage of islet function, patients exhibit large blood glucose variability and significantly increased risk of hypoglycemia and continue to need long-term therapy of insulin replacement. Therefore, it is necessary to comprehensively understand the characteristics of blood glucose variability through various monitoring techniques including self-monitoring of blood glucose (SMBG) and continuous glucose monitoring (CGM) technology in particular, in order to optimize the hypoglycemic regimen.

15.1 Overview of Fulminant Type 1 Diabetes Mellitus

15.1.1 The Concept of Fulminant Type 1 Diabetes

The 1997 American Diabetes Association (ADA) and the 1999 World Health Organization (WHO) have proposed the classification of diabetes mellitus [5–7], which divides diabetes into four types, namely, type 1 diabetes, type 2 diabetes, special types of diabetes, and gestational diabetes. Among them, type 1 diabetes is divided into two subtypes, namely, autoimmune-mediated diabetes (type 1A) and type 1B. Furthermore, three distinct stages of type 1 diabetes can be identified according to the latest ADA diabetes criteria (2017; Table 15.1) [8].

In 2000, Imagawa et al. [1] found a group of 11 patients with newly diagnosed type 1 diabetes that was characterized by a remarkably abrupt onset, the absence of insulitis and diabetes-related antibodies, and the high level of serum pancreatic enzyme concentrations. This was referred to a special type of type 1 diabetes and named "fulminant type 1 diabetes".

J. Zhou
Department of Endocrinology and Metabolism, Shanghai Clinical Center for Diabetes, Shanghai Diabetes Institute, Shanghai Jiao Tong University Affiliated Sixth People's Hospital, Shanghai, China
e-mail: zhoujian@sjtu.edu.cn

W. Jia (ed.), *Continuous Glucose Monitoring*, https://doi.org/10.1007/978-981-10-7074-7_15

Table 15.1 Staging of type 1 diabetes [8] (Reprinted with permission from *Diabetes Care*)

	Stage 1	Stage 2	Stage 3
Stage	• Autoimmunity • Normoglycemia • Presymptomatic	• Autoimmunity • Dysglycemia • Presymptomatic	• New-onset hyperglycemia • Symptomatic
Diagnostic criteria	• Multiple autoantibodies • No IGT or IFG	• Multiple autoantibodies • Dysglycemia: IFG and/or IGT • FPG 5.6–6.9 mmol/L (100–125 mg/dL) • 2hPG 7.8–11.0 mmol/L (140–199 mg/dl) • HbA_{1c} 5.7–6.4% (39–47 mmol/mol) or ≥10% increase in HbA_{1c}	• Clinical symptoms • Diabetes by standard criteria

IGT impaired glucose tolerance, *IFG* impaired fasting glucose, *FPG* fasting plasma glucose, *2hPG* 2-hour postload glucose

15.1.2 Diagnostic Criteria for Fulminant Type 1 Diabetes

There is no uniform diagnosis criterion of fulminant type 1 diabetes. The 2012 Japan Diabetes Society (JDS) criteria (Table 15.2) are commonly used for the diagnosis of fulminant type 1 diabetes, which include the screening criteria and diagnostic criteria [9].

For the diagnosis of fulminant type 1 diabetes, the following aspects need to be supplemented:

1. For patients with impaired glucose regulation, their HbA_{1c} level is relatively high. Thus, the cutoff point [HbA_{1c} < 8.7% (72 mmol/mol) (NGSP)] is not applicable to such patients.
2. For patients with the manifestations of diabetic ketosis or ketoacidosis, fulminant type 1 diabetes should be routinely screened. Further tests for islet autoantibody, HbA_{1c}, islet function, and liver function are required in patients with suspected fulminant type 1 diabetes.
3. Fulminant type 1 diabetes can be diagnosed if three of the JDS diagnostic criteria are met; the diagnosis is highly suspected if two of the diagnostic criteria are met with a disease course exceeding 1 week.
4. The onset of fulminant type 1 diabetes is often preceded by influenza-like symptoms or gastrointestinal symptoms and, thus, is often misdiagnosed as acute respiratory infection or acute gastroenteritis. Therefore, improvements are needed in the early detection, early diagnosis, and early treatment of fulminant type 1 diabetes.

15.1.3 Epidemiology of Fulminant Type 1 Diabetes

According to the previous case reports, fulminant type 1 diabetes most commonly occurs in Asian countries, with the highest incidence in Japan, followed by China and South Korea. It is rarely reported in Europe and the USA. Preliminary epidemiological studies show that the ketosis-onset fulminant type 1 diabetes accounted for 19.4% (43/222) [10] and 7.1% (7/99) [11] of cases of type 1 diabetes in Japan and South Korea. The prevalence rate in China was 9.1% among type 1 diabetes patients, accounting for 14.0% of type 1 diabetes with ketosis or ketoacidosis-onset over 18 years of age.

The existing evidence shows that fulminant type 1 diabetes has the following epidemiological characteristics:

1. Sporadic distribution.
2. Racial and ethnic variations in incidence rates. The incidence is higher in Asians than in Caucasians, with no reports so far in African American.
3. Average age at onset of 39.1 years (most cases over 20 years old). Women showed a younger age at onset than men.
4. No significant difference in the morbidity between men and women, although morbidity increases with age in males.
5. Greater morbidity associated with pregnancy.

Table 15.2 Criteria for definite diagnosis of fulminant type 1 diabetes mellitus (2012) [9] (Reprinted from *Journal of Diabetes Investigation*)

Criteria for screening: 1. Ketosis or ketoacidosis within 1 week after the onset of hyperglycemic symptoms 2. Plasma glucose level ≥16.0 mmol/L (≥288 mg/dL) at first visit
Criteria for definite diagnosis: 1. Occurrence of diabetic ketosis or ketoacidosis soon (approximately 7 days) after the onset of hyperglycemic symptoms (elevation of urinary and/or serum ketone bodies at first visit) 2. Plasma glucose level ≥16.0 mmol/L (≥288 mg/dL) and glycated hemoglobin A_{1c} level <8.7% (NGSP value) [72 mmol/mol (IFCC value)][a] at first visit 3. Urinary C-peptide excretion <10 μg/day or fasting serum C-peptide level <0.3 ng/mL (<0.10 nmol/L) and <0.5 ng/mL (<0.17 nmol/L) after intravenous glucagon (or after meal) load at onset
Other findings in fulminant type 1 diabetes mellitus: 1. Islet-related autoantibodies, such as antibodies to glutamic acid decarboxylase antibody (GAD-Ab), islet-associated antigen 2 (IA-A2) and insulin, are undetectable in general 2. Duration of the disease before the start of insulin treatment can be 1–2 weeks 3. Elevation of serum pancreatic enzyme levels (amylase, lipase, or elastase-1) is observed in 98% of the patients 4. Flu-like symptoms (fever, upper respiratory symptoms, etc.) or gastrointestinal symptoms (upper abdominal pain, nausea and/or vomiting, etc.) precede the disease onset in 70% of patients 5. The disease can occur during pregnancy or just after delivery 6. Association with HLA *DRB1*0405-DQB1*0401* is reported

HLA human leukocyte antigen, *NGSP* National Glycohemoglobin Standardization Program, *IFCC* International Federation of Clinical Chemistry

[a]This value is not applicable for patients with previously diagnosed glucose intolerance

15.1.4 Etiology of Fulminant Type 1 Diabetes

The etiology and pathogenesis of fulminant type 1 diabetes are not yet clear and are currently thought to be associated with genetic, environmental (viral infection), and autoimmune factors (Fig. 15.1).

15.1.4.1 Genetic Susceptibility

The results of previous studies have shown that a genetic polymorphism of human leukocyte antigen II (HLA-II) is associated with the occurrence of fulminant type 1 diabetes (Table 15.3). The results indicate that HLA *DR4-DQ4* is associated with the onset of Japanese fulminant type 1 diabetes mellitus, especially the *DRB1*0405-DQB1*0401*, *DQA1*0303-DQB1*0401* and *DQA1*0302-DQB1*0303* haplotypes. Tsutsumi et al. [12] found that 32.6% of fulminant type 1 diabetes patients carried the *DRB1*0405-DQB1*0401* genotype, which was significantly higher than 14.2% of individuals in the normal control group. Therefore, the 2012 JDS diagnostic criteria for diagnosis of fulminant type 1 diabetes mellitus include the characteristic of "association with HLA *DRB1*0405-DQB1*0401*" [9]. Moreover, studies have shown that HLA *DRB1*0405-DQB1*0401* is a susceptibility gene in Japanese patients with negative GAD-Ab, whereas the HLA *DRB1*0901-DQB1*0303* genotype is more common in GAD-Ab positive and fulminant type 1 diabetes associated with pregnancy [12, 13]. The results of a study in South Korea also showed the involvement of HLA *DRB1*0405-DQB1*0401* in fulminant type 1 diabetes [14]. HLA *DQA1*0102-DQB1*0601* may be a susceptibility gene for the Chinese population [15].

In addition, there is evidence for genetic heterogeneity in fulminant type 1 diabetes. A pair of twins in South Korea had the same HLA *DR-DQ* haplotype but different phenotypes, namely, fulminant type 1 diabetes and autoimmune-mediated diabetes, type 1A [16].

15.1.4.2 Viral Infection

Most fulminant type 1 diabetes patients have a history of infection 2 weeks before onset, suggestive of an association between viral infection and the onset of fulminant type 1 diabetes. A Japanese national survey showed that 71.7% of fulminant type 1 diabetes patients had influenza-like symptoms before the onset and 72.5% had abdominal symptoms [17]. Also, some

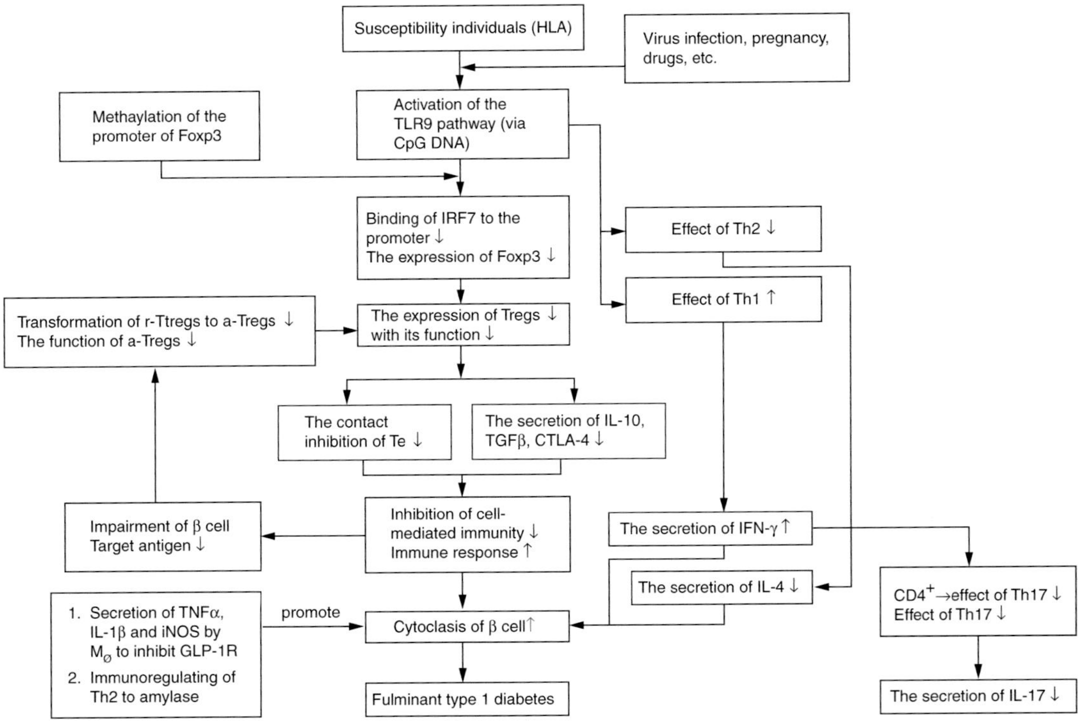

Fig. 15.1 The etiology and pathogenesis of fulminant type 1 diabetes. *HLA* human leukocyte antigen, *Foxp3* forkhead box protein 3, *IRF7* interferon regulatory factor 7, *CTLA-4* cytotoxic T-lymphocyte antigen 4, *Th1* helper T cell 1, *Th2* helper T cell 2, *Th17* helper T cell 17, M_D macrophage, *IL-1β* interleukin-1β, *IL-4* interleukin-4, *IL-10* interleukin-10, *IL-17* interleukin-17, *TNFα* tumor necrosis factor α, *TGFβ* transforming growth factor β, *iNOS* inducible nitric oxide synthase, *CpG DNA* non-methylated DNA, *TLR9* Toll-like receptor 9, *Te* effector T cell, *GLP-1R* glucagon like peptide-1 receptor, T_{regs} regulatory T cell, *a-*T_{regs} activated regulatory T cell, *r-*T_{regs} rest regulatory T cell

Table 15.3 Fulminant type 1 diabetes mellitus-related HLA genotype

Japan
HLA *DRB1*0405-DQB1*0401* [mostly in GAD-Ab (−)]
HLA *DQA1*0303-DQB1*0401*
HLA *DQA1*0302-DQB1*0303*
HLA *DRB1*0901-DQB1*0303* [mostly in GAD-Ab (+) and PF]
China
HLA *DQA1*0102-DQB1*0601*
South Korea
HLA *DRB1*0405-DQB1*0401*

HLA human leukocyte antigen, *PF* fulminant type 1 diabetes associated with pregnancy, *GAD-Ab* glutamic acid decarboxylase antibody

patients had significantly high titers of IgA antibodies to enterovirus [18]. The common viruses identified are herpes simplex virus (HSV), human herpesvirus 6 (HHV6), cytomegalovirus (CMV), coxsackie virus, etc. (Table 15.4).

Imagawa et al. [19] found elevations in a variety of antibodies after viral infection, suggesting that the virus-induced immune response, rather than viruses themselves, triggered the fulminant type 1 diabetes. Tanaka et al. [20] found the presence of enterovirus in islet cells and exocrine tissues, and immune response to enterovirus infection might be involved in the onset of fulminant type 1 diabetes.

15.1.4.3 Autoimmunity

At the initial discovery of fulminant type 1 diabetes, Imagawa et al. [1] found that islet autoantibody was negative in 11 fulminant type 1 diabetes patients and, thus, eliminated an association of fulminant type 1 diabetes with autoimmune disease, which distinguished it from type 1A diabetes. However,

Table 15.4 Fulminant type 1 diabetes mellitus-related virus

	Cases in China	Cases in other countries
Herpes simplex virus 1 (HSV1)	Zhou ZG, et al. Chinese Journal of Endocrinology and Metabolism, 2010	Nagaoka T, et al. Tonyobyo (J Japan Diab Soc), 2001
Human herpesvirus 6 (HHV6)	–	Imagawa A, et al. Tonyobyo (J Japan Diab Soc), 2008
Cytomegalovirus (CMV)	Liu F, et al. Chinese Journal of Endocrinology and Metabolism, 2009	Imagawa A, et al. Tonyobyo (J Japan Diab Soc), 2008
Coxsackie virus (A4.5.6, B3.4)	Zhou ZG et al. Chinese Journal of Endocrinology and Metabolism, 2010	Nishida W, et al. Tonyobyo (J Japan Diab Soc), 2005
Chlamydia	Liu F, et al. Chinese Journal of Endocrinology and Metabolism, 2009	–
ECHO virus	–	Vreugdenhill GR, et al. Clin Infect Dis, 2008
Influenza virus	Liu F, et al. Chinese Journal of Endocrinology and Metabolism, 2009	Sano H, et al. Diabetes Res Clin Pract, 2008
Rotavirus	–	Imagawa A, et al. Tonyobyo (J Japan Diab Soc), 2008
Parvovirus B19	–	Nishiumi T, et al. J Diabetes Investig, 2014
Epstein-Barr virus	Wang T, et al. Chin Med J (Engl), 2008	Sekine N, et al. JAMA, 2001
Mumps virus	–	Goto A, et al. Endocr J, 2008
Norovirus	–	Koyano HM, et al. Intern Med, 2013
Encephalomyocarditis virus (EMV)	–	Sano H, et al. Biochem Biophys Res Commun, 2011
Parainfluenza virus	–	Ohara N, et al. Int Heart J, 2015
Hepatitis A virus	–	Hwang YC, et al. Diabet Med, 2010

the follow-up study found some fulminant type 1 diabetes patients were positive for GAD-Ab or also had Graves' disease or Hashimoto's thyroiditis. A small number of patients presented with lymphocyte infiltration in pancreatic tissues [10, 21]. These data suggest that immune factors are involved in the occurrence of this disease.

A subsequent study has confirmed cellular or humoral immune abnormalities in a portion of fulminant type 1 diabetes patients. Aida et al. [22] found T cell and macrophage infiltration in and around the islets in three cases of fulminant type 1 diabetes, suggesting that both innate and acquired immunity are involved in the occurrence of this disease. It has also been reported that macrophage-mediated insulitis may be a more important cause of β-cell damage than T cells ($CD8^+$ T cells were originally thought to cause fulminant type 1 diabetes) [23, 24].

Moreover, the recent study showed that the Toll-like receptor-9/interferon regulatory factor-7 (TLR9/IRF7) pathway is involved in the occurrence of fulminant type 1 diabetes, mainly through cytotoxic T-lymphocyte-associated protein 4 (CTLA-4) and transcription factor forkhead box P3 (Foxp3). Zhou et al. [25] found that Foxp3 promoter hypermethylation in human peripheral blood mononuclear cells prevented IRF-7 binding to the Foxp3 promoter, downregulated the expression of TLR9 and Foxp3, and thus impaired the function of regulatory T cells (T_{reg}) and decreased CTLA-4. T_{reg} immunodeficiency in peripheral blood and islets resulted in failure of the body to produce effective immune tolerance, which triggered a sustained autoimmune destruction of β-cells and finally led to fulminant type 1 diabetes.

15.1.4.4 Pregnancy

The fulminant type 1 diabetes can be divided into pregnancy-related fulminant type 1 diabetes and nonpregnancy-related fulminant type 1 diabetes according to its relationship with pregnancy. The study performed by Imagawa et al. [1] showed that almost all cases of abrupt onset of type 1 diabetes during pregnancy are fulminant type 1 diabetes, mostly occurring during late pregnancy or 2 weeks after delivery. Shimizu et al. [13] compared the clinical characteristics of the two types of the disease and found that fulminant type 1 diabetes associated with pregnancy might be related to the hormone levels and metabolic disorders of pregnant women: sex hormones during pregnancy can promote the Th2-type immune response and antagonize the Th1-type immune reaction. In addition, there is a case report of fulminant type 1 diabetes occurring 10 days after artificial abortion, revealing that abortion may also increase the risk of fulminant type 1 diabetes.

15.1.4.5 Others

Some medications (carbamazepine, mexiletine, ibuprofen, tegafur-uracil, pembrolizumab, etc.) may be involved in the occurrence of this disease by drug-induced hypersensitivity syndrome [26–28]. Onuma et al. [29] reported that compared with general population, patients with drug-induced hypersensitivity syndrome had a higher probability of developing fulminant type 1 diabetes, with a susceptibility gene HLA-B62, suggesting that in addition to genetic susceptibility, the use of specific drugs is associated with the occurrence of this disease.

15.1.5 Clinical Characteristics of Fulminant Type 1 Diabetes

Most fulminant type 1 diabetes patients are adults with no difference in the incidence between men and women. Pregnant women are at higher risk of this disease. Compared with type 1A diabetes, fulminant type 1 diabetes has the following clinical characteristics:

1. Prodromal symptoms. Patients often develop prodromal symptoms 2 weeks before the onset of fulminant type 1 diabetes, for instance, influenza-like symptoms (fever, upper respiratory tract infection, etc.) or gastrointestinal symptoms (diarrhea, nausea, vomiting, etc.), with fever (60%) being most common.
2. Hyperglycemia and ketoacidosis. The onset is very sudden, with typically <1 week from the presentation of typical hyperglycemic symptoms (polyuria, polyphagia, polydipsia, and weight loss) to the occurrence of ketosis or ketoacidosis. Sekine et al. [30] reported a case of a patient who had blood glucose within normal range 1 day before the onset, followed by a sudden increase in blood glucose and a sudden drop in C-peptide level the next day. Some researchers have even observed hypoglycemic events before the onset, probably due to a rapid release of synthesized insulin into the blood resulting from the rapid destruction of islets. As the course of the disease is very short, the HbA_{1c} at onset is close to normal or only mildly increased.
3. Severe metabolic disorders. Approximately 90% of fulminant type 1 diabetes begins with ketosis or ketoacidosis and half with disturbance of consciousness. At the onset, hyperglycemia, ketoacidosis, and electrolyte imbalance are more serious than type 1A diabetes.
4. Almost complete, irreversible loss of islet function. The existing evidence shows permanent destruction of islet α- and β-cells in patients with fulminant type 1 diabetes.
5. Serious complications such as rhabdomyolysis, liver dysfunction, and kidney dysfunction. Some patients exhibit multiple organ dysfunction such as loss of liver, kidney, heart, and striated muscle function, as manifested by an elevation in hepatic enzymes, pancreatic enzymes (amylase, lipase, elastase, etc.), and myokinases, or severe conditions like rhabdomyolysis, acute renal failure, cerebral edema, and even cardiac arrest [2–4] (Table 15.5).
6. Others. Most cases of pregnancy-related type 1 diabetes are fulminant type 1 diabetes and mostly occur during the late pregnancy or 2 weeks after delivery [1, 17]. The clinical symptoms of fulminant type 1 diabetes associated with pregnancy appear to be much

Table 15.5 Complications, comorbidities and related disorders of fulminant type 1 diabetes mellitus

Complications/comorbidities	Cases in China	Cases in other countries
Rhabdomyolysis	Zhou J, et al. Chinese journal of internal medicine, 2007	–
Sjogren's syndrome	Zhang J, et al. Chin J Diabetes, 2013	–
Multiple organ failure (MOF)	Liang DC, et al. Chinese Critical Care Medicine, 2012	Ochi F, et al. Nihon Naika Gakkai Zasshi, 2008
Fetal death in utero (FDIU)	Zhang Z, et al. Chinese Journal of Perinatal Medicine, 2012	Bresson L, et al. J Gynecol Obstet Biol Reprod (Paris), 2010
Acute pancreatitis	Cao FL, et al. International Journal of Endocrinology and Metabolism, 2010	Tanaka S, et al. Endocrine J, 2013
Acute liver failure	Xiao J, et al. Journal of Internal Intensive Medicine, 2013	–
Myocarditis	Wei Q, et al. Jiangsu Med J, 2012	Makino K, et al. BMC Res Notes, 2013
Acute renal failure	–	Mizutani T, et al. Leg Med (Tokyo), 2011
Glycogen liver disease	–	Murata F, et al. Endocr J, 2012
Drug rash with eosinophilia and systemic symptoms (DRESS)	–	Dubois-Laforgue D, et al. Diabetes Care, 2013
Drug hypersensitivity syndrome (DHS)	–	Minegaki Y, et al. Int J Dermatol, 2013

Table 15.5 (continued)

Complications/comorbidities	Cases in China	Cases in other countries
Hashimoto's thyroiditis	–	Minegaki Y, et al. Int J Dermatol, 2013
Insulin autoimmune syndrome (IAS)	–	Kim HS, et al. Diabet Med, 2012
Thrombocytopenia	–	Yasuda H, et al. Diabet Med, 2012
Coronary microcirculation disorder	–	Yamada H, et al. J Diabetes Investig, 2014
Acanthosis nigricans	Lu ZY, et al. Chin J Diabetes, 2009	–
Encephaledema	Dong HM, et al. J Forensic Leg Med, 2014	–

more serious, with lower HbA_{1c} and arterial pH value. Fulminant type 1 diabetes associated with pregnancy can result in severe maternal and fetal complications, for instance, an extremely high incidence of abortion and stillbirth.

15.2 Treatment and Prognosis of Fulminant Type 1 Diabetes Mellitus

15.2.1 Treatment of Fulminant Type 1 Diabetes

At present, the evidence on the treatment of fulminant type 1 diabetes is mainly derived from case reports. According to its characteristics, the treatment is divided into acute-phase treatment and long-term insulin therapy.

15.2.1.1 Acute-Phase Treatment

Fulminant type 1 diabetes is characterized by an abrupt onset of the disease mostly with ketosis and ketoacidosis, accompanied by severe metabolic disorders and remarkably elevated blood glucose concentration. Once fulminant type 1 diabetes is suspected, the patient should be treated immediately for diabetic ketoacidosis including rehydration; small doses of intravenous insulin infusion; correction of electrolyte and acid-base imbalance, along with symptomatic and supportive treatment; and prevention and management of complications.

In addition, the following points need to be noted:

1. Given the acute onset with severe metabolic disorders, fulminant type 1 diabetes should be diagnosed and treated in a timely manner with (1) rapid establishment of two intravenous accesses, one for continuous intravenous insulin infusion and the other for rehydration and anti-infection treatment, and (2) due to severe dehydration and poor subcutaneous absorption of insulin, it is recommended to use intravenous insulin infusion rather than insulin pump therapy.
2. In serious cases, rhabdomyolysis and resultant acute renal failure may occur. (1) Pay attention to the presence or absence of muscle weakness, swelling, pain, and brown urine; (2) the serum creatine kinase level is the most specific indicator of rhabdomyolysis, which should be routinely tested and used for constant monitoring of dynamic changes during the early diagnosis and treatment of fulminant type 1 diabetes.
3. Fulminant type 1 diabetes associated with pregnancy can result in severe maternal complications and stillbirth. Key measures to save the fetus include shortening of hyperglycemia-lasting duration, timely correction of ketoacidosis, and performing a cesarean section in a timely manner.

15.2.1.2 Long-Term Insulin Therapy

As there is almost complete, irreversible destruction of islet α- and β-cells in fulminant type 1 diabetes, the patient usually has extremely poor islet function, large blood glucose variability, and increased incidence of hypoglycemia. Therefore, patients usually require four times of intensive treatment with subcutaneous rapid-acting or short-acting insulin combined with intermediate-acting or long-acting insulin. In addition, an insulin pump, which simulates the physiological insulin secretion, can be used to improve blood glucose control in patients [3]. It improves inter- and intra-day glucose variability [3, 31]. The use of an insulin pump as long-term insulin replacement therapy is suggested, with a significantly higher insulin dosage than that used for type 1A diabetes [32].

15.2.2 Prognosis of Fulminant Type 1 Diabetes

Due to the sudden onset and severe metabolic disorders of fulminant type 1 diabetes, the mortality rate is high in the absence of early diagnosis and timely treatment. After correction of ketosis or ketoacidosis, abnormal hepatic enzyme, pancreatic enzyme, and myokinase levels will return to normal within 2–3 weeks; however, fulminant type 1 diabetes causes permanent destruction of islet α- and β-cells, which requires long-term insulin replacement therapy. Compared with type 1A diabetes, fulminant type 1 diabetes results in worse islet function, more severe β-cell destruction, higher insulin requirement, and increased risk of hypoglycemia and diabetic microvascular diseases. However, Koyano et al. [33] reported the partial recovery of pancreatic α-cells after treatment from fulminant type 1 diabetes in a case of 34-year-old male, but his serum C-peptide level was still under the detection limit. Also, it was reported that early intensive treatment achieved partial recovery of β-cell function in a 44-year-old female patient who developed acute pancreatitis and concomitant fulminant type 1 diabetes [34]. Recently, a case of idiopathic type 1 diabetes with subsequent recovery of β-cell function has also been reported [35].

15.3 Use of CGM for Patients with Fulminant Type 1 Diabetes

Due to the almost complete destruction of islet β-cells, the blood glucose level is more easily influenced by exogenous insulin, and the patients exhibit large blood glucose variability and increased risks of hypoglycemia and diabetic microvascular diseases. Thus, glucose monitoring is particularly important.

At present, SMBG and CGM are commonly used glucose monitoring methods for diabetes patients. HbA_{1c}, glycated albumin (GA), and other indicators can also reflect the recent glycemic control. SMBG represents the glucose concentration at a specific time-point, and it cannot reflect continuous, dynamic changes in blood glucose. CGM can detect occult hypoglycemia and hyperglycemia, which may be not easily detected by traditional methods. Thus, CGM is an effective supplement to traditional glucose monitoring methods. Moreover, CGM facilitates the understanding of trends in blood glucose variability and determination of the influences of meal uptake, exercise, and medication on blood glucose, so as to guide better improvements in lifestyle and adjustment of the treatment regimen. According to the Chinese clinical guideline for CGM (2012), CGM is desirable for type 1 diabetes patients [36]. Given that fulminant type 1 diabetes is a subtype of type 1 diabetes, CGM is also applicable to fulminant type 1 diabetes patients. CGM supports the management of type 1 diabetes by effectively detecting hyperglycemic and hypoglycemic events, providing data for blood glucose variability, and guiding the adjustment of treatment plan.

15.3.1 CGM Is an Effective Tool for Detecting Blood Glucose Variability

15.3.1.1 Detection of Hyperglycemic and Hypoglycemic Events

The results of the study performed by Melki et al. [37] showed that two-thirds of daily utilization of CGM was applied to monitor asymptomatic nocturnal hypoglycemia. Accumulating evidence has shown that CGM can detect asymptomatic nocturnal hypoglycemic events. Cheyne et al. [38] conducted a CGM study in ten type 1 diabetes patients with poor glycemic control and found that eight patients experienced asymptomatic hypoglycemia with blood glucose <3 mmol/L. For children with type 1 diabetes, CGM measurements suggested that about 70% of subjects had nocturnal hypoglycemia and 20% experienced nocturnal hypoglycemia for three consecutive nights [39]. CGM not only detects nocturnal hypoglycemia but also contributes to the detection of asymptomatic hypoglycemia during daytime [38, 39].

CGM also helps to detect postprandial hyperglycemia [40]. SMBG only represents the glucose concentration at a specific time-point, not the blood glucose levels throughout the day. Thus, it cannot detect all hyperglycemic events in a timely manner, especially postprandial hyperglycemia. Boland et al. [39] emphasized that CGM is an effective tool for detecting postprandial hyperglycemia in patients who only monitor fasting and bedtime blood glucose. Schaepelynck-Bélicar et al. [41] applied CGM in 12 patients with poor glycemic control and found that there were 24 postprandial hyperglycemic episodes in ten patients; five patients experienced prolonged nocturnal hyperglycemia; and four had the dawn phenomenon. Also, CGM facilitates the distinction between asymptomatic hypoglycemia and the dawn phenomenon [42].

15.3.1.2 Comprehensive Understanding of Glucose Variability

CGM not only detects hyperglycemic and hypoglycemic events but also contributes to the understanding of the characteristics of blood glucose variability [40–43]. Bhide et al. [44] believe that the biggest advantage of CGM is that it is capable of revealing the dynamic trends of blood glucose concentration so that practitioners can guide the adjustment of the treatment plan accordingly. Moreover, CGM also provides information about the causes of glycemic variability in diabetes patients.

15.3.2 Use of CGM to Guide Adjustments to Therapy

In clinical practice, CGM can be used to monitor the detailed changes in blood glucose variability throughout the day. It can improve the management of blood glucose levels and reduce hypoglycemic events by guiding the fine regulation of blood glucose. Long-term use of CGM helps improving the HbA_{1c} [45–51]. However, improper use of CGM may also have a potentially negative impact: CGM provides interstitial fluid glucose readings, which lag behind capillary glucose levels. Moreover, overtreatment of hyperglycemia or hypoglycemia may increase blood glucose variability.

Fulminant type 1 diabetes developed rapidly and accompanied with more severe dysfunction of islets when compared with type 1A diabetes mellitus resulted in dramatic glycemic variability. However, HbA_{1c} levels are more commonly normal at the early stage of the disease. Thus, the application of CGM mainly focuses on improving and maintaining the stability of blood glucose levels at the initial stage. CGM can also help improving the HbA_{1c} when HbA_{1c} is markedly elevated.

In our previous study, we analyzed the CGM results of three patients with fulminant type 1 diabetes who were treated in our hospital from January 2007 to March 2008, and the therapeutic regimens were adjusted accordingly (Table 15.6) [3].

Case 1 (Fig. 15.2): A patient treated with subcutaneous insulin injection four times daily with insulin dose of 0.67 U/(kg·d). The mean blood glucose (MBG) was 8.9 mmol/L, and standard deviation of blood glucose (SDBG) was 3.6 mmol/L, indicating the presence of high glycemic variability. The patient also had hypoglycemia, and the percentage of time (PT) spent with glucose ≤3.9 mmol/L was 4% with no time spent with blood glucose ≤2.8 mmol/L (Fig. 15.2a). Six months later, the glucose variation was still quite large (SDBG was 3.0 mmol/L), and MBG decreased to 6.5 mmol/L. Thus, the patient had a potentially increased risk of hypoglycemia. The PT spent with glucose ≤3.9 mmol/L and ≤2.8 mmol/L were 21% and 6%, respectively (Fig. 15.2b).

Case 2 (Fig. 15.3): A patient was treated with an insulin pump with insulin dose of 0.57 U/(kg·d). CGM revealed good glycemic control. The MBG was 6.3 mmol/L, SDBG was 2.2 mmol/L, and the PT spent with glucose ≤3.9 mmol/L was 10%

Table 15.6 Clinical characteristics of three cases of fulminant type 1 diabetes [3] (Reprinted with permission from *Chinese Journal of Diabetes Mellitus*)

Cases	Gender	Age (year)	BMI (kg/m^2)	Duration (day)	Glucose (mmol/L)	Urine ketone	Arterial blood pH	BE (mmol/L)
1	Male	31	23.3	4	38.9	+++	7.25	−17.0
2	Male	43	21.5	2	>38.9	+++	7.14	−25.2
3	Male	29	22.3	2	60.5	++++	7.02	−24.0

Cases	ALT (U/L)	AST (U/L)	Cr (μmol/L)	Na$^+$ (mmol/L)	K$^+$ (mmol/L)	CK (U/L)	LDH (U/L)	CK-MB (ng/ml)
1	293	366	230	117	7.3	11,754	1461	114.43
2	64	27	300	134	9.2	1,283	561	6.59
3	449	801	255	131	8.6	12,239	2147	42.71
Reference value	0–65	8–37	53–115	135–155	3.5–5.5	21–190	313–618	0–5

Cases	cTn (ng/ml)	Mb (ng/ml)	AMY (U/L)	UAMY (U/L)	Lipase (U/L)	HbA_{1c} (%[mmol/mol])	GA (%)	GAD-Ab (U/ml)
1	8.29	961.90	263	1015	830	6.2 (44)	22	0
2	0.118	–	387	>1300	812	6.3 (45)	24	3.6
3	1.27	>1000	2319	859	859	6.2 (44)	15	0
Reference value	0–1.5	0–110	30–110	32–641	0–190	4.3–6.5 (23–48)	11–17	0–7.5

Cases	IA_2-Ab (U/ml)	OGTT CP_0 (ng/ml)	OGTT CP_{30} (ng/ml)	OGTT CP_{120} (ng/ml)	Arginine stimulating test CP_0 (ng/ml)	Arginine stimulating test CP_2 (ng/ml)	Arginine stimulating test CP_4 (ng/ml)	Arginine stimulating test CP_6 (ng/ml)
1	0	0.01	0.02	0.05	0.08	0.22	0.14	0.21
2	0	0.01	0.01	0.01	0.01	0.01	0.01	0.01
3	0	0.01	0.02	0.11	0.01	0.01	0.01	0.01
Reference value	0–7.5	0.5–1.5	–	–	0.5–1.5	–	–	–

a

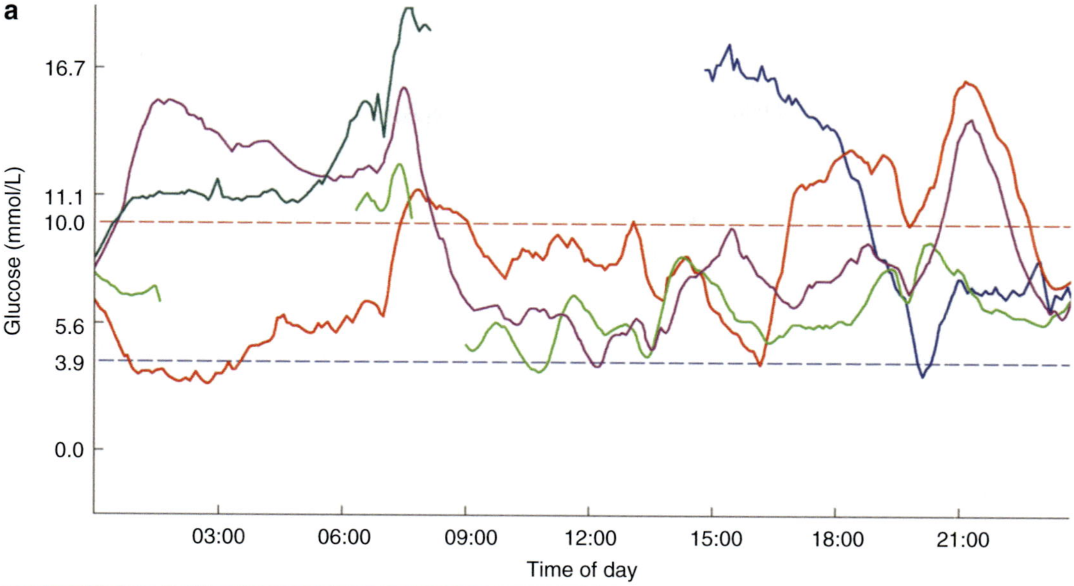

GLUCOSE EXPOSURE	GLUCOSE VARIABILITY	Dangerously Low	Low	GLUCOSE RANGES In Target Range	High	High
MBG mmol/L	SDBG mmol/L	≤ 2.8 mmol/L	≤ 3.9 mmol/L	3.9< GLUCOSE <10.0 mmol/L	≥ 10.0 mmol/L	≥ 11.1 mmol/L
8.9	**3.6**	**0%**	**4%**	**60%**	**36%**	**28%**

b

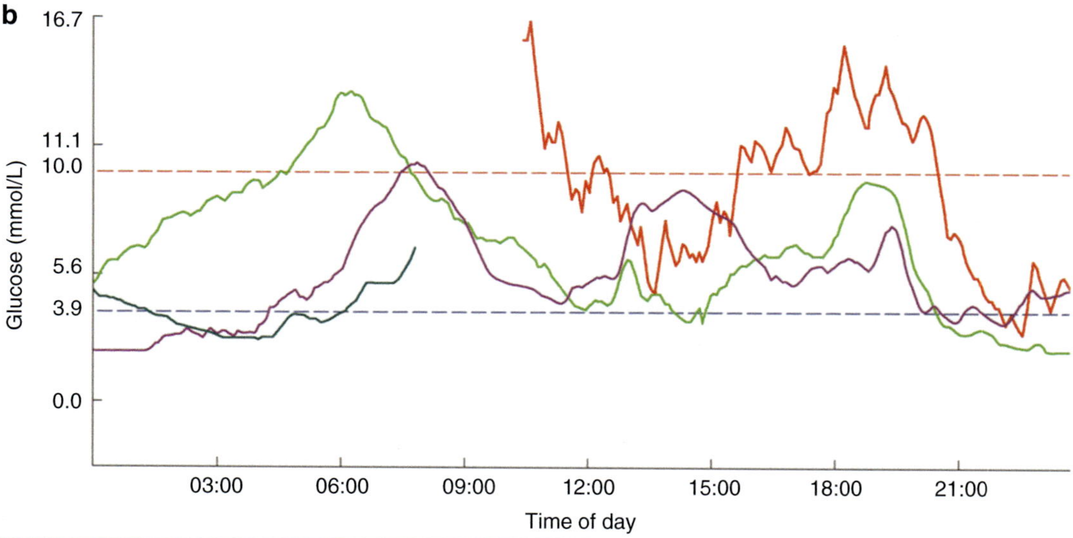

GLUCOSE EXPOSURE	GLUCOSE VARIABILITY	Dangerously Low	Low	GLUCOSE RANGES In Target Range	High	High
MBG mmol/L	SDBG mmol/L	≤ 2.8 mmol/L	≤ 3.9 mmol/L	3.9< GLUCOSE <10.0 mmol/L	≥ 10.0 mmol/L	≥ 11.1 mmol/L
6.5	**3.0**	**6%**	**21%**	**65%**	**14%**	**9%**

Fig. 15.2 Case 1: The CGM profiles of one case of fulminant type 1 diabetes treated with four-time daily subcutaneous insulin injections before and 6 months later

with no time spent with blood glucose ≤2.8 mmol/L (Fig. 15.3a). After follow-up for 6 months, the MBG was reduced to 5.5 mmol/L, and the SDBG was unchanged (2.2 mmol/L). Thus, the PT spent with glucose ≤3.9 mmol/L and ≤2.8 mmol/L were 27% and 9%, respectively, indicating an increased duration of hypoglycemic events, which were mainly concentrated in the period after dinner and before bedtime (Fig. 15.3b). These data demonstrated that hypoglycemia was associated with MBG, and a lower blood glucose level caused an increased risk of hypoglycemia, if the blood glucose fluctuation was basically unchanged. In conclusion, the blood glucose level of the patient was kept too low. Thus, we adjusted the therapy by reducing

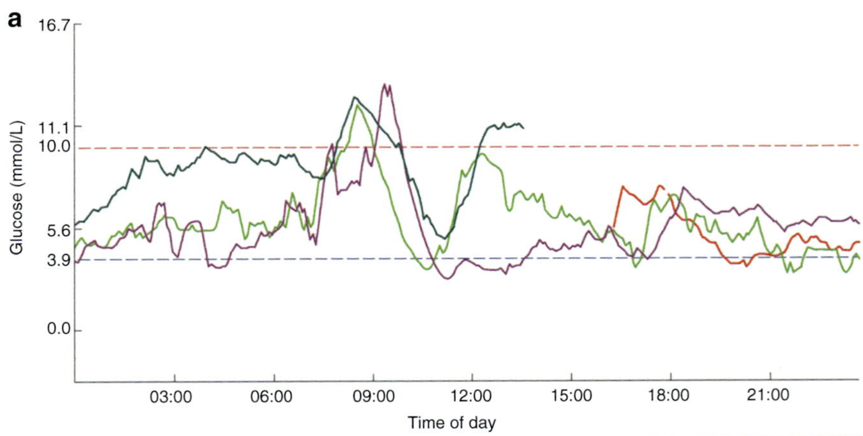

GLUCOSE EXPOSURE	GLUCOSE VARIABILITY	Dangerously Low	Low	GLUCOSE RANGES In Target Range	High	High
MBG mmol/L	SDBG mmol/L	≤ 2.8 mmol/L	≤ 3.9 mmol/L	3.9< GLUCOSE <10.0 mmol/L	≥ 10.0 mmol/L	≥ 11.1 mmol/L
6.3	**2.2**	**0%**	**10%**	**83%**	**7%**	**3%**

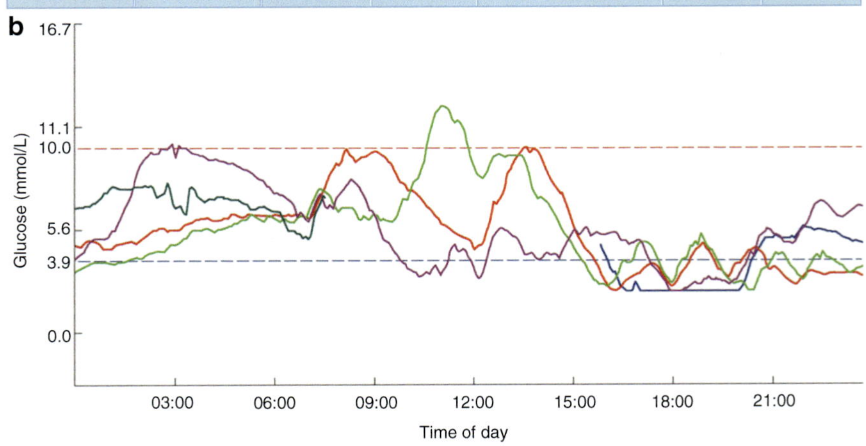

GLUCOSE EXPOSURE	GLUCOSE VARIABILITY	Dangerously Low	Low	GLUCOSE RANGES In Target Range	High	High
MBG mmol/L	SDBG mmol/L	≤ 2.8 mmol/L	≤ 3.9 mmol/L	3.9< GLUCOSE <10.0 mmol/L	≥ 10.0 mmol/L	≥ 11.1 mmol/L
5.5	**2.2**	**9%**	**27%**	**71%**	**2%**	**1%**

Fig. 15.3 Case 2: The CGM profiles of one case of fulminant type 1 diabetes treated with an insulin pump before and 6 months later

the basal rate of the insulin pump from before dinner to bedtime, in order to increase the target glucose level.

Case 3 (Fig. 15.4): A patient was initially treated with four times daily subcutaneous insulin injections with insulin dose of 0.95 U/(kg·d),

a

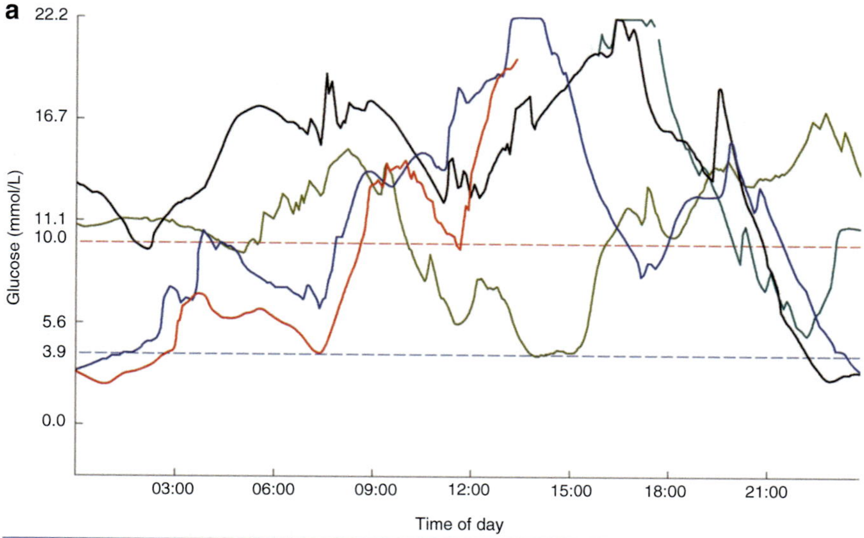

GLUCOSE EXPOSURE	GLUCOSE VARIABILITY	Dangerously Low	Low	GLUCOSE RANGES In Target Range	High	High
MBG mmol/L	SDBG mmol/L	≤ 2.8 mmol/L	≤ 3.9 mmol/L	3.9< GLUCOSE <10.0 mmol/L	≥ 10.0 mmol/L	≥ 11.1 mmol/L
11.5	**5.0**	**2%**	**7%**	**29%**	**64%**	**54%**

b

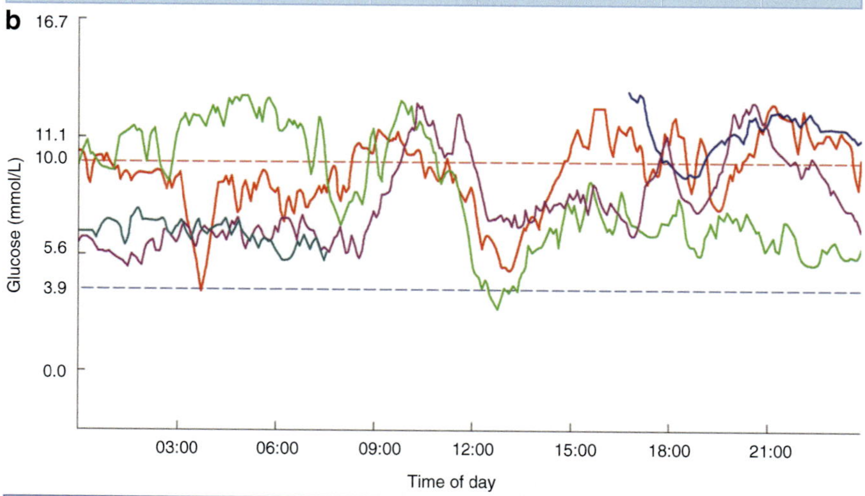

GLUCOSE EXPOSURE	GLUCOSE VARIABILITY	Dangerously Low	Low	GLUCOSE RANGES In Target Range	High	High
MBG mmol/L	SDBG mmol/L	≤ 2.8 mmol/L	≤ 3.9 mmol/L	3.9< GLUCOSE<10.0 mmol/L	≥ 10.0 mmol/L	≥ 11.1 mmol/L
8.7	**2.3**	**0%**	**1%**	**66%**	**33%**	**20%**

Fig. 15.4 Case 3: The CGM profiles of a fulminant type 1 diabetes patient changing from subcutaneous insulin injection to insulin pump therapy

but the patient had poor control of blood glucose, with MBG of 11.5 mmol/L, SDBG of 5.0 mmol/L, and largest amplitude of glycemic excursion (LAGE) of 6.1 mmol/L (reference range < 1.4 mmol/L), and the occurrence of asymptomatic nocturnal hypoglycemia (Fig. 15.4a). After transferring to insulin pump treatment with an insulin dose of 0.9 U/(kg·d), there were significant improvements in the blood glucose levels and the degree of variability. The MBG was 8.7 mmol/L, SDBG was 2.3 mmol/L, and LAGE was decreased to 2.9 mmol/L (Fig. 15.4b). The results showed that the CGM facilitated the understanding of the patient's blood glucose variability, and the insulin pump might help to control blood glucose variability in fulminant type 1 diabetes patients, thereby reducing the incidence of hypoglycemia and achieving satisfactory glycemic control.

Statement on Consent for Participation

All the clinical trials carried out by the authors in this book have been reported to the Ethics Committee of Shanghai Jiao Tong University Affiliated Sixth People's Hospital already and were in accordance with the Good Clinical Practice and Standards of China Association for Ethical Studies (approval number: 2007-45).

References

1. Imagawa A, Hanafusa T, Miyagawa J, Matsuzawa Y. A novel subtype of type 1 diabetes mellitus characterized by a rapid onset and an absence of diabetes-related antibodies. Osaka IDDM Study Group. N Engl J Med. 2000;342:301–7. https://doi.org/10.1056/NEJM200002033420501.
2. Deng D, Xia L, Chen M, Xu M, Wang Y, Wang C. A case of fulminant type 1 diabetes associated with acute renal failure. Neuro Endocrinol Lett. 2015;36:115–8.
3. Zhou J, Bao YQ, Li M, Liu F, Chen HB, Han JF, Lu W, Ma XJ, Hu C, Xiang KS, Jia WP. Fulminant type 1 diabetes: the clinical features and treatment strategy. Chin J Diabetes Mellitus. 2009;1:34–8. https://doi.org/10.3760/cma.j.issn.1674-5809.2009.01.011.
4. Dong H, Liu L, Zhou Y, Mu J, Zhang J. Sudden death of a 15-year-old girl due to fulminant type 1 diabetes mellitus-diabetic ketoacidosis induced cerebral edema? J Forensic Legal Med. 2014;26:5–9. https://doi.org/10.1016/j.jflm.2014.05.001.
5. Expert Committee on the Diagnosis and Classification of Diabetes Mellitus. Report of the expert committee on the diagnosis and classification of diabetes mellitus. Diabetes Care. 2003;26(Suppl 1):5–20.
6. The Expert Committee on the Diagnosis and Classification of Diabetes Mellitus. Report of the expert committee on the diagnosis and classification of diabetes mellitus. Diabetes Care. 1997;20:1183–97.
7. Alberti KG, Zimmet PZ. Definition, diagnosis and classification of diabetes mellitus and its complications. Part 1: diagnosis and classification of diabetes mellitus provisional report of a WHO consultation. Diabet Med. 1998;15:539–53. https://doi.org/10.1002/(SICI)1096-9136(199807)15:7<539::AID-DIA668>3.0.CO;2-S.
8. American Diabetes Association. Standards of Medical Care in Diabetes-2017. Diabetes Care. 2017;40(Suppl 1):1–135.
9. Imagawa A, Hanafusa T, Awata T, Ikegami H, Uchigata Y, Osawa H, Kawasaki E, Kawabata Y, Kobayashi T, Shimada A, Shimizu I, Takahashi K, Nagata M, Makino H, Maruyama T. Report of the Committee of the Japan Diabetes Society on the research of fulminant and acute-onset type 1 diabetes mellitus: new diagnostic criteria of fulminant type 1 diabetes mellitus (2012). J Diabetes Investig. 2012;3:536–9. https://doi.org/10.1111/jdi.12024.
10. Imagawa A, Hanafusa T. Series: clinical study from Japan and its reflections; a nationwide survey of fulminant type 1 diabetes. Nippon Naika Gakkai Zasshi. 2013;102:1829–35.
11. Cho YM, Kim JT, Ko KS, Koo BK, Yang SW, Park MH, Lee HK, Park KS. Fulminant type 1 diabetes in Korea: high prevalence among patients with adult-onset type 1 diabetes. Diabetologia. 2007;50:2276–9. https://doi.org/10.1007/s00125-007-0812-z.
12. Tsutsumi C, Imagawa A, Ikegami H, Makino H, Kobayashi T, Hanafusa T, Japan Diabetes Society Committee on Type 1 Diabetes Mellitus Research. Class II HLA genotype in fulminant type 1 diabetes: a nationwide survey with reference to glutamic acid decarboxylase antibodies. J Diabetes Investig. 2012;3:62–9. https://doi.org/10.1111/j.2040-1124.2011.00139.x.
13. Shimizu I, Makino H, Imagawa A, Iwahashi H, Uchigata Y, Kanatsuka A, Kawasaki E, Kobayashi T, Shimada A, Maruyama T, Hanafusa T. Clinical and immunogenetic characteristics of fulminant type 1 diabetes associated with pregnancy. J Clin Endocrinol Metab. 2006;91:471–6. https://doi.org/10.1210/jc.2005-1943.
14. Kwak SH, Kim YJ, Chae J, Lee CH, Han B, Kim JI, Jung HS, Cho YM, Park KS. Association of HLA genotype and fulminant type 1 diabetes in Koreans. Genomics Inform. 2015;13:126–31. https://doi.org/10.5808/GI.2015.13.4.126.
15. Zheng C, Zhou Z, Yang L, Lin J, Huang G, Li X, Zhou W, Wang X, Liu Z. Fulminant type 1 diabetes mellitus exhibits distinct clinical and autoimmunity features from classical type 1 diabetes mellitus in Chinese.

Diabetes Metab Res Rev. 2011;27:70–8. https://doi.org/10.1002/dmrr.1148.

16. Jung JH, Hahm JR, Kim MA, Park MH, Kim DR, Jung TS, Chung SI. Fulminant autoantibody-negative and type 1A diabetes phenotypes in a Korean HLA identical dizygotic twin. Diabetes Care. 2005;28:2330–1.
17. Imagawa A, Hanafusa T, Uchigata Y, Kanatsuka A, Kawasaki E, Kobayashi T, Shimada A, Shimizu I, Toyoda T, Maruyama T, Makino H. Fulminant type 1 diabetes: a nationwide survey in Japan. Diabetes Care. 2003;26:2345–52.
18. Imagawa A, Hanafusa T, Makino H, Miyagawa JI, Juto P. High titres of IgA antibodies to enterovirus in fulminant type-1 diabetes. Diabetologia. 2005;48:290–3. https://doi.org/10.1007/s00125-004-1624-z.
19. Imagawa A, Hanafusa T. Fulminant type 1 diabetes--an important subtype in East Asia. Diabetes Metab Res Rev. 2011;27:959–64. https://doi.org/10.1002/dmrr.1236.
20. Tanaka S, Aida K, Nishida Y, Kobayashi T. Pathophysiological mechanisms involving aggressive islet cell destruction in fulminant type 1 diabetes. Endocr J. 2013;60:837–45.
21. Minegaki Y, Higashida Y, Ogawa M, Miyachi Y, Fujii H, Kabashima K. Drug-induced hypersensitivity syndrome complicated with concurrent fulminant type 1 diabetes mellitus and Hashimoto's thyroiditis. Int J Dermatol. 2013;52:355–7. https://doi.org/10.1111/j.1365-4632.2011.05213.x.
22. Aida K, Nishida Y, Tanaka S, Maruyama T, Shimada A, Awata T, Suzuki M, Shimura H, Takizawa S, Ichijo M, Akiyama D, Furuya F, Kawaguchi A, Kaneshige M, Itakura J, Fujii H, Endo T, Kobayashi T. RIG-I-and MDA5-initiated innate immunity linked with adaptive immunity accelerates beta-cell death in fulminant type 1 diabetes. Diabetes. 2011;60:884–9. https://doi.org/10.2337/db10-0795.
23. Mizutani T, Yoshimoto T, Kaneko R, Ishii A. Diagnosis of fulminant type 1 diabetes mellitus in an autopsy case with postmortem changes. Leg Med (Tokyo). 2011;13:250–3. https://doi.org/10.1016/j.legalmed.2011.05.007.
24. Shibasaki S, Imagawa A, Tauriainen S, Iino M, Oikarinen M, Abiru H, Tamaki K, Seino H, Nishi K, Takase I, Okada Y, Uno S, Murase-Mishiba Y, Terasaki J, Makino H, Shimomura I, Hyöty H, Hanafusa T. Expression of toll-like receptors in the pancreas of recent-onset fulminant type 1 diabetes. Endocr J. 2010;57:211–9.
25. Wang Z, Zheng Y, Hou C, Yang L, Li X, Lin J, Huang G, Lu Q, Wang CY, Zhou Z. DNA methylation impairs TLR9 induced Foxp3 expression by attenuating IRF-7 binding activity in fulminant type 1 diabetes. J Autoimmun. 2013;41:50–9. https://doi.org/10.1016/j.jaut.2013.01.009.
26. Adachi J, Mimura M, Gotyo N, Watanabe T. The development of fulminant type 1 diabetes during chemotherapy for rectal cancer. Intern Med. 2015;54:819–22. https://doi.org/10.2169/internalmedicine.54.3413.
27. Gaudy C, Clévy C, Monestier S, Dubois N, Préau Y, Mallet S, Richard MA, Grob JJ, Valéro R, Béliard S. Anti-PD1 pembrolizumab can induce exceptional fulminant type 1 diabetes. Diabetes Care. 2015;38:e182–3. https://doi.org/10.2337/dc15-1331.
28. Hughes J, Vudattu N, Sznol M, Gettinger S, Kluger H, Lupsa B, Herold KC. Precipitation of autoimmune diabetes with anti-PD-1 immunotherapy. Diabetes Care. 2015;38:e55–7. https://doi.org/10.2337/dc14-2349.
29. Onuma H, Tohyama M, Imagawa A, Hanafusa T, Kobayashi T, Kano Y, Ohashi J, Hashimoto K, Osawa H, Makino H, Japan Diabetes Society Committee on Type 1 Diabetes Mellitus Research, Japanese Dermatological Association. High frequency of HLA B62 in fulminant type 1 diabetes with the drug-induced hypersensitivity syndrome. J Clin Endocrinol Metab. 2012;97:E2277–81. https://doi.org/10.1210/jc.2012-2054.
30. Sekine N, Motokura T, Oki T, Umeda Y, Sasaki N, Hayashi M, Sato H, Fujita T, Kaneko T, Asano Y, Kikuchi K. Rapid loss of insulin secretion in a patient with fulminant type 1 diabetes mellitus and carbamazepine hypersensitivity syndrome. JAMA. 2001;285:1153–4. https://doi.org/10.1001/jama.285.9.1153.
31. Imagawa A, Hanafusa T. Fulminant type 1 diabetes mellitus. Endocr J. 2006;53:577–84.
32. Murase Y, Imagawa A, Hanafusa T, Iwahashi H, Uchigata Y, Kanatsuka A, Kawasaki E, Kobayashi T, Shimada A, Shimizu I, Maruyama T, Makino H. Fulminant type 1 diabetes as a high risk group for diabetic microangiopathy--a nationwide 5-year-study in Japan. Diabetologia. 2007;50:531–7. https://doi.org/10.1007/s00125-006-0575-y.
33. Koyano HM, Matsumoto T. Recovery from exocrine pancreatic insufficiency in a patient with fulminant type 1 diabetes. Intern Med. 2013;52:573–5. https://doi.org/10.2169/internalmedicine.52.9019.
34. Yamashita K, Sato Y, Seki K, Asano J, Funase Y, Yamauchi K, Aizawa T. Fulminant type 1 diabetes with robust recovery of insulin secretion: a case report. Diabetes Res Clin Pract. 2013;100:e34–8. https://doi.org/10.1016/j.diabres.2013.01.032.
35. Kaneko K, Satake C, Yamamoto J, Takahashi H, Sawada S, Imai J, Yamada T, Katagiri H. A case of idiopathic type 1 diabetes with subsequent recovery of endogenous insulin secretion despite initial diagnosis of fulminant type 1 diabetes. Endocr J. 2017;64:369–74. https://doi.org/10.1507/endocrj.EJ16-0245.
36. Chinese Diabetes Society. Chinese clinical guideline for continuous glucose monitoring (2012). Chin Med J. 2012;125:4167–74. https://doi.org/10.3760/cma.j.issn.0366-6999.2012.23.002.
37. Melki V, Ayon F, Fernandez M, Hanaire-Broutin H. Value and limitations of the Continuous Glucose Monitoring System in the management of type 1 diabetes. Diabetes Metab. 2006;32:123–9.
38. Cheyne EH, Kerr D. Making "sense" of diabetes: using a continuous glucose sensor in clinical practice.

Diabetes Metab Res Rev. 2002;18(Suppl 1):43–8. https://doi.org/10.1002/dmrr.209.
39. Boland E, Monsod T, Delucia M, Brandt CA, Fernando S, Tamborlane WV. Limitations of conventional methods of self-monitoring of blood glucose: lessons learned from 3 days of continuous glucose sensing in pediatric patients with type 1 diabetes. Diabetes Care. 2001;24:1858–62.
40. Edelman SV, Bailey TS. Continuous glucose monitoring health outcomes. Diabetes Technol Ther. 2009;11(Suppl 1):68–74. https://doi.org/10.1089/dia.2009.0012.
41. Schaepelynck-Bélicar P, Vague P, Simonin G, Lassmann-Vague V. Improved metabolic control in diabetic adolescents using the continuous glucose monitoring system (CGMS). Diabetes Metab. 2003;29:608–12.
42. Kaufman FR, Gibson LC, Halvorson M, Carpenter S, Fisher LK, Pitukcheewanont P. A pilot study of the continuous glucose monitoring system: clinical decisions and glycemic control after its use in pediatric type 1 diabetic subjects. Diabetes Care. 2001;24:2030–4.
43. Jensen MH, Christensen TF, Tarnow L, Seto E, Dencker Johansen M, Hejlesen OK. Real-time hypoglycemia detection from continuous glucose monitoring data of subjects with type 1 diabetes. Diabetes Technol Ther. 2013;15:538–43. https://doi.org/10.1089/dia.2013.0069.
44. Bhide M, Grey JM, Moser EG, Garg SK. A primary care perspective on the use of continuous glucose monitoring in clinical practice. Diabetes Technol Ther. 2013;15:533–7. https://doi.org/10.1089/dia.2013.0169.
45. Juvenile Diabetes Research Foundation Continuous Glucose Monitoring Study Group. Effectiveness of continuous glucose monitoring in a clinical care environment: evidence from the Juvenile Diabetes Research Foundation continuous glucose monitoring (JDRF-CGM) trial. Diabetes Care. 2010;33:17–22. https://doi.org/10.2337/dc09-1502.
46. Battelino T, Phillip M, Bratina N, Nimri R, Oskarsson P, Bolinder J. Effect of continuous glucose monitoring on hypoglycemia in type 1 diabetes. Diabetes Care. 2011;34:795–800. https://doi.org/10.2337/dc10-1989.
47. Sachedina N, Pickup JC. Performance assessment of the Medtronic-MiniMed Continuous Glucose Monitoring System and its use for measurement of glycaemic control in Type 1 diabetic subjects. Diabet Med. 2003;20:1012–5. https://doi.org/10.1046/j.1464-5491.2003.01037.x.
48. Juvenile Diabetes Research Foundation Continuous Glucose Monitoring Study Group, Tamborlane WV, Beck RW, Bode BW, Buckingham B, Chase HP, Clemons R, Fiallo-Scharer R, Fox LA, Gilliam LK, Hirsch IB, Huang ES, Kollman C, Kowalski AJ, Laffel L, Lawrence JM, Lee J, Mauras N, O'Grady M, Ruedy KJ, Tansey M, Tsalikian E, Weinzimer S, Wilson DM, Wolpert H, Wysocki T, Xing D. Continuous glucose monitoring and intensive treatment of type 1 diabetes. N Engl J Med. 2008;359:1464–76. https://doi.org/10.1056/NEJMoa0805017.
49. Garg SK, Voelmle MK, Beatson CR, Miller HA, Crew LB, Freson BJ, Hazenfield RM. Use of continuous glucose monitoring in subjects with type 1 diabetes on multiple daily injections versus continuous subcutaneous insulin infusion therapy: a prospective 6-month study. Diabetes Care. 2011;34:574–9. https://doi.org/10.2337/dc10-1852.
50. Juvenile Diabetes Research Foundation Continuous Glucose Monitoring Study Group, Beck RW, Buckingham B, Miller K, Wolpert H, Xing D, Block JM, Chase HP, Hirsch I, Kollman C, Laffel L, Lawrence JM, Milaszewski K, Ruedy KJ, Tamborlane WV. Factors predictive of use and of benefit from continuous glucose monitoring in type 1 diabetes. Diabetes Care. 2009;32:1947–53. https://doi.org/10.2337/dc09-0889.
51. Bergenstal RM, Tamborlane WV, Ahmann A, Buse JB, Dailey G, Davis SN, Joyce C, Peoples T, Perkins BA, Welsh JB, Willi SM, Wood MA, STAR 3 Study Group. Effectiveness of sensor-augmented insulin-pump therapy in type 1 diabetes. N Engl J Med. 2010;363:311–20. https://doi.org/10.1056/NEJMoa1002853.

Using Continuous Glucose Monitoring for Diabetes Mellitus in Pregnancy

16

X. J. Ma and J. Zhou

Pregnancy associated with diabetes includes pregestational diabetes mellitus and gestational diabetes mellitus. Pregestational diabetes mellitus refers to those diagnosed with diabetes prior to pregnancy, or those whose glucose levels are found to be above the diabetes diagnostic criteria for the first time. Gestational diabetes mellitus refers to those with abnormal glucose metabolism during pregnancy. It is noted that patients whose glucose levels are high enough to be considered as diabetes mellitus for the first time during pregnancy should be diagnosed with pregestational diabetes mellitus rather than gestational diabetes mellitus [1]. In both cases, hyperglycemia has a serious adverse effect on pregnancy and is related to adverse maternal and neonatal outcomes [2]. With the increasing incidence of diabetes mellitus, glycemic management during pregnancy has drawn a considerable attention among clinical practitioners. Comprehensive monitoring of glycemic variability in pregnant patients with diabetes is of great clinical significance to optimize the hypoglycemic treatment regimen. Continuous glucose monitoring (CGM) technology helps us to continuously monitor glucose levels in patients, therefore tracking the trend of glycemic variability throughout the day. Also, CGM can detect hyperglycemia and hypoglycemia which are not easily identified with the traditional methods. This is conducive to glycemic management of pregnant women with diabetes and thereby improves the outcome of pregnancy.

X. J. Ma · J. Zhou (✉)
Department of Endocrinology and Metabolism, Shanghai Clinical Center for Diabetes, Shanghai Diabetes Institute, Shanghai Jiao Tong University Affiliated Sixth People's Hospital, Shanghai, China
e-mail: zhoujian@sjtu.edu.cn

16.1 Clinical Characteristics of Diabetes Mellitus in Pregnancy

The incidence of diabetes mellitus in pregnancy has been increasing due to the global epidemic of diabetes mellitus and the improved screening for obstetric conditions such as gestational diabetes mellitus. A majority of diabetes mellitus in pregnancy is diagnosed as gestational diabetes mellitus, accounting for 80–90%, with the remainder pregestational diabetes mellitus, accounting for 10–20%.

Gestational hyperglycemia causes a serious adverse effect on the pregnancy outcome [3, 4]. If a mother's glucose levels were poorly controlled before or during early stages of pregnancy, the risk of fetal congenital malformations will be increased [5]. If this occurs during second or third trimester, the fetal is inclined to grow excessively large or fast, which increases the risks of birth injury and cesarean section [6, 7]. Other adverse outcomes include stillbirth, neonatal hypoglycemia, and neonatal respiratory distress syndrome. In addition, diabetes in pregnancy may increase the risk of type 2 diabetes mellitus in offspring when they grow up.

W. Jia (ed.), *Continuous Glucose Monitoring*, https://doi.org/10.1007/978-981-10-7074-7_16

16.2 Diagnostic Criteria of Diabetes Mellitus in Pregnancy

For patients already diagnosed with diabetes mellitus before pregnancy, their diagnosis is relatively easy to make (Table 16.1) [1, 8]. In contrast, pregnant women with gestational diabetes mellitus usually have no symptoms, and the fasting plasma glucose (FPG) in most of them is also normal. Therefore, misdiagnosis is not uncommon if the diagnosis is based on the FPG examination alone. In 2001, the National Institutes of Health sponsored a global multicenter prospective study [2], i.e., the "Hyperglycemia and Adverse Pregnancy Outcomes study." This study involved a total of 25,305 pregnant women in 15 medical centers in 9 countries (Asia included). All the pregnant women underwent a 75-g oral glucose tolerance test (OGTT) at 24–32 weeks' gestation. The results showed that with the increase of maternal glucose level, the risks of adverse outcomes such as birth weight that is large for gestational age (LGA), fetal hyperinsulinemia, and excess fetal adiposity also increased. Even higher glucose levels (lower than those diagnostic of diabetes mellitus) are associated with increased risks of fetal macrosomia. Based on the above results, the International Association of Diabetes and Pregnancy Study Groups (IADPSG) updated the diagnosis criteria for gestational diabetes mellitus in 2010 (Table 16.2) [9].

Table 16.1 Diagnostic criteria for pregestational diabetes mellitus [1] (Reprinted with permission from Chinese Journal of Obstetrics and Gynecology)

Classification	FPG (mmol/L)	2-h 75-g OGTT plasma glucose (mmol/L)	HbA_{1c} (%[mmol/mol])
Normal glucose tolerance	<5.6	<7.8	<5.7 (39)
Impaired glucose tolerance	<5.6	7.8–11.0	5.7–6.4 (39–46)
Impaired fasting blood glucose	5.6–6.9	<7.8	5.7–6.4 (39–46)
Diabetes mellitus	≥7.0	or ≥11.1	≥6.5 (48)

Note: *FPG* fasting plasma glucose, *OGTT* oral glucose tolerance test, *HbA_{1c}* glycated hemoglobin A_{1c}

Table 16.2 Diagnostic criteria for gestational diabetes mellitus [9] (Reprinted with permission from Diabetes Care)

Diagnostic criteria	Plasma glucose values (mmol/L)
1. FPG or with the following	≥5.1
2. 1-h 75-g OGTT plasma glucose or with the following	≥10.0
3. 2-h 75-g OGTT plasma glucose	≥8.5

Note: *FPG* fasting plasma glucose, *OGTT* oral glucose tolerance test

For pregnant women with FPG values of not more than 4.4 mmol/L at 24–28 weeks' gestation in regions lacking medical resources, they can temporarily not undergo 75-g OGTT examination

The diagnosis of gestational diabetes mellitus is made when any one of the criteria in Table 16.2 is met

Since then, the American Diabetes Association (ADA) updated the diagnostic criteria for gestational diabetes mellitus in 2011 [10] and suggested that pregnant women at high risk of diabetes should undergo the glucose test in the initial prenatal checkup to rule out gestational diabetes mellitus. For those women who were not previously found to have overt diabetes mellitus or gestational diabetes mellitus, the IADPSG diagnostic criteria (2010) for gestational diabetes mellitus is recommended, and a 75-g OGTT, instead of 50-g glucose challenge test, at 24–28 weeks' gestation should be performed. In 2013, the World Health Organization (WHO) also accepted the diagnostic criteria proposed by IADPSG and ADA [11].

16.3 Glycemic Targets of Diabetes Mellitus in Pregnancy

Stringent glycemic control is the key to improve pregnancy outcomes. Both *Diagnosis and therapy guideline of pregnancy with diabetes mellitus (2014)* [1] and *Standards of Medical Care in*

Table 16.3 Glycemic targets of pregnant patients with diabetes

	FPG (mmol/L)	1-h postprandial blood glucose (mmol/L)	2-h postprandial blood glucose (mmol/L)	HbA_{1c} (%[mmol/mol])
2014 Chinese criteria				
Gestational diabetes mellitus	≤5.3	≤7.8	≤6.7	<5.5 (37)
Pregestational diabetes mellitus	3.3–5.6	5.6–7.1	5.6–7.1	<6.0 (42)
2016 ADA criteria				
Gestational diabetes mellitus	≤5.3	≤7.8	≤6.7	
Pregestational diabetes mellitus	≤5.0	7.2–7.8	≤6.7	
2017 ADA criteria				
Gestational diabetes mellitus/ pregestational diabetes mellitus	≤5.3	≤7.8	≤6.7	6.0–6.5 (42–48)[a]

[a]In the second and third trimesters, a target of 6.0–6.5% (42–48 mmol/mol) is recommended but 6.0% (42 mmol/mol) may be optimal as pregnancy progresses

Note: *FPG* fasting plasma glucose, *HbA_{1c}* glycated hemoglobin A_{1c}, *ADA* American Diabetes Association

Diabetes (2016) [12] by ADA have recommended appropriate glycemic targets in women with gestational diabetes mellitus and pregestational diabetes mellitus. In *Standards of Medical Care in Diabetes (2017)* [13], ADA has revised the glycemic targets for pregnant women with pregestational diabetes mellitus (the same for gestational diabetes mellitus) (Table 16.3).

16.4 The Application of CGM in Diabetes Mellitus in Pregnancy

Achieving near-normal glucose levels is the target for women with gestational diabetes mellitus or with pregestational diabetes mellitus. In the clinical practice, self-monitoring of blood glucose (SMBG) and CGM over three consecutive days are widely used. SMBG is the basic form of glucose monitoring. However, the data it collects is inherently momentary and is thus unable to reflect continuous and dynamic changes of blood glucose. On the other hand, CGM can track the blood glucose changes over 3 consecutive days and effectively complement SMBG.

CGM technology has been used in China since the year of 2001. Great progress in the clinical practice and research has been made. In recent years, real-time CGM technology has also been widely used. In 2012, the Chinese Diabetes Society (CDS) revised the *Chinese Clinical Guideline for Continuous Glucose Monitoring (2012)* [14] based on the 2009 edition. According to the guideline, CGM is recommended for pregnant women with diabetes mellitus.

Recently, researchers from China and overseas have conducted many studies on CGM technology in pregnant women with diabetes mellitus and achieved some progress [15].

16.4.1 Application of CGM to Detect Glycemic Variability in Pregnant Women with Diabetes Mellitus

Generally, a wide glycemic fluctuation is likely to appear in pregestational diabetes mellitus patients, among whom pregestational type 1 diabetes patients (Fig. 16.1) have a larger glycemic variability than those with pregestational type 2 diabetes (Fig. 16.2), while glycemic variability in patients with gestational diabetes mellitus is relatively small (Figs. 16.3 and 16.4) [12]. CGM provides continuous, comprehensive, and reliable information on glucose levels. By using CGM, the amplitude and trend of glycemic variability in short period can be detected, and quantitative assessments of glycemic variability can be achieved by calculating some indicators such as mean amplitude of glycemic excursion (MAGE),

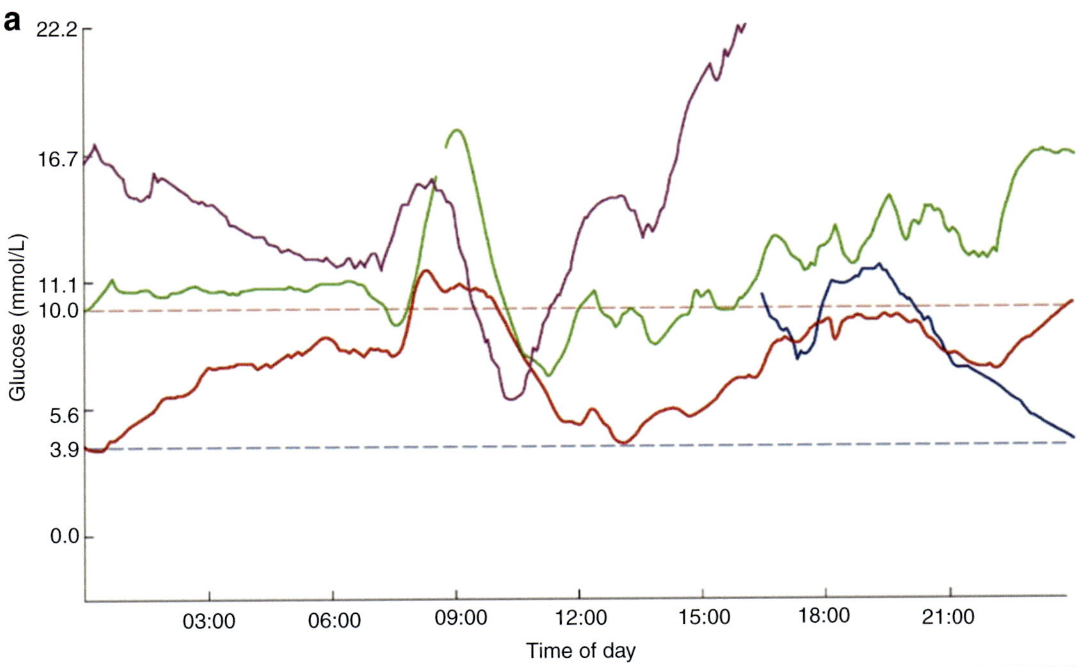

GLUCOSE EXPOSURE	GLUCOSE VARIABILITY	Dangerously Low	Low	GLUCOSE RANGES In Target Range	High	High
MBG mmol/L	SDBG mmol/L	≤ 2.8 mmol/L	≤ 3.9 mmol/L	3.9< GLUCOSE<10.0 mmol/L	≥ 10.0 mmol/L	≥ 11.1 mmol/L
10.3	**3.5**	**0%**	**1%**	**47%**	**52%**	**34%**

Fig. 16.1 CGM profiles of a patient with pregestational type 1 diabetes mellitus. Note: A 28-year-old female at 12 weeks' gestation was diagnosed as type 1 diabetes 4 years ago. The patient was given subcutaneous injections of insulin four times a day including short-acting insulin three times and intermediate-acting insulin once. The patient's glycemic control was poor. The patient had HbA_{1c} concentration of 12.5% (113 mmol/mol) and large glycemic variability as well as high mean blood glucose by CGM. Also, the patient presented with irregular nocturnal hyperglycemia and hypoglycemia. The use of an insulin pump for treatment was considered (**a**). After the patient switched to an insulin pump for 2 weeks, the patient was followed up with CGM. The glycemic control was significantly improved. Three-day CGM profile showed frequent hypoglycemia before lunch, and the basal rate of the insulin pump was adjusted accordingly (**b**). In addition, the patient presented hypoglycemia on the first day of glucose monitoring and even had asymptomatic hypoglycemia which lasted for up to 4 h at night. The basal rate of the insulin pump at night was reduced subsequently, and there was no hypoglycemia detected during nighttime on the third and fourth days of monitoring (**c**)

b

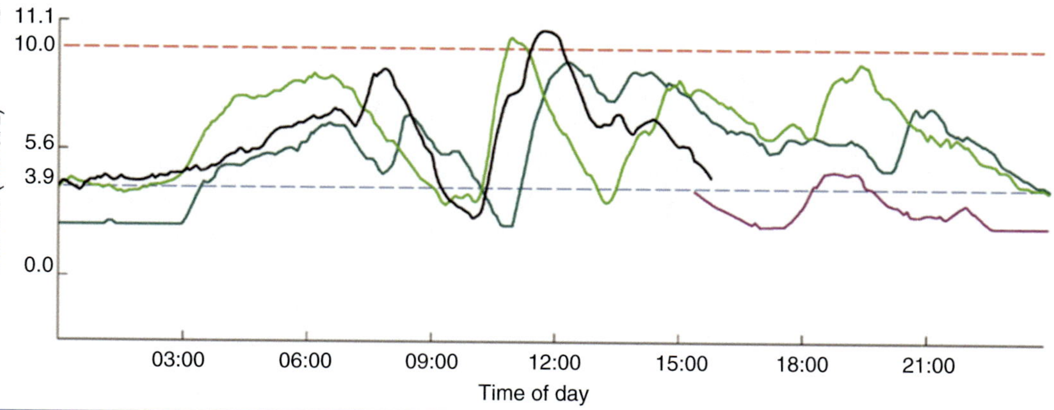

GLUCOSE EXPOSURE	GLUCOSE VARIABILITY	Dangerously Low	Low	GLUCOSE RANGES In Target Range	High	High
MBG mmol/L	SDBG mmol/L	≤ 2.8 mmol/L	≤ 3.9 mmol/L	3.9< GLUCOSE <10.0 mmol/L	≥ 10.0 mmol/L	≥ 11.1 mmol/L
5.6	**2.1**	**11%**	**21%**	**77%**	**2%**	**0%**

c

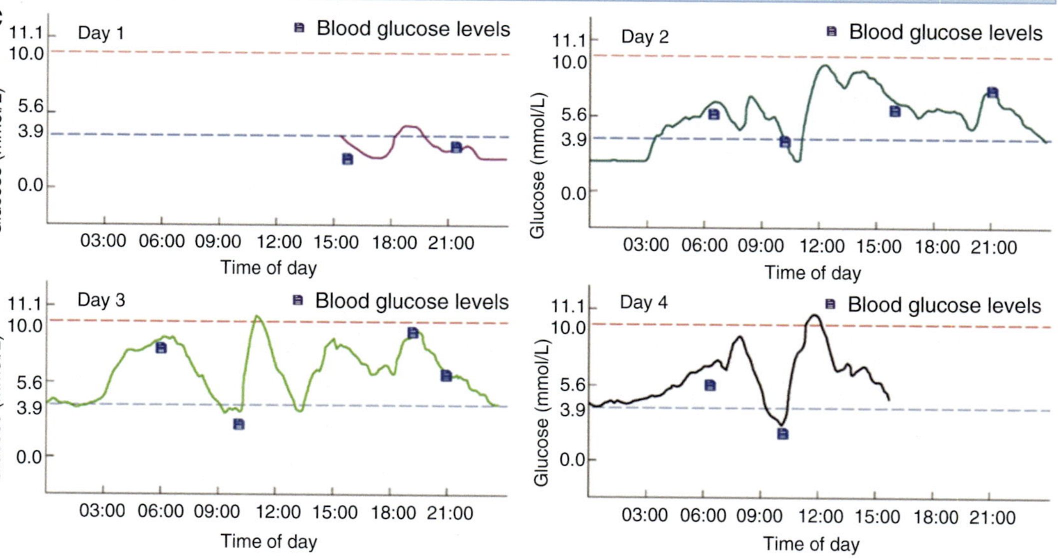

Fig. 16.1 (continued)

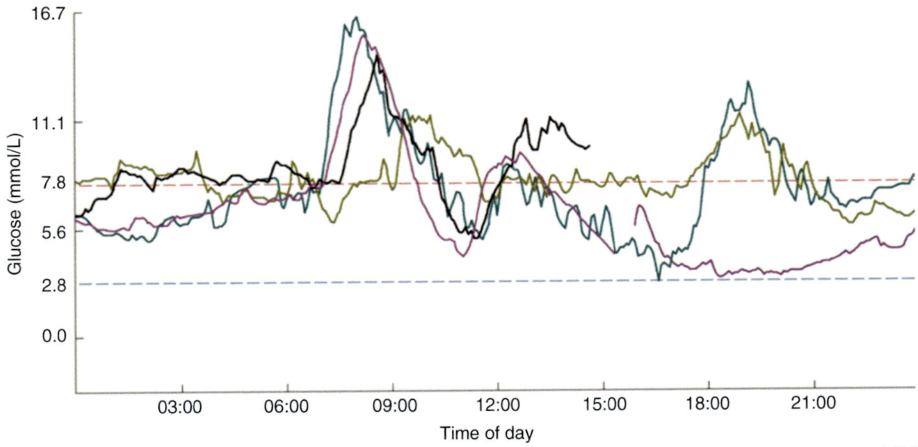

GLUCOSE EXPOSURE	GLUCOSE VARIABILITY	Dangerously Low	Low	GLUCOSE RANGES In Target Range	High	High
MBG mmol/L	SDBG mmol/L	≤ 2.8 mmol/L	≤ 3.9 mmol/L	3.9< GLUCOSE <10.0 mmol/L	≥ 10.0 mmol/L	≥ 11.1 mmol/L
7.5	**2.3**	**0%**	**7%**	**81%**	**12%**	**6%**

Fig. 16.2 CGM profiles of a patient with pregestational type 2 diabetes mellitus. Note: A 31-year-old female patient with pregestational type 2 diabetes mellitus was treated with insulin therapy. The HbA_{1c} concentration was 5.6% (38 mmol/mol), and the glycated albumin (GA) concentration was 14.0% (a false low result). But the CGM result suggested poor glycemic control. Further treatment adjustment was needed

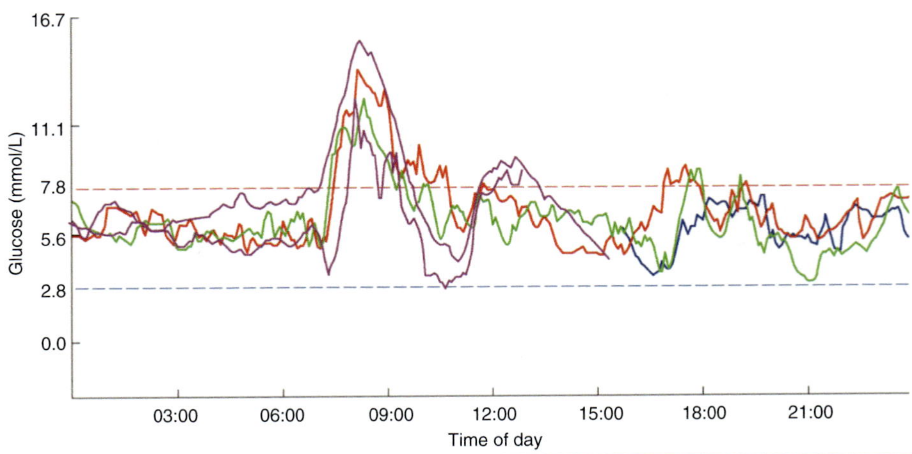

GLUCOSE EXPOSURE	GLUCOSE VARIABILITY	Dangerously Low	Low	GLUCOSE RANGES In Target Range	High	High
MBG mmol/L	SDBG mmol/L	≤ 2.8 mmol/L	≤ 3.9 mmol/L	3.9< GLUCOSE <10.0 mmol/L	≥ 10.0 mmol/L	≥ 11.1 mmol/L
6.3	**1.7**	**0%**	**5%**	**91%**	**4%**	**3%**

Fig. 16.3 CGM profiles of a gestational diabetes mellitus patient. Note: A 35-year-old female at 24 weeks' gestation underwent a 75-g OGTT examination. Fasting plasma glucose, 1-h 75-g OGTT plasma glucose, and 2-h 75-g OGTT plasma glucose were 5.6 mmol/L, 11.4 mmol/L, and 8.9 mmol/L, respectively. The HbA_{1c} concentration was 4.8% (29 mmol/mol), and the GA concentration was 15.0%. The CGM result showed that the patient had fewer glycemic fluctuations than pregestational diabetes mellitus patients. In addition, all cases above suggested that during pregnancy, the concentrations of HbA_{1c} and GA were falsely reduced, which could not timely reflect the real situation

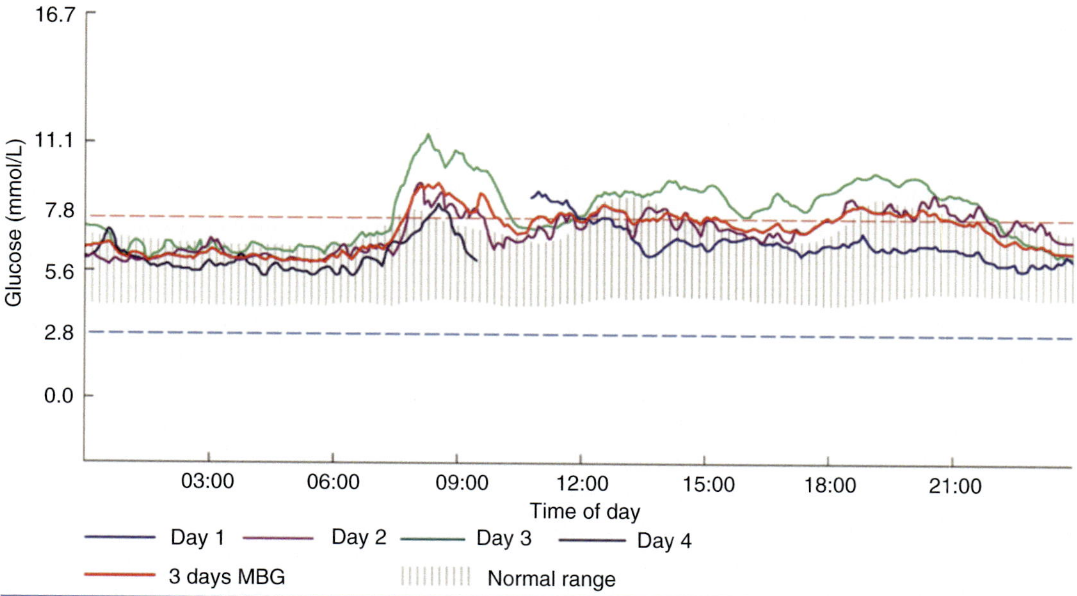

GLUCOSE EXPOSURE	GLUCOSE VARIABILITY	Dangerously Low	Low	GLUCOSE RANGES In Target Range	High	High
MBG mmol/L	SDBG mmol/L	≤ 2.8 mmol/L	≤ 3.9 mmol/L	3.9< GLUCOSE <10.0 mmol/L	≥ 10.0 mmol/L	≥ 11.1 mmol/L
7.2	**1.2**	**0%**	**0%**	**98%**	**2%**	**0%**

Fig. 16.4 The comparison of CGM profiles between a gestational diabetes mellitus patient and a normal control. Note: A 22-year-old female at 30 weeks' gestation was diagnosed with gestational diabetes mellitus. Her CGM profile presented a pattern of increasing postprandial glucose levels, especially after breakfast, when compared with the normal reference values established by our clinical center (the shadow area)

standard deviation of blood glucose (SDBG), and mean of daily differences (MODD) [14].

In recent years, some researchers have used CGM to compare and analyze glycemic variability in pregnant women with diabetes mellitus. In 2007, Murphy et al. [16] followed up 57 women with pregestational type 1 (n = 40) or type 2 (n = 17) diabetes mellitus with 7-day CGM system during each trimester. The study showed that the percentage of time (PT) while blood glucose over 7.8 mmol/L decreased with advancing gestation for women with both types of diabetes, while the rate of decrease was significantly greater in subjects with type 2 than type 1 diabetes. Moreover, women with type 2 diabetes spent approximately 33% less time hyperglycemic (>7.8 mmol/L) throughout pregnancy than those with type 1 diabetes. Although women with type 2 diabetes spent less overall time hypoglycemic, their risk of nocturnal hypoglycemia was equivalent to that of women with type 1 diabetes. In 2013, Dalfrà et al. [17] conducted CGM on 50 pregnant women (20 with pregestational type 1 diabetes mellitus, 20 with gestational diabetes mellitus, and 10 healthy controls) in all 3 trimesters of pregnancy. MAGE, SDBG, and other parameters were used for evaluation. It was found that women with pregestational type 1 diabetes mellitus showed higher glycemic variability than healthy pregnant women and gestational diabetes mellitus ones. In 2016, Tonoike et al. [18] also found that compared to women without glucose intolerance (both pregnant and nonpregnant), pregnant women with glucose intolerance exhibited greater glucose fluctuations with relativity higher MAGE and SDBG values.

16.4.2 Application of CGM in Guiding Antidiabetic Therapy in Pregnant Women with Diabetes Mellitus

Although optimal glycemic target can be achieved by lifestyle intervention (diet control and exercise) alone in some pregnant women, insulin therapy is still needed in a majority of gestational diabetes mellitus and pregestational diabetes mellitus patients. Two types of insulin regimens are commonly used. One is multiple daily injections of prandial insulin and basal insulin, and the other is continuous subcutaneous insulin infusion (CSII), which is also known as insulin pump therapy. Real-time CGM is helpful in adjusting insulin treatment regimen. The combination of real-time CGM and CSII can be used in two ways [19]. One is "open-loop," whereby the patient reads the CGM values and manually adjusts the CSII pump, or "closed-loop," whereby the CGM values are fed electronically directly into the pump with a personalized algorithm. The latter methodology, or "artificial pancreas," which is mainly composed of three parts, a glucose sensor, a feedback regulator system, and an insulin infusion system, is considered as the goal of further development.

In 2011, Petrovski et al. [20] evaluated the role of real-time CGM in guiding insulin pump therapy. The study included 25 women with type 1 diabetes with newly diagnosed pregnancy treated with insulin pump therapy for at least 1 year. All subjects were randomized into two groups: constant CGM group (n = 12) and intermittent CGM group (n = 13; 14 days/month). Both groups achieved good glycemic control during their pregnancies, and there was no significant difference in pregnancy outcomes, such as HbA_{1c} levels, fetal macrosomia, cesarean section, and severe hypoglycemia. The study indicated that CSII therapy together with constant or intermittent CGM could improve glycemic control and pregnancy outcomes in type 1 diabetes mellitus. However, the limitation of this study included the small sample size, as well as the lack of pump-only control group.

Albeit lacking sufficient clinical data, the closed-loop system has a similar effect of the "artificial pancreas" and a great prospect in the management of pregnant women with diabetes mellitus. In 2011, Murphy et al. [21] evaluated closed-loop insulin delivery with a model predictive control (MPC) algorithm over 24 h during early (12–16 weeks) and late gestation (28–32 weeks) in 10 pregnant women with pregestational type 1 diabetes mellitus. Based on real-time CGM results, the basal insulin infusion rate was adjusted every 15 min. Results showed that during closed-loop insulin delivery, median plasma glucose levels were 6.5 mmol/L in early and 7.0 mmol/L in late gestation. Overnight mean time spent with hyperglycemic (>7.8 mmol/L) was 7% in early and 0% in late pregnancy. No nocturnal hypoglycemia occurred. Postprandial glycemic control was not as ideal as overnight glycemic control. The duration of hyperglycemia was 13% in early and 5% in late gestation. Conclusively, the researchers demonstrated that overnight closed-loop insulin delivery with MPC algorithm could be used safely during pregnancy in pregestational diabetes mellitus. More work is needed to achieve optimal postprandial glycemic control. Subsequently, Murphy et al. [22] conducted a randomized controlled trial including 12 women with pregestational type 1 diabetes. Subjects were randomly allocated to closed-loop or conventional CSII. In closed-loop group, basal insulin infusion rates were manually adjusted at 15-min intervals according to CGM glucose levels and the algorithm advice. In conventional CSII group, subjects set temporary basal rates and used correction boluses according to capillary glucose measurements. After analysis, the study showed that closed-loop insulin delivery was as effective as conventional CSII but potentially safer, with reduced extent and duration of hypoglycemia. But on the other hand, some studies reported that hybrid closed-loop automated insulin delivery was associated with few serious or device-related adverse events, so it is worth noting that although this technology is now commercially available as a "hybrid closed-loop", it is not yet suitable for pregnancy because the target glucose of 6.7 mmol/L (120.6 mg/dL) is too high for pregnancy [23, 24].

16.4.3 Application of CGM to Improve Pregnancy Outcomes in Pregnant Women with Diabetes Mellitus

Previous study has shown that poor glycemic control before and during pregnancy in pregnant patients with diabetes is closely related to the occurrence of adverse pregnancy outcomes [25]. Stringent glycemic control during pregnancy plays a pivotal role in minimizing adverse pregnancy outcomes [26]. However, stringent glycemic control increases the risk of severe hypoglycemia [27], thus influencing glycemic control in patients [28]. Therefore, the optimal glucose range remains undetermined [29]. In recent years, quite a lot studies focus on the application of CGM in pregnant patients, hoping that stringent glycemic control will have advantages over gestation outcomes.

In 2008, Murphy et al. [30] conducted a prospective randomized controlled trial to evaluate the effectiveness of retrospective CGM during pregnancy on maternal glycemic control in women with type 1 and type 2 diabetes. A total of 71 women with type 1 diabetes ($n = 46$) or type 2 diabetes ($n = 25$) were allocated to antenatal care plus CGM ($n = 38$) or to standard antenatal care with SMBG ($n = 33$). CGM was performed in the retrospective CGM group for 5–7 days at intervals of 4–6 weeks. The study showed that women randomized into CGM had lower mean HbA_{1c} levels from 32 to 36 weeks' gestation compared with women randomized to standard antenatal care. Compared with infants of mothers in the control arm, those of mothers in the intervention arm had a reduced risk of macrosomia. There was no significant intergroup differences in terms of other outcomes, such as modes of delivery and neonatal morbidity.

In 2012, Voormolen et al. [31] applied retrospective CGM in 150 pregnant patients with diabetes for 5–7 days every 6 weeks. The researchers adjusted the insulin treatment regimen based on CGM results and gave dietary recommendations. Results showed that compared with the control group that received routine care alone, the use of CGM improved pregnancy outcomes, such as fetal macrosomia. In 2014, Secher et al. [32] found that the use of real-time CGM from early pregnancy onwards could help prevent severe hypoglycemia in a subpopulation of women with type 1 diabetes with a documented high risk of severe hypoglycemia in early pregnancy. Among 28 women with a recent history of severe hypoglycemia, 12 used real-time CGM. Among these 12 women, 8 experienced a total of 34 severe hypoglycemic events in the year before pregnancy and 9 experienced 23 events early in pregnancy. After initiation of real-time CGM, only two (17%) women experienced one event each.

Although a relatively large amount of evidences support that the use of CGM could effectively achieve glycemic control, improve fetal macrosomia, and reduce the occurrence of severe hypoglycemia and other adverse pregnancy outcomes, a few studies failed to confirm this result. In 2013, Secher et al. [33] conducted a randomized controlled trial to evaluate the effectiveness of real-time CGM. A total of 154 patients with pregestational type 1 or 2 diabetes mellitus were randomly assigned to use routine care only ($n = 75$) or real-time CGM ($n = 79$). Women assigned to the real-time CGM group used intermittently real-time CGM at 8, 12, 21, 27, and 33 gestational weeks. Results showed that there was no difference of HbA_{1c} values between both groups until the 33 weeks of pregnancy. The incidences of adverse pregnancy outcomes, such as hypoglycemic events, preeclampsia, cesarean section, neonatal hypoglycemia, were also similar in both groups. In addition, there was no significant intergroup difference in the incidence of fetal macrosomia either. Cordua et al. [34] also conducted a randomized controlled trial to explore whether the use of real-time CGM could reduce the prevalence of neonatal hypoglycemia [2-h plasma glucose (2hPG) <2.5 mmol/L]. Eighty-six patients with pregestational type 1 diabetes were divided randomly into two groups: a SMBG group ($n = 59$) and a real-time CGM group ($n = 27$). In the SMBG group, capillary glucose measuring was conducted every hour. In the real-time CGM group, capillary glucose level was also measured while using CGM. Results showed no significant difference in the incidence of neonatal hypoglycemia between these two groups. In 2016, Wei et al. [35] randomly assigned 106 women with gestational diabetes mellitus at 24–28 weeks' gestation to the CGM group or the SMBG group. The authors also found that there was no significant difference between two groups in terms of the incidence of adverse outcomes.

Therefore, the results of clinical trials are inconsistent, and these may be associated with different study subjects, type of diabetes mellitus, course of disease, etc. Multicentered, randomized controlled trials of large samples are needed before the extensive use of CGM in pregnant women with diabetes.

16.5 Summary and Prospective

Stringent glycemic control during pregnancy in pregnant women with diabetes is very necessary to improve maternal and fetal outcomes. CGM can monitor the postprandial hyperglycemia and nocturnal hypoglycemia which cannot be detected by traditional methods of glucose monitoring, which is effective for glycemic management in pregnant women with diabetes. Real-time CGM technology allows clinicians to timely adjust treatment regimen based on blood glucose variations in patients, thus providing information for optimizing glycemic control and helping to reduce the incidence of adverse pregnancy outcomes. Combined with CSII, the closed-loop system which resembles an "artificial pancreas," with a promising potential, has been applied in the clinical practice.

Currently, most researches published on CGM and diabetes in pregnancy are primarily clinical observations, and few researches include cost-effectiveness analysis. Further studies are needed to explore whether pregnant women with diabetes can benefit from the use of CGM and which type of patients can benefit more from the retrospective CGM or real-time CGM. The future development of CGM technology should focus on the accuracy of probes, the patients' compliance, and the reduction of the cost of healthcare.

Statement on Consent for Participation
All the clinical trials carried out by the authors in this book have been reported to the Ethics Committee of Shanghai Jiao Tong University Affiliated Sixth People's Hospital already and were in accordance with the Good Clinical Practice and Standards of China Association for Ethical Studies (approval number: 2007-45).

References

1. Obstetrics Subgroup, Chinese Society of Obstetrics and Gynecology, Chinese Medical Association, Group of Pregnancy with Diabetes Mellitus, Chinese Society of Perinatal Medicine, Chinese Medical Association, Obstetrics Subgroup Chinese Society of Obstetrics and Gynecology Chinese Medical Association, Group of Pregnancy with Diabetes Mellitus Chinese Society of Perinatal Medicine Chinese Medical Association. Diagnosis and therapy guideline of pregnancy with diabetes mellitus. Zhonghua Fu Chan Ke Za Zhi. 2014;49:561–9. https://doi.org/10.3760/cma.j.issn.0529-567x.2014.08.001.
2. HAPO Study Cooperative Research Group, Metzger BE, Lowe LP, Dyer AR, Trimble ER, Chaovarindr U, Coustan DR, Hadden DR, McCance DR, Hod M, McIntyre HD, Oats JJ, Persson B, Rogers MS, Sacks DA. Hyperglycemia and adverse pregnancy outcomes. N Engl J Med. 2008;358:1991–2002. https://doi.org/10.1056/NEJMoa0707943.
3. Negrato CA, Mattar R, Gomes MB. Adverse pregnancy outcomes in women with diabetes. Diabetol Metab Syndr. 2012;4:41. https://doi.org/10.1186/1758-5996-4-41.
4. Catalano PM, McIntyre HD, Cruickshank JK, McCance DR, Dyer AR, Metzger BE, Lowe LP, Trimble ER, Coustan DR, Hadden DR, Persson B, Hod M, Oats JJ, HAPO Study Cooperative Research Group. The hyperglycemia and adverse pregnancy outcome study: associations of GDM and obesity with pregnancy outcomes. Diabetes Care. 2012;35:780–6. https://doi.org/10.2337/dc11-1790.
5. Bell R, Glinianaia SV, Tennant PW, Bilous RW, Rankin J. Peri-conception hyperglycaemia and nephropathy are associated with risk of congenital anomaly in women with pre-existing diabetes: a population-based cohort study. Diabetologia. 2012;55:936–47. https://doi.org/10.1007/s00125-012-2455-y.
6. Kerssen A, de Valk HW, Visser GH. Increased second trimester maternal glucose levels are related to extremely large-for-gestational-age infants in women

with type 1 diabetes. Diabetes Care. 2007;30:1069–74. https://doi.org/10.2337/dc05-1985.
7. Kc K, Shakya S, Zhang H. Gestational diabetes mellitus and macrosomia: a literature review. Ann Nutr Metab. 2015;66 Suppl 2:14-20. https://doi.org/10.1159/000371628.
8. Weng J, Ji L, Jia W, Lu J, Zhou Z, Zou D, Zhu D, Chen L, Chen L, Guo L, Guo X, Ji Q, Li Q, Li X, Liu J, Ran X, Shan Z, Shi L, Song G, Yang L, Yang Y, Yang W, Chinese Diabetes Society. Standards of care for type 2 diabetes in China. Diabetes Metab Res Rev. 2016;32:442–58. https://doi.org/10.1002/dmrr.2827.
9. International Association of Diabetes and Pregnancy Study Groups Consensus Panel, Metzger BE, Gabbe SG, Persson B, Buchanan TA, Catalano PA, Damm P, Dyer AR, Leiva AD, Hod M, Kitzmiler JL, Lowe LP, McIntyre HD, Oats JJ, Omori Y, Schmidt MI. International association of diabetes and pregnancy study groups recommendations on the diagnosis and classification of hyperglycemia in pregnancy. Diabetes Care. 2010;33:676–82. https://doi.org/10.2337/dc09-1848.
10. American Diabetes Association. Diagnosis and classification of diabetes mellitus. Diabetes Care. 2011;34 Suppl 1:62-9. https://doi.org/10.2337/dc11-S062.
11. WHO Guidelines Approved by the Guidelines Review Committee. Diagnostic criteria and classification of hyperglycaemia first detected in pregnancy. Geneva: World Health Organization; 2013.
12. American Diabetes Association. 12. Management of diabetes in pregnancy. Diabetes Care. 2016;39 Suppl 1:94-8. https://doi.org/10.2337/dc16-S015.
13. American Diabetes Association. 13. Management of diabetes in pregnancy. Diabetes Care. 2017;40 Suppl 1:114-9. https://doi.org/10.2337/dc17-S016.
14. Chinese Diabetes Society. Chinese clinical guideline for continuous glucose monitoring (2012). Chin Med J. 2012;125:4167–74. https://doi.org/10.3760/cma.j.issn.0366-6999.2012.23.002.
15. Hernandez TL, Barbour LA. A standard approach to continuous glucose monitor data in pregnancy for the study of fetal growth and infant outcomes. Diabetes Technol Ther. 2013;15:172–9. https://doi.org/10.1089/dia.2012.0223.
16. Murphy HR, Rayman G, Duffield K, Lewis KS, Kelly S, Johal B, Fowler D, Temple RC. Changes in the glycemic profiles of women with type 1 and type 2 diabetes during pregnancy. Diabetes Care. 2007;30:2785–91. https://doi.org/10.2337/dc07-0500.
17. Dalfrà MG, Chilelli NC, Di Cianni G, Mello G, Lencioni C, Biagioni S, Scalese M, Sartore G, Lapolla A. Glucose fluctuations during gestation: an additional tool for monitoring pregnancy complicated by diabetes. Int J Endocrinol. 2013;2013:279021. https://doi.org/10.1155/2013/279021.
18. Tonoike M, Kishimoto M, Yamamoto M, Yano T, Noda M. Continuous glucose monitoring in patients with abnormal glucose tolerance during pregnancy: a case series. Jpn Clin Med. 2016;7:1–8. https://doi.org/10.4137/JCM.S34825.
19. Combs CA. Continuous glucose monitoring and insulin pump therapy for diabetes in pregnancy. J Matern Fetal Neonatal Med. 2012;25:2025–7. https://doi.org/10.3109/14767058.2012.670409.
20. Petrovski G, Dimitrovski C, Bogoev M, Milenkovic T, Ahmeti I, Bitovska I. Is there a difference in pregnancy and glycemic outcome in patients with type 1 diabetes on insulin pump with constant or intermittent glucose monitoring? A pilot study. Diabetes Technol Ther. 2011;13:1109–13. https://doi.org/10.1089/dia.2011.0081.
21. Murphy HR, Elleri D, Allen JM, Harris J, Simmons D, Rayman G, Temple R, Dunger DB, Haidar A, Nodale M, Wilinska ME, Hovorka R. Closed-loop insulin delivery during pregnancy complicated by type 1 diabetes. Diabetes Care. 2011;34:406–11. https://doi.org/10.2337/dc10-1796.
22. Murphy HR, Kumareswaran K, Elleri D, Allen JM, Caldwell K, Biagioni M, Simmons D, Dunger DB, Nodale M, Wilinska ME, Amiel SA, Hovorka R. Safety and efficacy of 24-h closed-loop insulin delivery in well-controlled pregnant women with type 1 diabetes: a randomized crossover case series. Diabetes Care. 2011;34:2527–9. https://doi.org/10.2337/dc11-1430.
23. Bergenstal RM, Garg S, Weinzimer SA, Buckingham BA, Bode BW, Tamborlane WV, Kaufman FR. Safety of a hybrid closed-loop insulin delivery system in patients with type 1 diabetes. JAMA. 2016;316:1407–8. https://doi.org/10.1001/jama.2016.11708.
24. Garg SK, Weinzimer SA, Tamborlane WV, Buckingham BA, Bode BW, Bailey TS, Brazg RL, Ilany J, Slover RH, Anderson SM, Bergenstal RM, Grosman B, Roy A, Cordero TL, Shin J, Lee SW, Kaufman FR. Glucose outcomes with the in-home use of a hybrid closed-loop insulin delivery system in adolescents and adults with type 1 diabetes. Diabetes Technol Ther. 2017;19:155–63. https://doi.org/10.1089/dia.2016.0421.
25. Lowe LP, Metzger BE, Dyer AR, Lowe J, McCance DR, Lappin TR, Trimble ER, Coustan DR, Hadden DR, Hod M, Oats JJ, Persson B, HAPO Study Cooperative Research Group. Hyperglycemia and adverse pregnancy outcome (HAPO) study: associations of maternal A1C and glucose with pregnancy outcomes. Diabetes Care. 2012;35:574–80. https://doi.org/10.2337/dc11-1687.
26. Hewapathirana NM, O'Sullivan E, Murphy HR. Role of continuous glucose monitoring in the management of diabetic pregnancy. Curr Diab Rep. 2013;13:34–42. https://doi.org/10.1007/s11892-012-0337-9.
27. Ringholm L, Pedersen-Bjergaard U, Thorsteinsson B, Damm P, Mathiesen ER. Hypoglycaemia during pregnancy in women with type 1 diabetes. Diabet Med. 2012;29:558–66. https://doi.org/10.1111/j.1464-5491.2012.03604.x.
28. Secher AL, Mathiesen ER, Andersen HU, Damm P, Ringholm L. Severe hypoglycemia in pregnant

women with type 2 diabetes-A relevant clinical problem. Diabetes Res Clin Pract. 2013;102:e17–8. https://doi.org/10.1016/j.diabres.2013.09.011.
29. Skupień J, Cyganek K, Małecki MT. Diabetic pregnancy: an overview of current guidelines and clinical practice. Curr Opin Obstet Gynecol. 2014;26:431–7. https://doi.org/10.1097/GCO.0000000000000111.
30. Murphy HR, Rayman G, Lewis K, Kelly S, Johal B, Duffield K, Fowler D, Campbell PJ, Temple RC. Effectiveness of continuous glucose monitoring in pregnant women with diabetes: randomised clinical trial. BMJ. 2008;337:a1680. https://doi.org/10.1136/bmj.a1680.
31. Voormolen DN, DeVries JH, Franx A, Mol BW, Evers IM. Effectiveness of continuous glucose monitoring during diabetic pregnancy (GlucoMOMS trial); a randomised controlled trial. BMC Pregnancy Childbirth. 2012;12:164. https://doi.org/10.1186/1471-2393-12-164.
32. Secher AL, Stage E, Ringholm L, Barfred C, Damm P, Mathiesen ER. Real-time continuous glucose monitoring as a tool to prevent severe hypoglycaemia in selected pregnant women with type 1 diabetes-an observational study. Diabet Med. 2014;31:352–6. https://doi.org/10.1111/dme.12383.
33. Secher AL, Ringholm L, Andersen HU, Damm P, Mathiesen ER. The effect of real-time continuous glucose monitoring in pregnant women with diabetes: a randomized controlled trial. Diabetes Care. 2013;36:1877–83. https://doi.org/10.2337/dc12-2360.
34. Cordua S, Secher AL, Ringholm L, Damm P, Mathiesen ER. Real-time continuous glucose monitoring during labour and delivery in women with type 1 diabetes - observations from a randomized controlled trial. Diabet Med. 2013;30:1374–81. https://doi.org/10.1111/dme.12246.
35. Wei Q, Sun Z, Yang Y, Yu H, Ding H, Wang S. Effect of a CGMS and SMBG on maternal and neonatal outcomes in gestational diabetes mellitus: a randomized controlled trial. Sci Rep. 2016;6:19920. https://doi.org/10.1038/srep19920.

Using Continuous Glucose Monitoring for Steroid-Induced Diabetes

17

J. Y. Lu and W. Jia

Steroid diabetes, also known as steroid-induced diabetes or glucocorticoid-induced diabetes, refers to a disorder of glucose metabolism caused by administration of exogenous glucocorticoids [1, 2]. According to the 1999 World Health Organization (WHO) diagnostic and classification criteria of diabetes mellitus, steroid diabetes is regarded as a special type of diabetes. Supraphysiologic doses of glucocorticoids, which have various potent pharmacological effects including anti-inflammatory, anti-allergic, and immunosuppressive actions, are indispensably used for the treatment of kidney, rheumatic, respiratory, hematological, and other systemic diseases. However, the use of supraphysiologic doses of glucocorticoids inevitably causes osteoporosis, gastrointestinal ulcers, glucose metabolism disorder, and other adverse reactions. In the 1940s, Ingle et al. [3] observed that administration of glucocorticoids could significantly elevate the blood glucose levels in rats and was the first to put forward the concept of steroid diabetes. Steroid diabetes is not rare, and it is more likely to arise following long course and high dose of glucocorticoid treatment. Improper handling of the condition will not only increase the risk of diabetes-related complications but also hamper the treatment of primary diseases. Cushing's syndrome is the most common etiology for excessive endogenous glucocorticoid-induced diabetes, which is also within the scope of this chapter.

J. Y. Lu · W. Jia (✉)
Department of Endocrinology and Metabolism, Shanghai Clinical Center for Diabetes, Shanghai Diabetes Institute, Shanghai Jiao Tong University Affiliated Sixth People's Hospital, Shanghai, China
e-mail: wpjia@sjtu.edu.cn

17.1 Clinical Characteristics of Steroid Diabetes

17.1.1 The Epidemiology of Steroid Diabetes

Generally, 40–45% of patients with Cushing's syndrome were reported to develop diabetes, and a further 10–30% of patients have impaired glucose tolerance (IGT) [4]. The prevalence of steroid diabetes in individuals treated with exogenous glucocorticoids varies among studies due to the differences in age, primary disease, dosage and course of steroids, study design, and others. However, the incidence of steroid diabetes is generally high. Studies have shown that among patients receiving glucocorticoid therapy, the risk of newly onset diabetes mellitus increases by 36–131% [5, 6].

W. Jia (ed.), *Continuous Glucose Monitoring*, https://doi.org/10.1007/978-981-10-7074-7_17

17.1.2 The Pathogenesis of Steroid Diabetes

Similar to type 2 diabetes mellitus, the pathogenesis of glucocorticoid-induced diabetes involves insulin resistance and islet β-cell dysfunction. The resultant glucose metabolic disorder is mainly attributed to decreased sensitivity to insulin in the liver, skeletal muscle, and adipose tissue [1]. The main pathogenic mechanisms include the following:

1. In the liver, glucocorticoids promote gluconeogenesis by upregulating the expression and activity of phosphoenolpyruvate carboxylase and glucose-6-phosphatase [7, 8] and increase hepatic glucose output. Moreover, glucocorticoids accelerate protein and fat catabolism, and the resulting metabolites can be used as substrates in the process of hepatic gluconeogenesis [9]. In addition, glucocorticoids have a permissive and synergistic effect with glycemic counter-regulatory hormones including glucagon, epinephrine, and growth hormone, further leading to elevated blood glucose [10].
2. In the skeletal muscle, glucocorticoids can decrease insulin-stimulated glucose uptake by 30–50% and reduce glycogen synthesis by 70%, through interference with post-receptor insulin signaling and inhibition of glucose transporter 4 (GLUT4) expression and its translocation from intracellular vesicles to the cell membrane [11]. The catabolic action of glucocorticoids increases the concentration of nonesterified fatty acids and amino acids in plasma, further inhibiting glucose uptake by skeletal muscle [12, 13].
3. Excessive glucocorticoids (both endogenous and exogenous) can lead to fat redistribution, manifested as reduced subcutaneous fat and increased visceral fat, and exacerbate insulin resistance [14]. Adipose tissues may be involved in the regulation of glycolipid metabolism by secreting a variety of adipokines [15]. Studies have shown that glucocorticoids can upregulate the levels of resistin and leptin and simultaneously downregulate the level of adiponectin, thereby worsening insulin resistance [16].
4. In islets, glucocorticoids cause impaired glucose-stimulated insulin secretion via downregulation of glucose transporter 2 (GLUT2) and glucokinase expression in β-cells [17]. The data in vitro have shown that glucocorticoids are able to induce the apoptosis of islet β-cells [18].

17.1.3 The Glycemic Characteristics of Steroid Diabetes

At present, there has been no study reported on the use of continuous glucose monitoring (CGM) system in patients with Cushing's syndrome for analysis of intraday blood glucose variability. However, several studies have investigated the glycemic characteristics of steroid diabetes by oral glucose tolerance test (OGTT). Mancini et al. [19] performed OGTT in 49 patients with untreated Cushing's syndrome. They found that 46.8% of patients with Cushing's syndrome met the diagnostic criteria for diabetes. It is noteworthy that 64% of diabetic patients presented a fasting plasma glucose (FPG) <6.1 mmol/L, and they were correctly diagnosed only after the OGTT. Friedman et al. [20] observed 16 patients with Cushing's syndrome and found that, compared to healthy obese individuals (control), patients with Cushing's syndrome had significantly elevated glucose levels but no elevated insulin response to the OGTT after glucose loading, revealing impaired insulin secretion as the main mechanism of elevated blood glucose in patients with Cushing's syndrome. In a study of 41 cases of adrenal incidentaloma, Terzolo et al. [21] found that FPG and 30-min glucose levels did not differ between patients and controls (with nonfunctioning adenoma), whereas 60-, 90-, and 120-min glucose levels were significantly higher in individuals with adrenal incidentaloma during OGTT. Taken together, these findings indicate that excessive secretion of endogenous glucocorticoids results in elevated blood glucose, especially hyperglycemia after an oral glucose loading.

Glucocorticoids are classified as short-, intermediate-, or long-acting hormones, based on the duration of action. Short-acting glucocorticoids have relatively weaker anti-inflammatory and immunosuppressive capacity, whereas long-acting glucocorticoids possess a marked inhibitory effect on the hypothalamic-pituitary-adrenal (HPA) axis. Therefore, intermediate-acting glucocorticoids are most widely used, such as prednisone, prednisolone, and methylprednisolone. Taking prednisone, for instance, it exhibits a peak effect at 4–8 h after administration and the duration of action lasts 12–16 h [22]. With once-daily administration in the morning, blood glucose often increases significantly in afternoon and at bedtime, whereas FPG may remain normal or be slightly elevated [23]. We find that patients with long-course and high-dosage glucocorticoid treatment are likely to develop fasting and morning hypoglycemia due to attenuated effects of exogenous glucocorticoids, as a result of complete inhibition of endogenous cortisol secretion. On the other hand, if glucocorticoids are given twice or more times daily, hyperglycemia is likely to be persistent.

The impact of exogenous glucocorticoids on glucose metabolism is usually reversible. In most cases, the blood glucose gradually returns to normal with the tapering or withdrawal of drugs. However, there is a proportion of patients who develop permanent hyperglycemia after cessation of glucocorticoids. Currently, data from large population-based studies regarding the effects of glucocorticoids on insulin sensitivity, islet function, and the incidence of diabetes are limited.

17.1.4 The Diagnosis and Treatment of Steroid Diabetes

Patients who have no previous history of diabetes, present with elevated blood glucose, and meet the diagnostic criteria for diabetes after glucocorticoid treatment can be diagnosed with steroid diabetes. Notably, detecting FPG alone is likely to increase the rate of missed diagnosis because of the unique glycemic characteristics of steroid diabetes. Especially for patients with once-daily morning administration of glucocorticoids, detection of blood glucose after lunch and dinner is important to facilitate timely diagnosis.

A variety of factors should be considered for the comprehensive treatment of steroid diabetes, including the type, dosage, course, and route of administration of glucocorticoids, primary diseases, and comorbidities of patients. The management of steroid diabetes is generally similar to that of type 2 diabetes, including lifestyle intervention (diet and exercise therapy) and medications. All classic antidiabetic agents including metformin, insulin secretagogues, thiazolidinedione, and insulin are suitable for the treatment of steroid diabetes. These agents should be employed with strict reference to the indications and contraindications in light of a patient's underlying and concomitant diseases and physical condition. Glucagon-like peptide-1 (GLP-1) analogs and dipeptidyl peptidase-4 (DPP-4) inhibitors are relatively new antidiabetic agents with pleotropic actions such as stimulating insulin secretion, protecting islet β-cells, and delaying gastric emptying. It has been reported that injection of exenatide can significantly improve glucocorticoid-induced hyperglycemia by promoting insulin secretion and inhibiting glucagon [24], suggesting that this kind of drug could be a new option for the treatment of steroid diabetes.

17.2 Application of CGM in Steroid Diabetes

As mentioned above, patients with Cushing's syndrome are characterized by hyperglycemia after glucose loading, due to excessive secretion of endogenous glucocorticoids. Regarding steroid diabetes induced by exogenous glucocorticoids, the glycemic characteristics depend on the type, dosage, course, and route of administration of the glucocorticoids used. Unlike those with typical type 2 diabetes, some patients with steroid diabetes exhibit normal or mild elevated FPG, or even hypoglycemia in the morning, with blood glucose rising remarkably from the afternoon until bedtime, especially for postprandial blood glucose. This intraday blood glucose variability often cannot be fully recognized by self-monitoring of blood glucose (SMBG), resulting in delay in the diagnosis and treatment. Here are five typical examples to illustrate the specific application of CGM in glucocorticoid-induced diabetes.

Case 1 A 55-year-old male patient presented with overt "polyuria, polydipsia, polyphagia, and weight loss" in 2011 with a FPG of 16 mmol/L. He was diagnosed with diabetes and treated with subcutaneous injection of premixed insulin twice a day (BID), totaling 52 U/day, combined with oral administration of metformin and pioglitazone. The patient had sustained poor glycemic control despite therapy. After admission, his glycated hemoglobin A_{1c} (HbA_{1c}) was 10.8% (95 mmol/mol) and glycated albumin (GA) was 22.3%. After adjustment of hypoglycemic treatment, the CGM (Fig. 17.1) showed improved glycemic control with FBG achieving the target goal. However, the patient still had postprandial hyperglycemia in the morning, which is similar to that seen in type 2 diabetes. A few months later, the patient presented with physical signs of moon face, buffalo hump, central obesity, and plethoric appearance. Laboratory tests showed that basal plasma cortisol levels were increased, and the diurnal rhythm disappeared. The cortisol levels were not suppressed in either low- or high-dose dexamethasone suppression test. Radiology revealed a left adrenal adenoma, approximately 3.3 cm × 2.6 cm in size (Fig. 17.2). The patient was diagnosed with Cushing's syndrome and later transferred to the Department of Urology. After resection of the left adrenal adenoma, the patient was only treated with premixed insulin at the dose

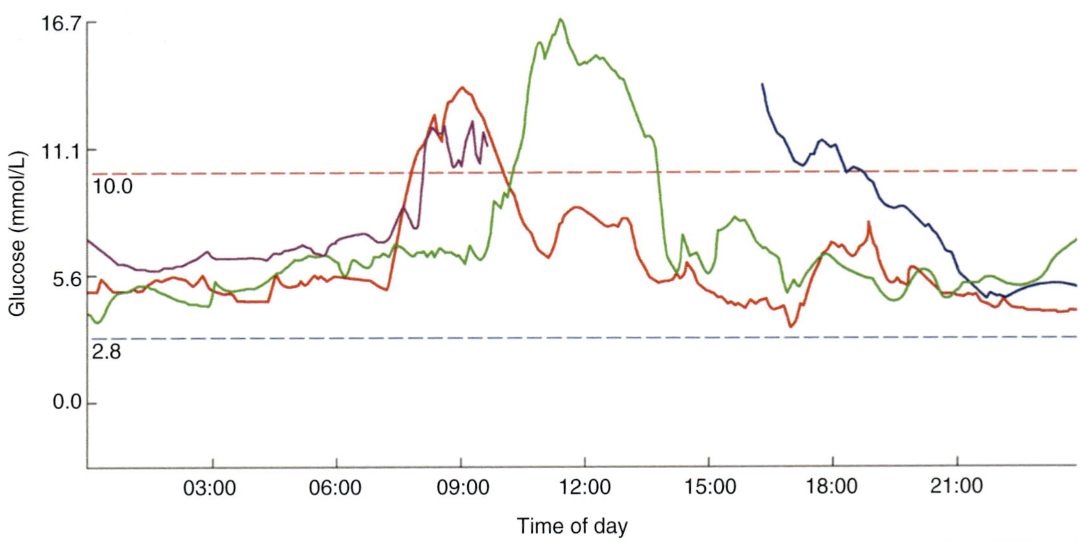

GLUCOSE EXPOSURE	GLUCOSE VARIABILITY	Dangerously Low	Low	GLUCOSE RANGES In Target Range	High	High
MBG mmol/L	SDBG mmol/L	≤ 2.8 mmol/L	≤ 3.9 mmol/L	3.9 < GLUCOSE < 10.0 mmol/L	≥ 10.0 mmol/L	≥ 11.1 mmol/L
6.8	**2.7**	**0%**	**1%**	**84%**	**15%**	**11%**

Fig. 17.1 Case 1: CGM profiles of a patient with Cushing's syndrome

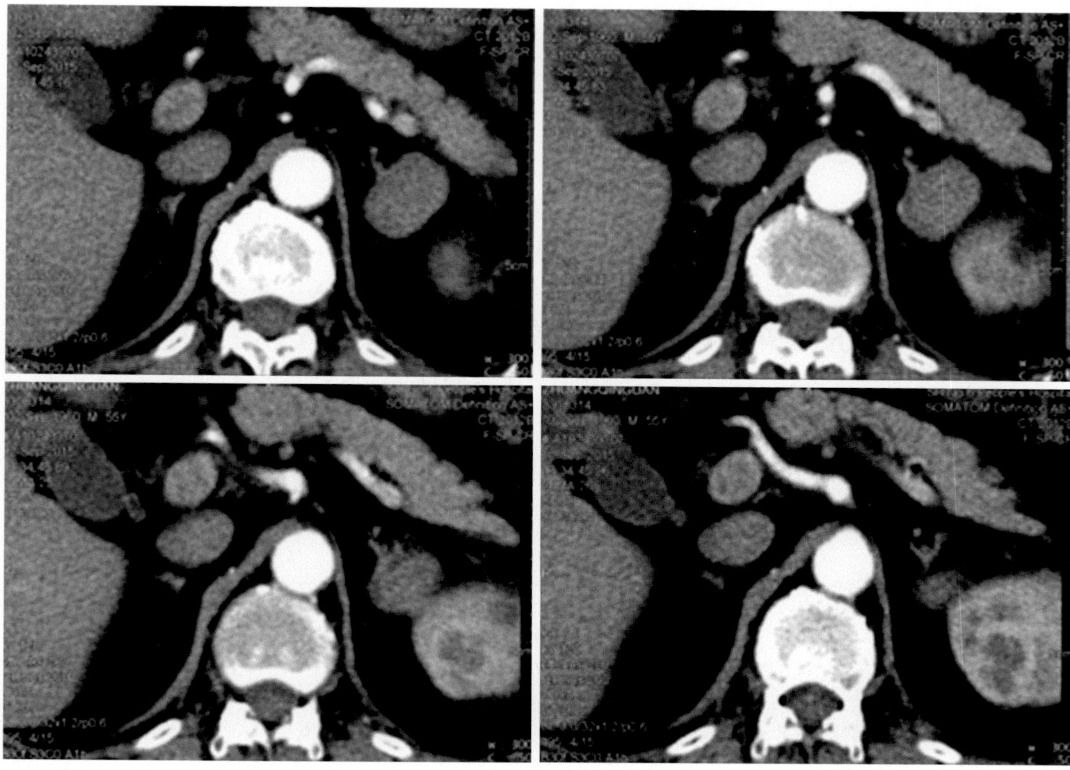

Fig. 17.2 Case 1: CT images from a patient with Cushing's syndrome. Notes: Red arrows indicate left adrenal adenoma

of 50 U/day, with FPG maintained between 7.7 and 8.3 mmol/L and 2-h postprandial glucose (2hPG) between 8.4 and 10.0 mmol/L.

Case 2 A 43-year-old female patient presented with repeated systemic edema and 2hPG >11.1 mmol/L in 2011. She was then diagnosed with diabetes and treated with metformin, acarbose, and glimepiride sequentially. Laboratory tests showed an HbA_{1c} of 7.5% (58 mmol/mol) and GA of 15.1%. The CGM (Fig. 17.3) showed poor control of postprandial blood glucose, similar to that in Case 1. The patient was diagnosed with Cushing's syndrome and left adrenal adenoma in 2014 during hospitalization due to persistent hypokalemia. After resection of the left adrenal adenoma, the systemic edema and persistent hypokalemia disappeared, and glucose metabolism was greatly improved.

Case 3 A 65-year-old female patient, who had no history of diabetes, had taken oral prednisone 20–30 mg once daily at 8:00 a.m. for the treatment of pulmonary fibrosis. Six months later, the patient developed thirst, polyuria, and polydipsia. FPG was 9.75 mmol/L and 2hPG was 14.34 mmol/L. The patient was diagnosed with diabetes. On examination, her body mass index (BMI) was 27.1 kg/m^2 and HbA_{1c} was 9.4% (79 mmol/mol). Biochemical parameters for kidney and liver function and electrolytes were all within normal range. Tests for glutamic acid decarboxylase antibody (GAD-Ab) and islet-associated antigen 2 antibody (IA2-Ab) were both negative. The serum insulin levels at 0, 2, 4, and 6 min during an arginine stimulation test were 8.93 mU/L, 45.77 mU/L, 32.06 mU/L, and 25.90 mU/L, respectively. The mean increase

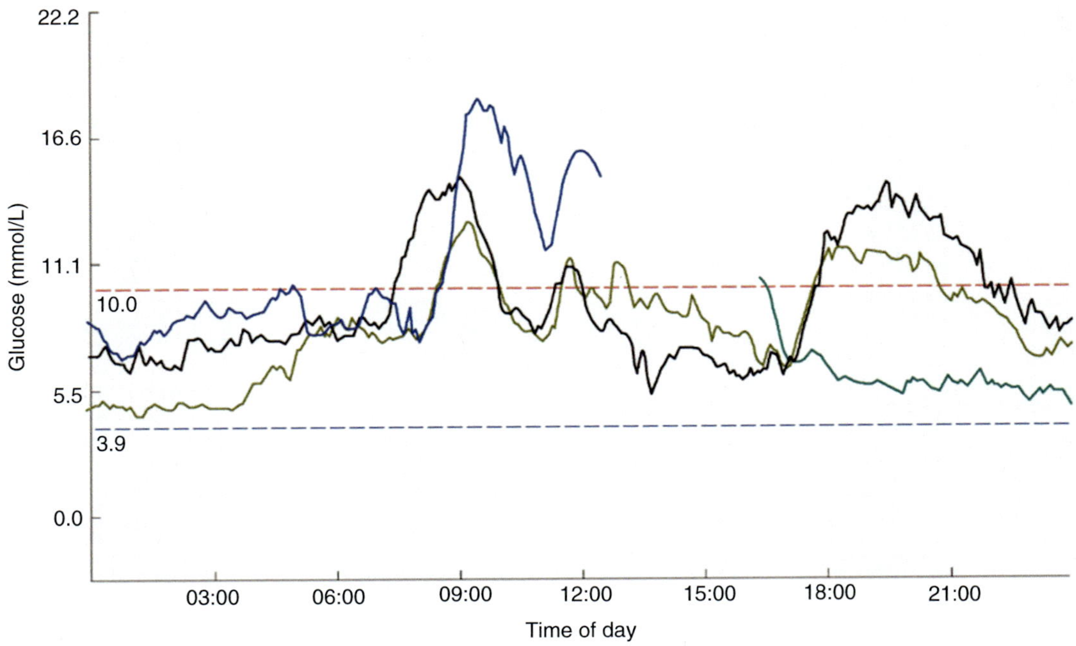

GLUCOSE EXPOSURE	GLUCOSE VARIABILITY	Dangerously Low	Low	GLUCOSE RANGES In Target Range	High	High
MBG mmol/L	SDBG mmol/L	≤ 2.8 mmol/L	≤ 3.9 mmol/L	3.9< GLUCOSE <10.0 mmol/L	≥ 10.0 mmol/L	≥ 11.1 mmol/L
8.8	**2.8**	**0%**	**0%**	**75%**	**25%**	**19%**

Fig. 17.3 Case 2: CGM profiles of a patient with Cushing's syndrome

of insulin (vs. 0 min) was 25.38 mU/L (normal reference value ≥10.46 mU/L), suggesting normal acute-phase insulin secretion. The CGM showed the features of the blood glucose profile (Fig. 17.4): predominant postprandial hyperglycemia after lunch and dinner, as manifested by the area under the curve (AUC), and the incremental area under the curve of postprandial blood glucose (AUCpp) after lunch and dinner were both significantly greater than those after breakfast. And the peak postprandial glucose and postprandial glucose excursion (PPGE) reached maximum levels after lunch (Table 17.1).

Summary The patient used intermediate-acting glucocorticoid (prednisone) once daily in the early morning. The glucose level increases after lunch until bedtime and is significantly higher than the level after breakfast. This feature is contrary to that of the common type of diabetes, which is characterized by postprandial hyperglycemia after breakfast (because the hyperglycemic action of glucocorticoids normally peaks in the early morning). This case emphasized that for patients with glucocorticoid treatment, in addition to FPG, efforts should be made to strengthen monitoring of postprandial blood glucose after lunch and dinner to raise the detection rate of steroid diabetes.

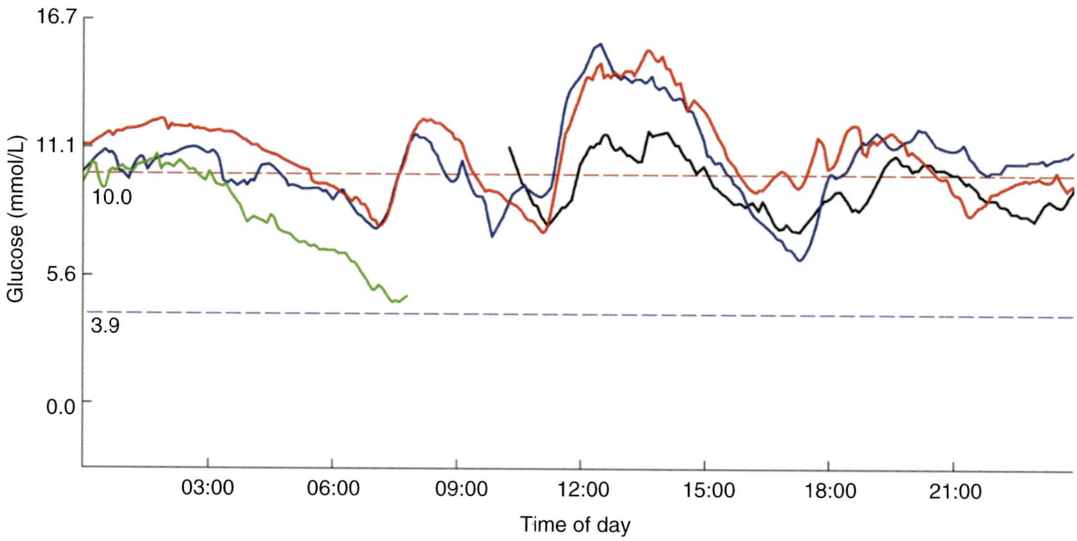

GLUCOSE EXPOSURE	GLUCOSE VARIABILITY	Dangerously Low	Low	GLUCOSE RANGES In Target Range	High	High
MBG mmol/L	SDBG mmol/L	≤2.8 mmol/L	≤3.9 mmol/L	3.9< GLUCOSE <10.0 mmol/L	≥10.0 mmol/L	≥11.1 mmol/L
10.1	**1.9**	**0%**	**0%**	**47%**	**53%**	**26%**

Fig. 17.4 Case 3: CGM profiles of a patient with new-onset exogenous glucocorticoid-induced diabetes

Table 17.1 Case 3: Postprandial blood glucose characteristics of a patient with newly diagnosed exogenous glucocorticoid-induced diabetes

PPG (mmol/L)			PPGE (mmol/L)		
Breakfast	Lunch	Dinner	Breakfast	Lunch	Dinner
11.7	15.6	11.9	4.2	8.4	5.6
AUC of the postprandial blood glucose (mmol·d/L)			AUCpp (mmol·d/L)		
Breakfast	Lunch	Dinner	Breakfast	Lunch	Dinner
1.08	3.22	2.88	0.27	1.22	1.17

Notes: *PPG* peak postprandial glucose, *PPGE* postprandial glucose excursion, *AUC* area under the curve, *AUCpp* incremental area under the curve of postprandial blood glucose

Case 4 A 58-year-old female patient, who had no history of diabetes, developed diabetes 1 year after oral administration of prednisone 10 mg once daily at 8:00 a.m. for the treatment of systemic lupus erythematosus. On examination, her BMI was 26.0 kg/m^2 and HbA_{1c} was 10.5% (91 mmol/mol). Tests for GAD-Ab and IA2-Ab were both negative. An arginine stimulation test revealed normal acute-phase insulin secretion. The antidiabetic regimen was premixed insulin 30R 20 U before breakfast and 16 U before dinner. The CGM displayed (Fig. 17.5) (1) an aver-

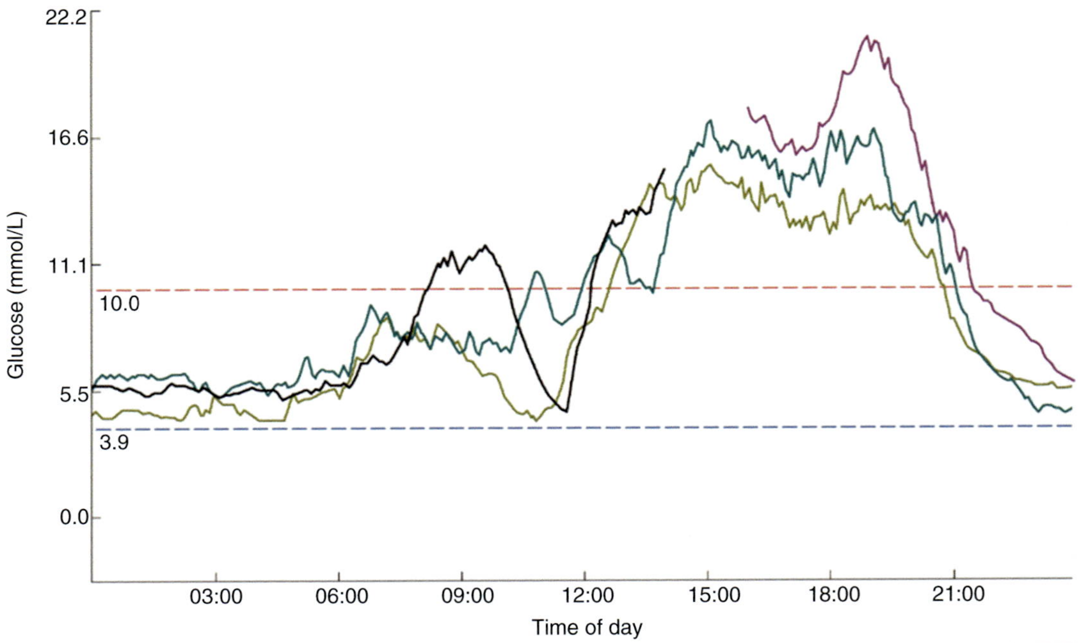

GLUCOSE EXPOSURE	GLUCOSE VARIABILITY	Dangerously Low	Low	GLUCOSE RANGES In Target Range	High	High
MBG mmol/L	SDBG mmol/L	≤ 2.8 mmol/L	≤ 3.9 mmol/L	3.9< GLUCOSE <10.0 mmol/L	≥ 10.0 mmol/L	≥ 11.1 mmol/L
9.4	**4.2**	**0%**	**0%**	**62%**	**38%**	**33%**

Fig. 17.5 Case 4: CGM profiles of a patient with exogenous glucocorticoid-induced diabetes who was treated with subcutaneous premixed insulin BID

age 24-h mean blood glucose (MBG) of 8.5 mmol/L with maximum and minimum values of 15.4 mmol/L and 4.2 mmol/L occurring after lunch and at night, respectively, and (2) further analysis of the blood glucose level in each period showed that glucose increased after lunch until bedtime, and FBG and postprandial blood glucose after breakfast were under good control.

Summary The patient used intermediate-acting glucocorticoid (prednisone) once daily in the early morning. The glucose level increases after lunch until bedtime. The antidiabetic regimen should be adjusted accordingly. Taking insulin, for instance, the dosage before lunch should be greater than those before dinner and breakfast, and insulin should be used at the lowest dose or even withdrawn at bedtime.

Case 5 A 56-year-old female patient developed diabetes after oral administration of prednisone BID (25 mg at 8:00 a.m. and 10 mg at 02:00 p.m.) for the treatment of polychondritis for 6 months. The antidiabetic regimen was Novolin R 6 U before breakfast, 4 U before lunch, and 4 U before dinner. HbA_{1c} was 6.5% (48 mmol/mol). Based on the measurements from the CGM system (Fig. 17.6), although the patient did not use insulin before bedtime, she experienced asymptomatic hypoglycemia (blood glucose

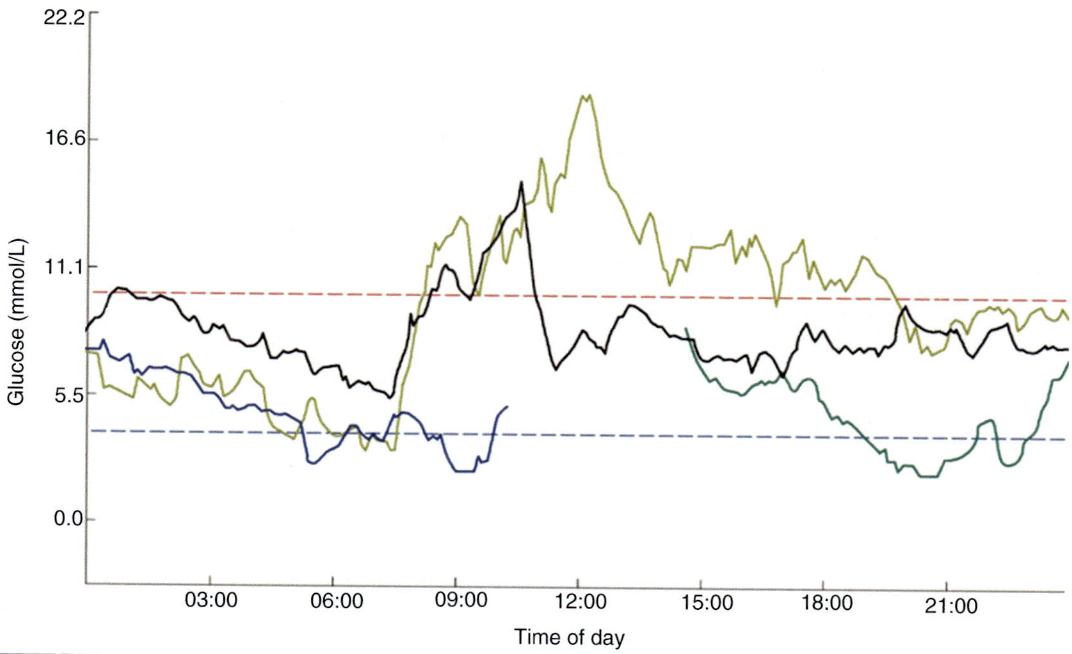

GLUCOSE EXPOSURE	GLUCOSE VARIABILITY	Dangerously Low	Low	GLUCOSE RANGES In Target Range	High	High
MBG mmol/L	SDBG mmol/L	≤ 2.8 mmol/L	≤ 3.9 mmol/L	3.9< GLUCOSE <10.0 mmol/L	≥ 10.0 mmol/L	≥ 11.1 mmol/L
7.7	**3.2**	**4%**	**13%**	**66%**	**21%**	**15%**

Fig. 17.6 Case 5: CGM profiles of an insulin-treated patient with steroid diabetes before adjustment of oral prednisone intake time

≤3.9 mmol/L) in the early morning for 115 min, with the lowest blood glucose level of 3.6 mmol/L. On the basis of the glycemic characteristics of the patient, oral prednisone was adjusted to prednisone three times a day (TID) (morning 20 mg, afternoon 10 mg, and bedtime 5 mg). A week later, the CGM revealed no occurrence of hypoglycemia and no changes in the AUC for blood glucose >7.8 mmol/L (Fig. 17.7). Further analysis showed that there was significant improvement in intraday blood glucose variability, manifested as significantly decreased mean amplitude of glycemic excursion (MAGE) and standard deviation of blood glucose (SDBG, Table 17.2).

Summary The patient used glucocorticoid (prednisone) at a dosage of 35 mg/day for a course of more than 1 year. The patient developed hypoglycemia in the early morning because of a weakened effect of exogenous prednisone and inhibited endogenous glucocorticoids secretion. When administration of prednisone was changed from twice a day (morning and afternoon) to three times a day (morning, afternoon, and bedtime) with the total dose unchanged, hypoglycemia significantly improved due to the persistent action of prednisone that covered the morning period. This example suggests that, in addition to antidiabetic agents, the use of glucocorticoids should be individualized (including

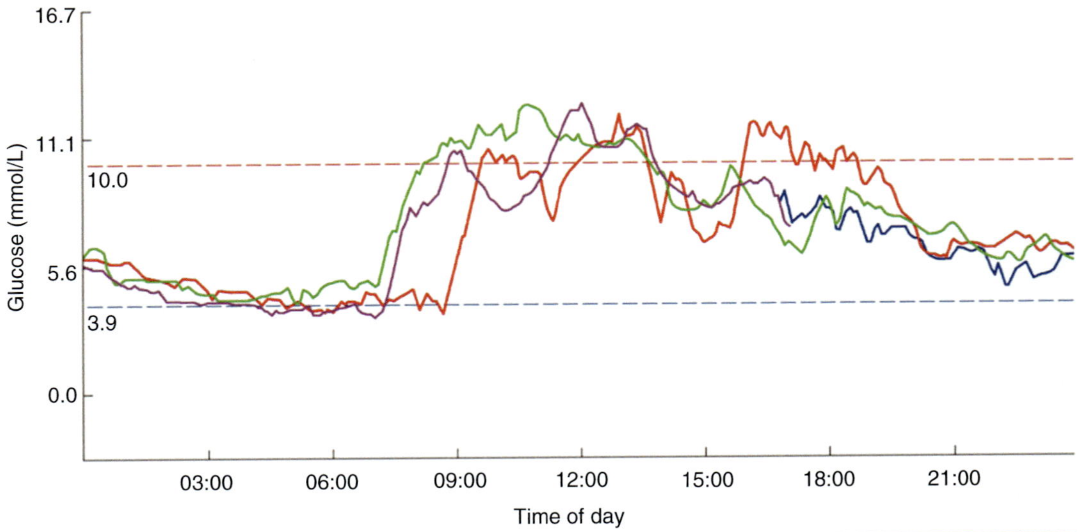

GLUCOSE EXPOSURE	GLUCOSE VARIABILITY	Dangerously Low	Low	GLUCOSE RANGES In Target Range	High	High
MBG mmol/L	SDBG mmol/L	≤ 2.8 mmol/L	≤ 3.9 mmol/L	3.9< GLUCOSE <10.0 mmol/L	≥ 10.0 mmol/L	≥ 11.1 mmol/L
7.1	**2.5**	**0%**	**6%**	**76%**	**18%**	**7%**

Fig. 17.7 Case 5: CGM profiles of an insulin-treated patient with steroid diabetes after adjustment of oral prednisone intake time

Table 17.2 Case 5: Comparison of CGM parameters before and after adjustment of treatment in a patient with steroid diabetes

	24-h MBG (mmol/L)	SDBG (mmol/L)	PPG breakfast (mmol/L)	PPG lunch (mmol/L)	PPG dinner (mmol/L)
Before adjustment	7.1	2.5	10.6	12.0	11.7
After adjustment	8.4	1.6	14.8	9.5	9.7
	MAGE (mmol/L)	PT 3.9 (%)	PT 7.8 (%)	PT 11.1 (%)	AUC of blood glucose >7.8 mmol/L (mmol·d/L)
Before adjustment	5.57	8	37	6	0.8
After adjustment	4.58	0	58	6	0.9

Notes: *MBG* mean blood glucose, *SDBG* standard deviation of blood glucose, *PPG* peak postprandial glucose, *MAGE* mean amplitude of glycemic excursion, *PT 3.9* percentage of time of blood glucose <3.9 mmol/L, *PT 7.8* percentage of time of blood glucose >7.8 mmol/L, *PT 11.1* percentage of time of blood glucose >11.1 mmol/L, *AUC* area under the curve dose, timing, routine, course of administration, etc.) in order to minimize the side effects of glucocorticoids. In addition, the patient experienced hypoglycemia without the presentation of clinical symptoms, that is, asymptomatic hypoglycemia. Asymptomatic hypoglycemia is difficult to treat and is a serious life-threatening condition, especially for the elderly and patients with cardiovascular and cerebrovascular diseases. Asymptomatic nocturnal hypoglycemia is usually not detected by SMBG, whereas the CGM system has a unique advantage to greatly facilitate the detection of asymptomatic hypoglycemia.

Statement on Consent for Participation
All the clinical trials carried out by the authors in this book have been reported to the Ethics Committee of Shanghai Jiao Tong University Affiliated Sixth People's Hospital already and were in accordance with the Good Clinical Practice and Standards of China Association for Ethical Studies (approval number: 2007-45).

References

1. Xiang KS. Special types of diabetes mellitus. Shanghai: Shanghai Scientific and Technical; 2011.
2. Hwang JL, Weiss RE. Steroid-induced diabetes: a clinical and molecular approach to understanding and treatment. Diabetes Metab Res Rev. 2014;30:96–102. https://doi.org/10.1002/dmrr.2486.
3. Ingle DJ, Winter HA, Li CH, Evans HM. Production of glycosuria in normal rats by means of adrenocorticotrophic hormone. Science. 1945;101:671–2. https://doi.org/10.1126/science.101.2635.671.
4. Munir A, Newell-Price J. Management of diabetes mellitus in Cushing's syndrome. Neuroendocrinology. 2010;92(Suppl 1):82–5. https://doi.org/10.1159/000314316.
5. Blackburn D, Hux J, Mamdani M. Quantification of the risk of corticosteroid-induced diabetes mellitus among the elderly. J Gen Intern Med. 2002;17:717–20. https://doi.org/10.1046/j.1525-1497.2002.10649.x.
6. Gulliford MC, Charlton J, Latinovic R. Risk of diabetes associated with prescribed glucocorticoids in a large population. Diabetes Care. 2006;29:2728–9. https://doi.org/10.2337/dc06-1499.
7. Jin JY, DuBois DC, Almon RR, Jusko WJ. Receptor/gene-mediated pharmacodynamic effects of methylprednisolone on phosphoenolpyruvate carboxykinase regulation in rat liver. J Pharmacol Exp Ther. 2004;309:328–39. https://doi.org/10.1124/jpet.103.061515.
8. Vander Kooi BT, Onuma H, Oeser JK, Svitek CA, Allen SR, Vander Kooi CW, Chazin WJ, O'Brien RM. The glucose-6-phosphatase catalytic subunit gene promoter contains both positive and negative glucocorticoid response elements. Mol Endocrinol. 2005;19:3001–22. https://doi.org/10.1210/me.2004-0497.
9. Kraus-Friedmann N. Hormonal regulation of hepatic gluconeogenesis. Physiol Rev. 1984;64:170–259.
10. Dirlewanger M, Schneiter PH, Paquot N, Jequier E, Rey V, Tappy L. Effects of glucocorticoids on hepatic sensitivity to insulin and glucagon in man. Clin Nutr. 2000;19:29–34. https://doi.org/10.1054/clnu.1999.0064.
11. Ruzzin J, Wagman AS, Jensen J. Glucocorticoid-induced insulin resistance in skeletal muscles: defects in insulin signalling and the effects of a selective glycogen synthase kinase-3 inhibitor. Diabetologia. 2005;48:2119–30. https://doi.org/10.1007/s00125-005-1886-0.
12. Krebs M, Krssak M, Bernroider E, Anderwald C, Brehm A, Meyerspeer M, Nowotny P, Roth E, Waldhäusl W, Roden M. Mechanism of amino acid-induced skeletal muscle insulin resistance in humans. Diabetes. 2002;51:599–605.
13. Perseghin G, Petersen K, Shulman GI. Cellular mechanism of insulin resistance: potential links with inflammation. Int J Obes Relat Metab Disord. 2003;27(Suppl 3):6–11. https://doi.org/10.1038/sj.ijo.0802491.
14. Ibrahim MM. Subcutaneous and visceral adipose tissue: structural and functional differences. Obes Rev. 2010;11:11–8. https://doi.org/10.1111/j.1467-789X.2009.00623.x.
15. Fasshauer M, Paschke R. Regulation of adipocytokines and insulin resistance. Diabetologia. 2003;46:1594–603. https://doi.org/10.1007/s00125-003-1228-z.
16. Ouchi N, Parker JL, Lugus JJ, Walsh K. Adipokines in inflammation and metabolic disease. Nat Rev Immunol. 2011;11:85–97. https://doi.org/10.1038/nri2921.
17. Penfornis A, Kury-Paulin S. Immunosuppressive drug-induced diabetes. Diabetes Metab. 2006;32:539–46. https://doi.org/10.1016/s1262-3636(06)72809-9.
18. Ranta F, Avram D, Berchtold S, Düfer M, Drews G, Lang F, Ullrich S. Dexamethasone induces cell death in insulin-secreting cells, an effect reversed by exendin-4. Diabetes. 2006;55:1380–90.
19. Mancini T, Kola B, Mantero F, Boscaro M, Arnaldi G. High cardiovascular risk in patients with Cushing's syndrome according to 1999 WHO/ISH guidelines. Clin Endocrinol. 2004;61:768–77. https://doi.org/10.1111/j.1365-2265.2004.02168.x.

20. Friedman TC, Mastorakos G, Newman TD, Mullen NM, Horton EG, Costello R, Papadopoulos NM, Chrousos GP. Carbohydrate and lipid metabolism in endogenous hypercortisolism: shared features with metabolic syndrome X and NIDDM. Endocr J. 1996;43:645–55.
21. Terzolo M, Pia A, Alì A, Osella G, Reimondo G, Bovio S, Daffara F, Procopio M, Paccotti P, Borretta G, Angeli A. Adrenal incidentaloma: a new cause of the metabolic syndrome? J Clin Endocrinol Metab. 2002;87:998–1003. https://doi.org/10.1210/jcem.87.3.8277.
22. Magee MH, Blum RA, Lates CD, Jusko WJ. Prednisolone pharmacokinetics and pharmacodynamics in relation to sex and race. J Clin Pharmacol. 2001;41:1180–94. https://doi.org/10.1177/00912700122012733.
23. Burt MG, Roberts GW, Aguilar-Loza NR, Frith P, Stranks SN. Continuous monitoring of circadian glycemic patterns in patients receiving prednisolone for COPD. J Clin Endocrinol Metab. 2011;96:1789–96. https://doi.org/10.1210/jc.2010-2729.
24. van Raalte DH, van Genugten RE, Linssen MM, Ouwens DM, Diamant M. Glucagon-like peptide-1 receptor agonist treatment prevents glucocorticoid-induced glucose intolerance and islet-cell dysfunction in humans. Diabetes Care. 2011;34:412–7. https://doi.org/10.2337/dc10-1677.

Using Continuous Glucose Monitoring for Patients with Insulinoma

18

J. F. Han and Y. Bao

18.1 Brief Introduction of Insulinoma

18.1.1 Basic Concept

An insulinoma is a tumor made up of specialized pancreatic islet β-cells that accounts for 70–80% of pancreatic endocrine tumors. The insulinoma is usually benign and only 5–11% is malignant. Insulinoma most commonly occurs in young and middle-aged population. The incidence of insulinoma is 1–5 per million, and women have a slight higher morbidity than men. Approximately 10% are multiple, 10% are related to type 1 multiple endocrine neoplasia (MEN), and only 10% are larger than 2.0 cm in diameter [1]. Malignant insulinomas are generally more than 3.0 cm in diameter, accompanied by metastasis to liver or adjacent tissues [2]. Insulinomas are mostly located in the pancreas, with approximately one-third located in the head of the pancreas, one-third in the body, and one-third in the tail. In few cases, insulinoma can occur in extrapancreatic locations, particularly the stomach, duodenum, and upper jejunum [3]. Insulinomas are generally small, round, or oval with smooth surface and have pink or dark-red appearance. The texture is usually soft or relative hard, and there is a clear boundary around the lesion. Insulinoma is characteristic of recurrent fasting hypoglycemia, along with inappropriate secretion of high levels of insulin and/or proinsulin. The clinical manifestations vary among patients, and some cases begin with neurological and psychiatric disorders, which are easily misdiagnosed. Because glucose metabolism provides energy for maintaining physiological brain function, long-term recurrent hypoglycemia can cause damage to the central nervous system and even mental disorders, epilepsy, dementia, etc., which are often misdiagnosed as mental illness or other functional diseases. Thus, early detection and diagnosis of insulinoma is essential to avoid severe, irreversible brain and nerve damage resulting from recurrent hypoglycemia.

J. F. Han · Y. Bao (✉)
Department of Endocrinology and Metabolism, Shanghai Clinical Center for Diabetes, Shanghai Diabetes Institute, Shanghai Jiao Tong University Affiliated Sixth People's Hospital, Shanghai, China
e-mail: yqbao@sjtu.edu.cn

18.1.2 Diagnosis of Insulinoma

The main clinical manifestations of insulinoma are the "Whipple triad," namely, typical hypoglycemic symptoms, measured hypoglycemia (blood glucose <2.8 mmol/L), and relief of symptoms when the glucose is raised to normal. Simultaneously, serum insulin level increases inappropriately, with a synchronous insulin level ≥ 6 μU/ml (43 pmol/L) and C peptide ≥0.6 ng/ml (200 pmol/L) [4]. The diagnosis of insulinoma needs to exclude other causes of

W. Jia (ed.), *Continuous Glucose Monitoring*, https://doi.org/10.1007/978-981-10-7074-7_18

symptoms such as pituitary dysfunction and insulin autoimmune syndrome. The hypoglycemic symptoms are mainly divided into two categories: (1) adrenergic symptoms, palpitation, trembling, pale, sweating, tachycardia, hunger, and others as a result from hypoglycemia-induced catecholamine release, and (2) neurologic symptoms, personality changes, insanity, seizures, coma, and others resulting from inadequate glucose supply to the brain. A small number of patients are misdiagnosed with epilepsy or mental illness. Calculation of the insulin release index (IRI) and C-peptide index at the onset of hypoglycemia in the fasting test helps to identify the causes of hypoglycemia. Generally, an IRI >0.4 is highly suspicious, and an IRI >1.0 can be diagnosed as insulinoma [5]. In our case-control study, we found that the measurements of glycated hemoglobin A_{1c} (HbA_{1c}) and fasting plasma glucose (FPG) during oral glucose tolerance test (OGTT), IRI, and C-peptide index all might be useful for the diagnosis of insulinoma [6].

However, there are still some challenges in clinical applications, which make diagnosis of insulinoma difficult. Currently, there is no consensus on the plasma glucose threshold for hypoglycemic symptoms. Some patients develop palpitations and sweating with a blood glucose above 3.0 mmol/L, whereas other patients have no subjective symptoms even with a glucose level below 2.0 mmol/L. Especially for patients with insulinoma, long-term recurrent hypoglycemia causes them to be insensitive to hypoglycemic insults, and their threshold of plasma glucose is lower than that of normal individuals. In addition, most hypoglycemic events occur during night or early morning in patients with insulinoma, which are difficult to detect at the early stage.

Once a clinical and biochemical diagnosis of insulinoma is made, a variety of imaging techniques can be used to localize the insulinoma and thus help guide treatment. These techniques have their own advantages. A combination of thin-slice computed tomography (CT) scanning and endoscopic ultrasonography can greatly improve the positive detection rate [7]. Magnetic resonance image (MRI) examination has a high sensitivity in distinguishing benign and malignant tumors and detecting metastasis to adjacent tissues [8]. It is usually difficult to detect a tumor <1 cm by conventional techniques. Multi-slice spiral CT perfusion imaging has good spatial and temporal resolution, by which three-dimensional data acquisition and reconstruction of thin slices can be completed within a short period of time for the abdomen. Its two phases of contrast-enhanced helical scanning are currently widely accepted, which can effectively improve the accuracy of topical diagnosis of insulinoma [9]. Therefore, combined detection technologies may be beneficial for complex lesions that cannot be detected by a single technique [10].

18.2 Application of CGM in Insulinoma

Continuous glucose monitoring (CGM) continuously monitors blood glucose fluctuations of patients and is capable of detecting hypoglycemia, especially nocturnal hypoglycemia, which cannot be detected by SMBG.

18.2.1 Use of CGM Facilitates the Detection of Nocturnal Hypoglycemia and Asymptomatic Hypoglycemia

It is difficult to assess the trends in blood glucose during hypoglycemia based on several glucose measurements at specific time points in patients with insulinoma. However, CGM can accurately reflect the fluctuation in blood glucose during hypoglycemia [11, 12]. Thus, CGM can be used as a valuable tool for the detection of asymptomatic hypoglycemia, especially in combination with the fasting test, which exhibits high value for the differential diagnosis of hypoglycemia [13]. Studies have shown that more than 50% of hypoglycemic events in patients with insulinoma occur during nighttime [14] and CGM is helpful for the detection and evaluation of nocturnal hypoglycemia [15].

18.2.2 Application of CGM Helps to Clarify the Causes of Hypoglycemia

Previously, we applied CGM to compare the glucose profiles among patients with insulinoma, diabetic patients with hypoglycemia, and individuals with normal glucose regulation. The results showed that (1) in normal individuals, the percentage of time (PT) spent in normoglycemia (3.9–7.8 mmol/L) was 99.2% and, in patients with insulinoma and diabetic patients with reactive hypoglycemia, the PT spent in normoglycemia was only 50%. Patients with insulinoma exhibited recurrent hypoglycemia and subsequent hyperglycemia caused by frequent glucose intake; and more than half of hypoglycemic events occur during nighttime. Reactive hypoglycemia mainly manifests as hyperglycemic symptoms, and the hypoglycemic events are usually mild and short period. (2) The M-value reflects glycemic information in terms of overall blood glucose levels and blood glucose fluctuations. Patients with hypoglycemia have an elevated M-value. With data of glycemic parameters like mean blood glucose (MBG), standard deviation of blood glucose (SDBG), and the PTs spent with different glucose concentrations, CGM can analyze the distribution, types, and causes of hypoglycemia and facilitate the clinical evaluation and etiologic diagnosis of insulinoma.

18.2.3 Use of CGM Contributes to Postoperative Evaluation of Insulinoma

CGM helps us develop a comprehensive understanding of postoperative blood glucose levels as well as to accurately assess surgical efficacy in patients with insulinoma.

18.3 Summary and Prospective

The main clinical manifestation of insulinoma is recurrent hypoglycemia. Before CGM, there was a lack of effective monitoring means for detecting asymptomatic hypoglycemia and nocturnal hypoglycemia. It should be noted that the CGM system is unable to measure glucose values below 2.2 mmol/L and it may overestimate the duration of hypoglycemia [16]. Thus, the severity of hypoglycemia should be judged based on specific clinical situations.

It is well known that the diagnosis of insulinoma relies on hypoglycemic episodes synchronized with inappropriately elevated serum insulin (or proinsulin) levels. Thus, a real-time CGM system with an alarm feature for detecting episodes of hypoglycemia and hyperglycemia is undoubtedly helpful for the diagnosis of insulinoma, especially for atypical cases. Here, two practical examples are illustrated to introduce the utilization of CGM for the diagnosis and treatment of insulinoma.

Case 1: A 46-year-old female patient had recurrent dizziness, fatigue, palpitation, hunger, sweating, and even disturbance of consciousness over a period of 6 years, with a frequency of 3–5 times a year. The above symptoms could be alleviated by food intake. Her blood glucose was 3 mmol/L when the symptoms occurred, and she had gained 15 kg of body weight since the onset of disease. She had no history of special medication use or gastrointestinal surgery. On physical examination, the patient was conscious, with a blood pressure of 140/80 mmHg, body mass index (BMI) of 36.7 kg/m^2, and no palpable thyroid nodules. Her heart rate was 78 beats/min, and there were no special abnormalities on physical examination of the cardiopulmonary system. Her abdomen was soft, without masses or tenderness, and no swelling was observed in the lower extremities.

The CGM results after admission showed (1) based on 871 CGM measurements over 3 days, the mean absolute difference (MAD) of consecutive glucose values was 12.9% and the mean, maximum, and minimum glucose measurements were 4.8 mmol/L, 10.8 mmol/L, and 2.2 mmol/L, respectively. (2) The patient experienced recurrent nocturnal and preprandial hypoglycemia, as well as postprandial hyperglycemia due to excessive meal intake (Fig. 18.1). The PT with blood glucose <2.8 mmol/L was 14% (595 min), and

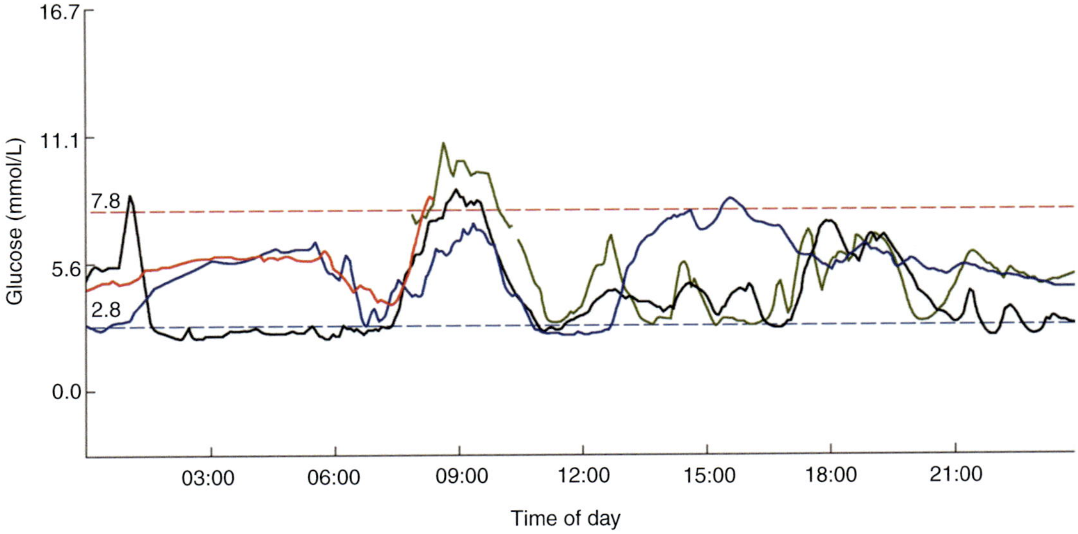

Fig. 18.1 Case 1: The CGM profiles of a patient with insulinoma

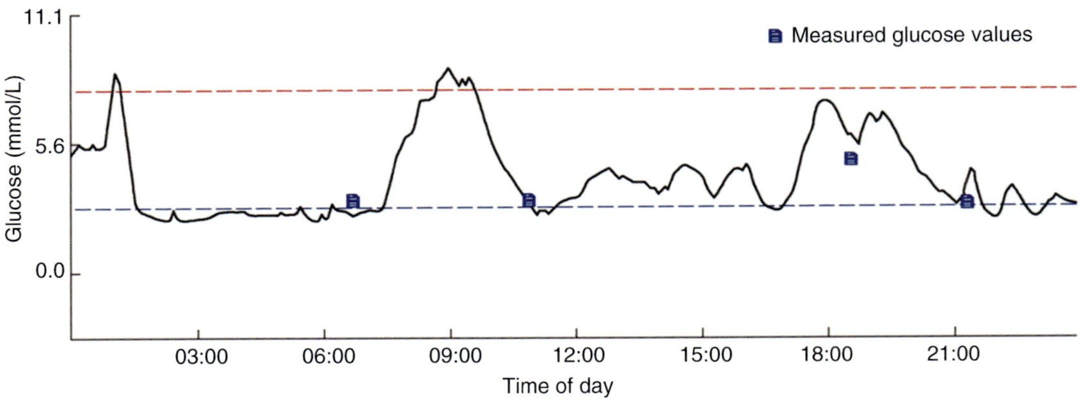

Fig. 18.2 Case 1: The preoperative CGM glucose profiles of a patient with insulinoma on day 2

the PT with blood glucose >7.8 mmol/L was 5% (215 min). (3) On the second day (Fig. 18.2), the patient felt fatigue and hunger in the morning with a blood glucose of 3.1 mmol/L, and the symptoms were relieved after food intake. The CGM demonstrated that the nocturnal hypoglycemia lasted for 345 min. The patient also experienced asymptomatic hypoglycemic events before lunch (35 min) and before dinner (25 min) for a short period of time. (4) On the third day (Fig. 18.3), the patient fasted after breakfast, and she developed hypoglycemic symptoms at 12:10 p.m., which lasted for 105 min. Analysis of venous blood showed a glucose concentration of 1.71 mmol/L, insulin concentration of 75.03 mU/L, C-peptide concentration of 6.63 μg/L (normal reference value, 0.8–4.0 μg/L), proinsulin concentration of 70.46 mU/L (normal reference value, 5–15 mU/L), and IRI of 2.44 at the onset of hypoglycemia. On radiological examination, abdominal ultrasound and thin-section CT revealed a lesion at the neck of the pancreas.

On exploratory laparotomy, a mass of 2.5 cm in diameter located at the top of the pancreatic neck below the hepatic artery was noted. No mass or lesion was detected in the pancreatic body or tail by intraoperative ultrasonography.

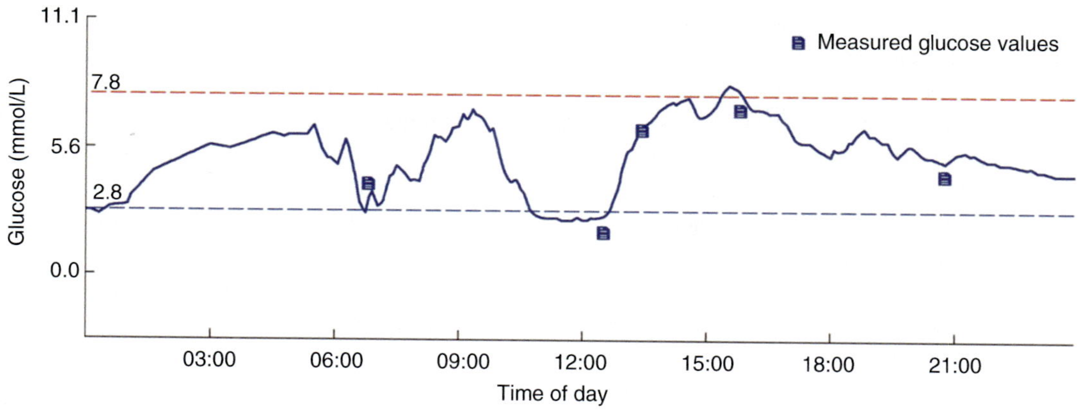

Fig. 18.3 Case 1: The preoperative CGM glucose profiles of a patient with insulinoma on day 3

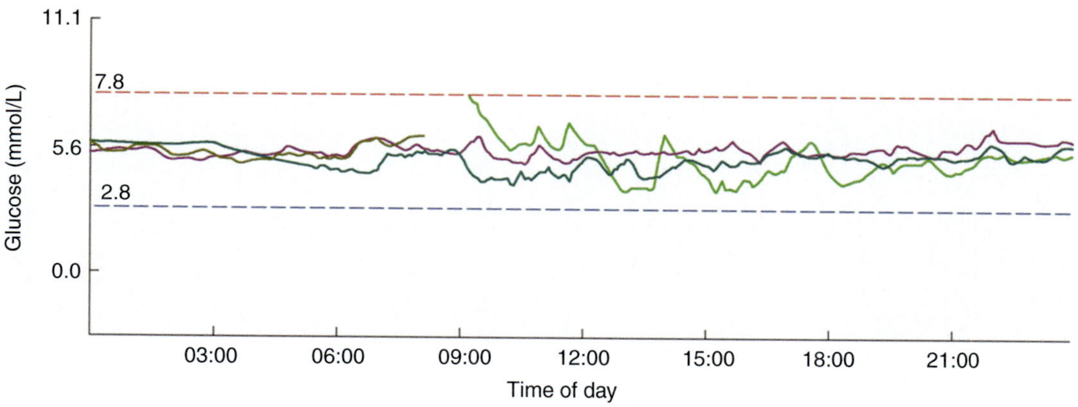

Fig. 18.4 Case 1: The postoperative CGM glucose profiles of a patient with insulinoma

Thirty minutes after resection of the tumor, the patient's blood glucose was increased from 3.1 mmol/L to 5.1 mmol/L, and blood glucose was 5.3 mmol/L at 60 min and 6.6 mmol/L at 150 min postoperatively. Pathological analysis of the lesion confirmed the diagnosis of insulinoma, with immunohistochemically staining showing the tissue was positive for insulin, chromogranin, synaptophysin, and neuron-specific enolase and weakly positive for somatostatin. The patient never suffered hypoglycemia after surgery, with a FPG of 4.68 mmol/L, insulin concentration of 23.98 mU/L, and IRI of 0.28. Consistently, CGM revealed the absence of hypoglycemia and postprandial hyperglycemia during monitoring period, and the blood glucose fluctuated within the range of 3.5–7.7 mmol/L, with an average concentration of 5.1 mmol/L (Fig. 18.4).

Case 2: A 37-year-old male patient was admitted due to "repeated palpitation, sweating, and hunger for 14 years with an aggravation of symptoms for the most recent 2 years." Fourteen years previously, the patient suffered symptoms such as sweating, palpitation, hunger, dizziness, blurred consciousness, and limb weakness when he worked in a fasting state, and the symptoms could be relieved after intake of food. The blood glucose was not measured at that time. The symptoms repeatedly occurred thereafter, 1–2 times a year and mostly at 3 h after meals. Ten years previously, the symptoms occurred again in a fasting state, while he was working. The venous blood glucose concentration was 2.8 mmol/L after admission. In the most recent 2 years, the above symptoms had become increasingly aggravated with a frequency of 3–5 times a day, manifesting as loss of consciousness and limb convulsion lasting for 5–10 min, without incontinence, nausea, vomiting, chest tightness or pain, abdominal pain, and diarrhea. The symptoms were relieved after meal intake. He had gained 5–6 kg of body weight since the onset of disease. The patient denied a history of diabetes.

On physical examination, the patient's temperature was 37 °C, his heart rate was 80 beats/min, breathing was 20 times/min, blood pressure was 120/70 mmHg, and BMI was 27.2 kg/m^2. The patient was conscious, and there were no special abnormalities on physical examination of the cardiopulmonary system and abdomen.

During the 72 h before surgery, the PT spent with glucose ≤2.8 mmol/L was 11% (470 min), and half of this period occurred between 01:00 a.m. and 06:00 a.m. The patient did not undergo fasting test due to recurrent hypoglycemic events. During the nighttime, he was given a 10–20% glucose intravenous infusion continuously. The IRI was calculated as >0.4 (maximum up to 5.54), and the prolonged OGTT test also yielded similar results. Although upper abdominal CT did not find evidence of insulinoma (Fig. 18.5a), insulinoma was highly suspected based on examinations. The diagnosis was further confirmed by ultrasound angiography (Fig. 18.5b), dynamic enhanced CT (Fig. 18.5c), and selective intra-arterial calcium stimulation with hepatic venous sampling for insulin secretion (Fig. 18.5d). The patient underwent enucleation of the insulinoma under general anes-

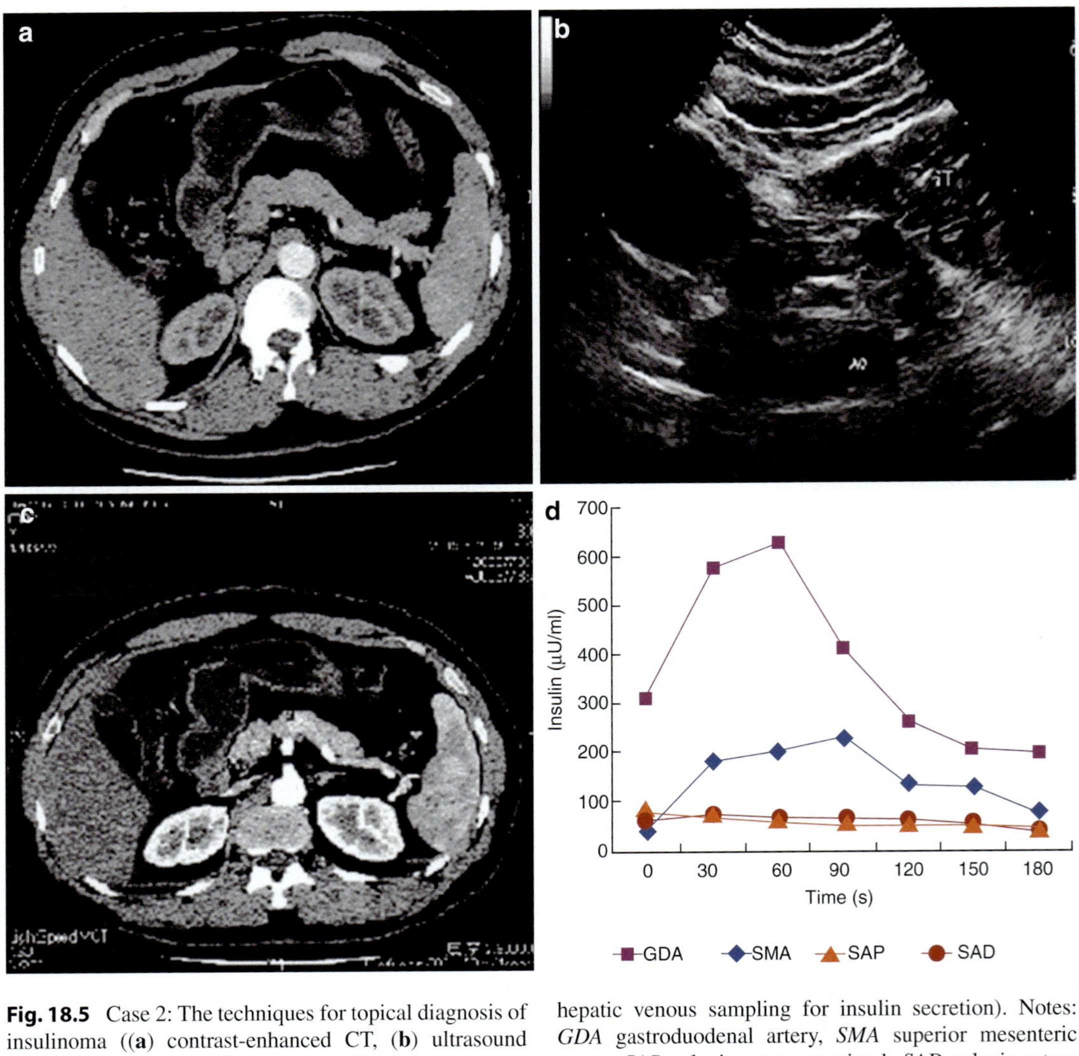

Fig. 18.5 Case 2: The techniques for topical diagnosis of insulinoma ((**a**) contrast-enhanced CT, (**b**) ultrasound angiography, (**c**) dynamic enhanced CT of the pancreas, (**d**) selective intra-arterial calcium stimulation with hepatic venous sampling for insulin secretion). Notes: *GDA* gastroduodenal artery, *SMA* superior mesenteric artery, *SAP* splenic artery proximal, *SAD* splenic artery distal

thesia. The blood glucose checked on arrival at the operating room was 2.3 mmol/L, and he was given continuous 20% dextrose intravenous infusion at 50 mL/h. A mass 2.0 cm × 1.2 cm × 1.0 cm with a hard texture and complete capsule was excised from the body of the pancreas. The glucose infusion was immediately discontinued after resection, and the blood glucose gradually rose from 4.2 mmol/L before resection to 8 mmol/L at 2 h after resection (Fig. 18.6). Intraoperative frozen sectioning revealed "neuroendocrine tumor with mild atypical cell, nodular tumor growth, no obvious capsule" (Fig. 18.7); the final pathological diagnosis was a pancreatic neuroendocrine tumor.

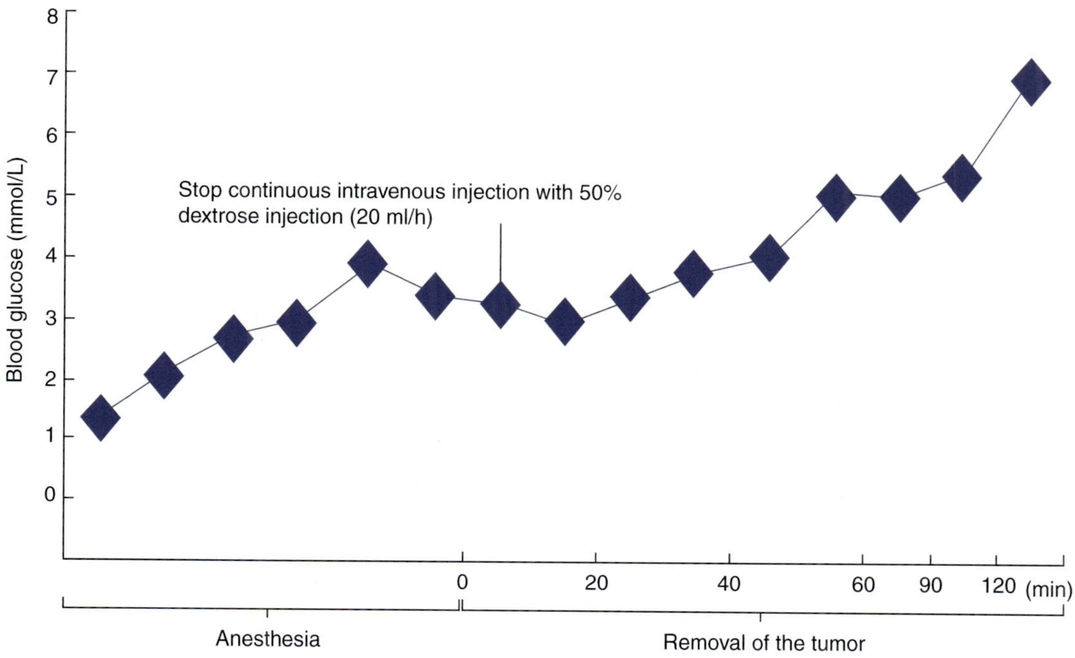

Fig. 18.6 Case 2: Intraoperative blood glucose monitoring results of a patient with insulinoma

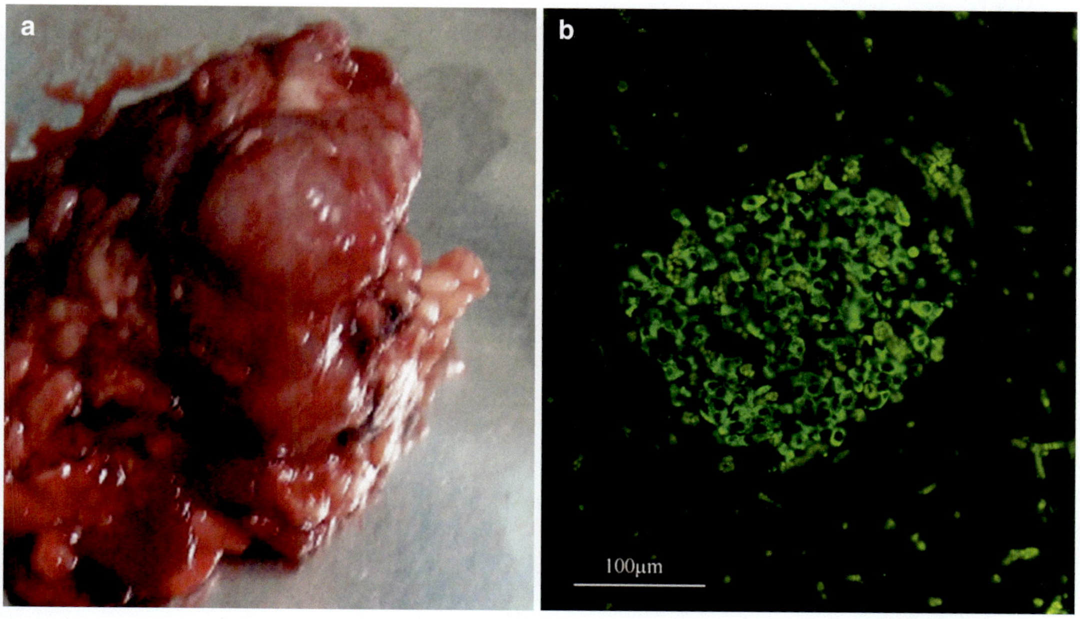

Fig. 18.7 Case 2: The tumor specimen (**a**) and immunofluorescence results (**b**) of a patient with insulinoma

The patient exhibited significantly higher postoperative blood glucose levels than that before surgery, without hypoglycemia. The OGTT revealed impaired glucose tolerance at 15 days postoperatively. Although the OGTT at 42 days postoperatively still revealed a 2-h glucose >7.8 mmol/L, this level was significantly lower than before. In addition, the IRI and modified IRI at all-time points were decreased as compared with that before surgery (Fig. 18.8). Postoperative CGM data revealed no hypoglycemia thereafter (Figs. 18.9, 18.10, 18.11, and 18.12).

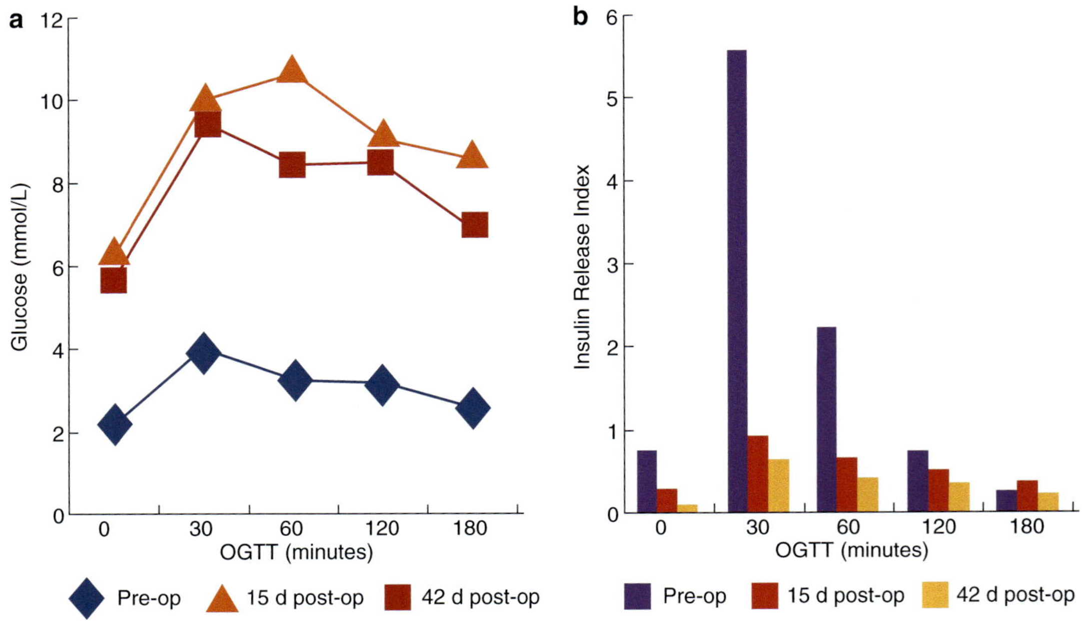

Fig. 18.8 Case 2: OGTT results before and after surgery (**a**) and changes in IRI at different time points (**b**) in patients with insulinoma

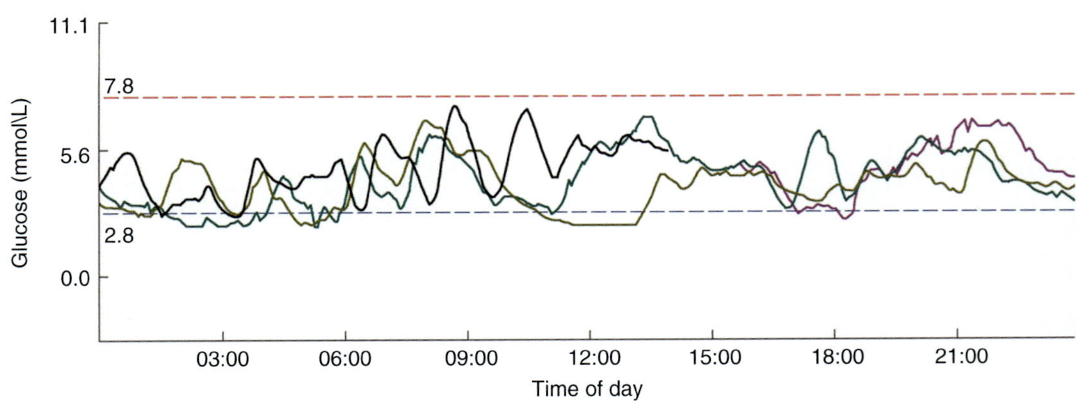

GLUCOSE EXPOSURE	GLUCOSE VARIABILITY	Dangerously Low	Low	GLUCOSE RANGES In Target Range	High	High
MBG mmol/L	SDBG mmol/L	≤ 2.8 mmol/L	≤ 3.9 mmol/L	3.9< GLUCOSE <10.0 mmol/L	≥ 10.0 mmol/L	≥ 11.1 mmol/L
4.3	**1.2**	**11%**	**39%**	**61%**	**0%**	**0%**

Fig. 18.9 Case 2: The preoperative CGM data of a patient with insulinoma

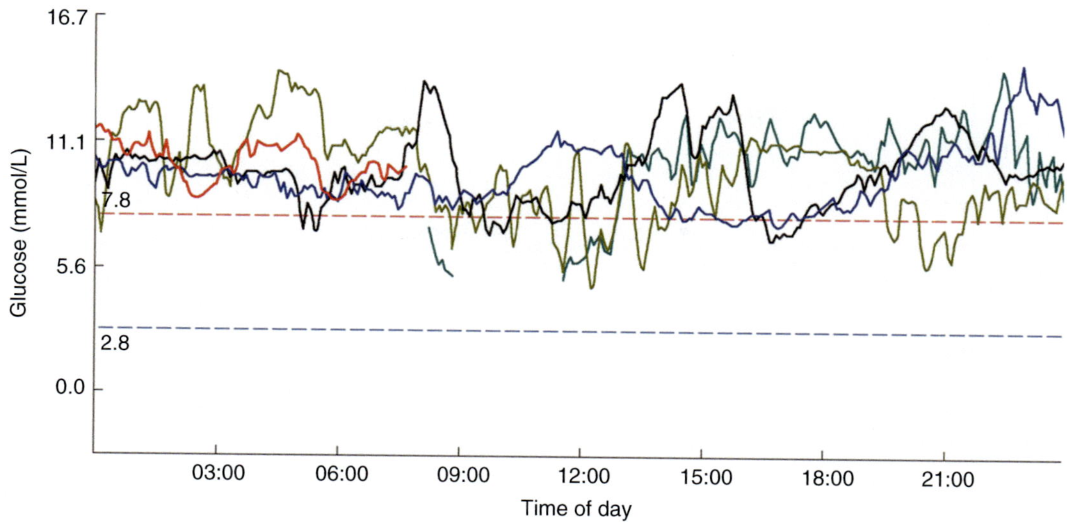

GLUCOSE EXPOSURE	GLUCOSE VARIABILITY	Dangerously Low	Low	GLUCOSE RANGES In Target Range	High	High
MBG mmol/L	SDBG mmol/L	≤ 2.8 mmol/L	≤ 3.9 mmol/L	3.9< GLUCOSE <10.0 mmol/L	≥ 10.0 mmol/L	≥ 11.1 mmol/L
9.8	**1.7**	**0%**	**0%**	**53%**	**47%**	**19%**

Fig. 18.10 Case 2: The CGM profiles of a patient with insulinoma at 3 days postoperatively

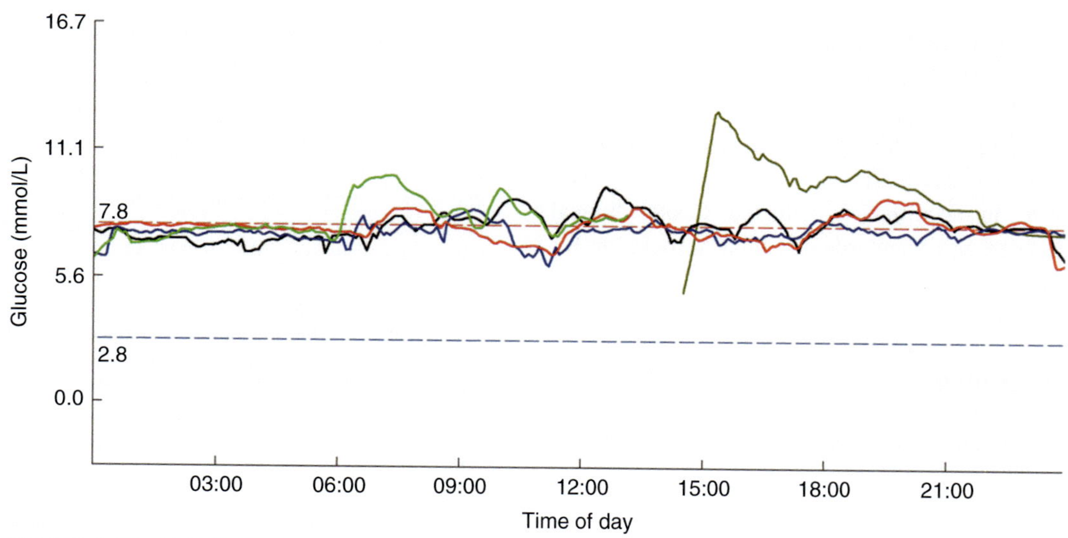

GLUCOSE EXPOSURE	GLUCOSE VARIABILITY	Dangerously Low	Low	GLUCOSE RANGES In Target Range	High	High
MBG mmol/L	SDBG mmol/L	≤ 2.8 mmol/L	≤ 3.9 mmol/L	3.9< GLUCOSE <10.0 mmol/L	≥ 10.0 mmol/L	≥ 11.1 mmol/L
7.9	**0.9**	**0%**	**0%**	**97%**	**3%**	**1%**

Fig. 18.11 Case 2: The CGM profiles of a patient with insulinoma at 1 week postoperatively

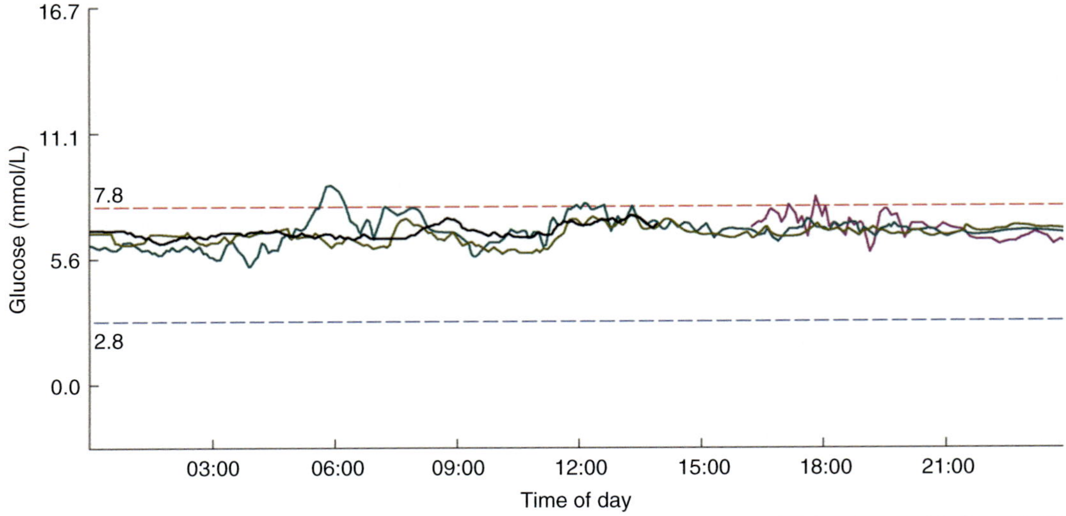

GLUCOSE EXPOSURE	GLUCOSE VARIABILITY	Dangerously Low	Low	GLUCOSE RANGES In Target Range	High	High
MBG mmol/L	SDBG mmol/L	≤ 2.8 mmol/L	≤ 3.9 mmol/L	3.9< GLUCOSE <10.0 mmol/L	≥ 10.0 mmol/L	≥ 11.1 mmol/L
6.7	**0.5**	**0%**	**0%**	**100%**	**0%**	**0%**

Fig. 18.12 Case 2: The CGM profiles of a patient with insulinoma at 6 weeks postoperatively

Statement on Consent for Participation
All the clinical trials carried out by the authors in this book have been reported to the Ethics Committee of Shanghai Jiao Tong University Affiliated Sixth People's Hospital already and were in accordance with the Good Clinical Practice and Standards of China Association for Ethical Studies (approval number: 2007-45).

References

1. Calledder GG, Rich TA, Perrier ND. Multiple endocrine neoplasia syndromes. Surg Clin North Am. 2008;88:863–95. https://doi.org/10.1016/j.suc.2008.05.001.
2. Muro S, Nasu J, Harada R, Matsubara M, Nakarai A, Kanzaki H, Tsutsumi K, Kato H, Tanaka T, Fujiwara H, Uno M, Okada H, Yamamoto K. Prompt resolution of hypoglycemia by hepatic transarterial embolization for malignant insulinoma with multiple liver metastases. Acta Med Okayama. 2014;68:303–6. https://doi.org/10.18926/AMO/52900.
3. Varas M, Gornals J, Ponseti JM, Alastruè A, Durán C, Llevaria C, Ballesta C, Díez-Caballero A, Artigas V. Pancreatic endocrine tumors or apudomas. Rev Esp Enferm Dig. 2011;103:184–90.
4. Grant CS. Insulinoma. Best Pract Res Clin Gastroenterol. 2005;19:783–98. https://doi.org/10.1016/j.bpg.2005.05.008.
5. Ito T, Igarashi H, Jensen RT. Pancreatic neuroendocrine tumors: clinical features, diagnosis and medical treatment: advances. Best Pract Res Clin Gastroenterol. 2012;26:737–53. https://doi.org/10.1016/j.bpg.2012.12.003.
6. Han JF, Zhang F, Bao YQ, Zhou J, Lu W, Lu JX, Jia WP. Diagnostic value of parameters of glucose metabolism as screening tests for insulinoma. Zhonghua Yi Xue Za Zhi. 2010;90:1093–6. https://doi.org/10.3760/cma.j.issn.0376-2491.2010.16.005.
7. Vaidakis D, Karoubalis J, Pappa T, Piaditis G, Zografos GN. Pancreatic insulinoma: current issues and trends. Hepatobiliary Pancreat Dis Int. 2010;9:234–41.
8. Patel S, Narwari M, Parekh D, Shah V. Insulinoma: case report and review of diagnostic and treatment modalities. J Assoc Physicians India. 2013;61:423–6.
9. Anakal MG, Kalra P, Dharmalingam M, Indushekhar S, Rao V, Prasanna Kumar KM. Insulinoma case series: experience of a tertiary care center. Indian J Endocrinol Metab. 2014;18:858–62. https://doi.org/10.4103/2230-8210.141385.
10. Han JF, Zhang F, Bao YQ, Zhou J, Lu W, Lu JX, Zhao JG, Huang XY, Bao ZK, Hu B, Jia WP. A case with

insulinoma localized by combined use of various means. Chin Med J. 2011;124:476–9.

11. Monsod TP, Flanagan DE, Rife F, Saenz R, Caprio S, Sherwin RS, Tamborlane WV. Do sensor glucose levels accurately predict plasma glucose concentrations during hypoglycemia and hyperinsulinemia? Diabetes Care. 2002;25:889–93.
12. Caplin NJ, O'Leary P, Bulsara M, Davis EA, Jones TW. Subcutaneous glucose sensor values closely parallel blood glucose during insulin-induced hypoglycaemia. Diabet Med. 2003;20:238–41. https://doi.org/10.1046/j.1464-5491.2003.00837.x.
13. Wang X. Application of the continuous glucose monitoring system (CGMS) in the 72-hour fast test in two patients with hypoglycemia. Diabetes Technol Ther. 2004;6:883. https://doi.org/10.1089/dia.2004.6.883.
14. Zhou J, Jia WP, Bao YQ, Lu W, Ma XJ, Yu M, Pan JM, Hu C, Xiang KS. Characteristics and clinical significance of daily blood glucose profiles of insulinoma detected by continuous glucose monitoring system. J Shanghai Jiaotong Univ (Med Sci). 2007;27:781–4. https://doi.org/10.3969/j.issn.1674-8115.2007.07.006.
15. Munir A, Choudhary P, Harrison B, Heller S, Newell-Price J. Continuous glucose monitoring in patients with insulinoma. Clin Endocrinol. 2008;68:912–8. https://doi.org/10.1111/j.1365-2265.2007.03161.x.
16. Cheyne EH, Cavan DA, Kerr D. Performance of a continuous glucose monitoring system during controlled hypoglycaemia in healthy volunteers. Diabetes Technol Ther. 2002;4:607–13. https://doi.org/10.1089/152091502320798222.

Using Continuous Glucose Monitoring for Patients Who Have Undergone Metabolic Surgery

19

H. Y. Yu and Y. Bao

Diabetes, cardiovascular disease, cancer, and chronic respiratory disease are the four main non-communicable diseases proposed by the World Health Organization (WHO). The prevalence of diabetes is 9.7% among general population over 20 years old, with 10.6% in men and 8.8% in women in China [1]. Accordingly, there are about 92.4 million diabetes patients in China, and thus, diabetes poses a threat to the health of residents and brings a heavy economic burden to society and families. Obesity is an important risk factor for diabetes. The prevalence rates of overweight and obesity were reported to be 33.7% and 13.7% in adult males and 29.2% and 10.7% in adult females, respectively, in China [2]. In China, 12.8% of overweight individuals and 18.5% of obese individuals have diabetes.

Comprehensive medical management is the traditional mode of treatment for diabetics, including diet therapy, exercise, hypoglycemic agents, health education, and glucose monitoring. However, for obese patients with type 2 diabetes, it is difficult to achieve long-term, stable glycemic control and to prevent the occurrence and development of chronic complications only by conventional medical therapy. The use of bariatric surgery for treating diabetes was originated from the findings of Pories et al. [3], who performed Roux-en-Y gastric bypass (RYGB) to treat morbid obesity and incidentally found that RYGB corrected abnormal blood glucose in obese patients with comorbid diabetes. Also, it was even possible for some patients to discontinue their hypoglycemic agents. After nearly two decades of development, the long-term efficacy of bariatric surgery in type 2 diabetes has been demonstrated by several studies. Schauer et al. [4] compared the effects of intensive medical therapy, laparoscopic sleeve gastrectomy (SG), and RYGB in a randomized, controlled study. In their study, 150 obese patients with type 2 diabetes were randomly assigned to receive intensive medical therapy, SG, or RYGB. After 1 year of follow-up, the patients' body weights were decreased by 5.4 ± 8.0 kg, 25.1 ± 8.5 kg, and 29.4 ± 9.0 kg, respectively, and the glycated hemoglobin A_{1c} (HbA_{1c}) measurements were decreased to 7.5% ± 1.8% (58 ± 20 mmol/mol), 6.6% ± 1.0% (49 ± 11 mmol/mol), and 6.4% ± 0.9% (46 ± 10 mmol/mol), respectively, suggesting that both bariatric surgeries were superior to intensive medical therapy in achieving better therapeutic efficacy. In the study by Mingrone et al. [5], 60 obese patients with type 2 diabetes were randomly assigned to receive conventional medical therapy or undergo either RYGB or biliopancreatic diversion (BPD). After 2 years, diabetes remission had occurred in 75%

H. Y. Yu · Y. Bao (✉)
Department of Endocrinology and Metabolism, Shanghai Clinical Center for Diabetes, Shanghai Diabetes Institute, Shanghai Jiao Tong University Affiliated Sixth People's Hospital, Shanghai, China
e-mail: yqbao@sjtu.edu.cn

W. Jia (ed.), *Continuous Glucose Monitoring*, https://doi.org/10.1007/978-981-10-7074-7_19

in the RYGB group and 95% in the BPD group, but no patients in the medical therapy group had diabetes remission. The HbA_{1c} was 4.95% ± 0.49% (31 ± 5 mmol/mol) in the BPD group, which was superior to that in the RYGB group 6.35 ± 1.42% (46 ± 16 mmol/mol). Both surgical procedures resulted in better glucose control than medical therapy did [HbA_{1c}, 7.69 ± 0.57% (61 ± 6 mmol/mol)]. From the opinion of Italian scholar Rubino, RYGB and BPD have been shown to dramatically improve type 2 diabetes, although they were originally meant to treat morbid obesity. RYGB and BPD can lead to improvements in a variety of metabolic indicators and modulate the secretion of endocrine hormones as well. Thus, it is more appropriate to describe these surgical procedures as "metabolic surgery" [6]. In recent years, Chinese studies have also shown that metabolic surgery has a beneficial effect on metabolic syndrome [7], sleep apnea syndrome [8], diabetic nephropathy [9], and vascular lesions [10], which is superior to the effect of conventional medical therapy. Moreover, metabolic surgery can reduce long-term medical costs and improve the quality of life of patients, thereby resulting in a reduction in the socioeconomic burden for obese patients with diabetes [11].

Metabolic surgery for the treatment of diabetes has been gradually accepted because it offers many benefits to obese patients with diabetes based on improved metabolism. In 2009, the American Diabetes Association (ADA) formally recommended metabolic surgery as a treatment for obese patients with type 2 diabetes in the guidelines. In 2011, the International Diabetes Federation (IDF) officially recognized metabolic surgery as a treatment for obese patients with type 2 diabetes [12]. In May 2016, 48 medical experts from 45 regional or international diabetes academic organizations gathered in London and published a milestone joint statement, "Metabolic Surgery in the Treatment Algorithm for Type 2 Diabetes: A Joint Statement by International Diabetes Organizations" [13], once again affirming the clinical significance of metabolic surgery in the treatment of obesity and type 2 diabetes.

19.1 Common Surgical Procedures of Metabolic Surgery

Metabolic surgery includes a variety of procedures, which can be divided into restrictive procedures and restrictive combined with malabsorptive procedures, according to the purpose of the surgery. The former mainly includes SG and adjustable gastric banding (AGB); the latter includes RYGB, BPD, and others. RYGB is currently the most widely used clinical procedure. SG is usually performed for weight loss in patients with simple obesity or for treating type 2 diabetes with high body mass index (BMI) and short disease duration. BPD is used in obese patients with BMI >50 kg/m^2. However, this procedure is difficult to perform and is often associated with postoperative nutritional complications. Thus, it has not been reported in China. AGB has been carried out less often due to poor efficacy and high postoperative recurrence rate.

19.2 Changes in Glucose Variability Detected by CGM After Metabolic Surgery

Although metabolic surgery can significantly improve the overall glucose level and reduce the HbA_{1c} value in obese patients with type 2 diabetes, the therapeutic efficacy on glucose variability differs among different surgical procedures. Generally, for the restrictive procedures SG and AGB, gastric emptying is not affected by preserving normal pyloric function, and thus, the fluctuations in blood glucose are small postoperatively. In contrast, after RYGB surgery, due to a short circuit from the stomach to the jejunum, food intake, especially high carbohydrate food, is dumped too quickly into the small intestine and makes dumping syndrome more likely. This can cause rapid elevation followed by a drop in postprandial blood glucose and dramatic fluctuations in blood glucose [14]. Continuous glucose monitoring (CGM) can continuously record glucose changes for 72 h or longer. It can accurately assess the magnitude and frequency of fluctuations in blood glucose and detect asymptomatic hypoglycemic events. Thus, it can be used as an effective means in evaluating postoperative glucose variability after metabolic surgery.

To this date, there are limited studies about using CGM to evaluate glucose variability before and after metabolic surgery, and most studies focus on RYGB procedures. Hanaire et al. [15] compared the glucose variability by CGM in a mixed meal test among diabetes patients who underwent RYGB, control diabetes patients who did not undergo surgery, and healthy controls ($n = 10$ each group). The results showed that patients treated with RYGB had a significantly lower mean blood glucose (MBG) level than control diabetes patients that did not receive surgery (6.2 ± 0.9 mmol/L vs. 7.7 ± 2.0 mmol/L, $P = 0.002$). However, the mean amplitude of glycemic excursions (MAGE) was not significantly improved in the RYGB group vs. the diabetes without surgery control group (4.8 ± 3.2 mmol/L vs. 3.7 ± 1.3 mmol/L, $P = 0.82$). The time to the postprandial peak glucose was significantly less in patients treated with RYGB than in control diabetes patients (42.8 ± 6.0 min vs. 82.2 ± 11.1 min, $P = 0.0002$); five cases (50%) in the RYGB group experienced postprandial hyperglycemia and hypoglycemia (the mean maximum and minimum glucose levels were 17.0 ± 3.3 mmol/L and 2.9 ± 0.6 mmol/L, respectively). In the study conducted by Kefurt et al. [16], a 5-day CGM was performed in 51 nondiabetic obese subjects at a mean of 86 months after RYGB to assess the incidence of hypoglycemic episodes in a mixed meal test. CGM revealed that hypoglycemic episodes occurred (defined as glucose <3.05 mmol/L) in 75% of the patients and 38% of patients experienced nocturnal hypoglycemic episodes. A mean of 3 ± 1 hypoglycemic episodes per patient with a mean duration of 71 ± 25 min of hypoglycemia was observed by CGM. Abrahamsson et al. [17] made a comparison of the therapeutic efficacy of the RYGB procedure ($n = 15$) versus the BPD procedure ($n = 15$) on glycemic variability and found that BPD yielded both a lower HbA_{1c} value [4.8% (29 mmol/mol) vs. 5.4% (36 mmol/mol), $P < 0.05$] and MAGE value (1.5 mmol/L vs. 3.2 mmol/L, $P < 0.05$) as compared with RYGB. However, there was no significant difference in the duration of hypoglycemia between two groups. Marfella et al. [18] also found that at 1 month after BPD surgery, obese patients with type 2 diabetes ($n = 36$) exhibited a significant decrease in MAGE (3.4 ± 0.7 mmol/L vs. 1.9 ± 0.7 mmol/L, $P < 0.01$) as well as the degree of oxidative stress as compared with that before surgery.

Based on the criteria for postoperative remission of diabetes in "*Standards of care for type 2 diabetes in China (2013)*" [19] and normal reference values for CGM parameters in Chinese subjects [20], we have put forward the concept of "dual-remission," which requires achievement of targets for both glucose level and variability. In our previous study, among 43 type 2 diabetes patients who underwent RYGB, complete diabetes remission was achieved in 27 patients (62.8%) 1 year after RYGB (Fig. 19.1). However, no change was observed in MAGE before and after surgery (5.4 ± 2.3 mmol/L vs. 5.9 ± 2.4 mmol/L, $P = 0.282$). Also, only 18.6% of patients ($n = 8$) achieved "dual-remission" [21] (Fig. 19.2). Thus, although RYGB is currently the most widely used metabolic procedure and allows for achievement of HbA_{1c} target goal in most patients, it has shortcomings and defects with respect to improving glucose variability.

The main reasons for inferior improvement in glucose variability after RYGB are related to the changes of gastrointestinal anatomy: (1) Accelerated gastric emptying and shortened intestinal transit time after food intake result in a glucose peak when monosaccharides rapidly pass into the jejunum. (2) Animal studies [22] showed that intestinal villus length increased by 38% with an increase in goblet cell numbers in both crypt and villus after RYGB surgery, which resulted in the increase in villus surface area and resultant rapid and abundant intestinal glucose absorption. (3) RYGB can induce increased expression of some glucose transporters such as sodium-glucose cotransporter-1, 2, and glucose transporter 2 (GLUT2) [23]. In short, RYGB-mediated postprandial hyperglycemia is related to shortened intestinal transit time and enhanced intestinal absorption after food intake. In addition, postprandial hyperglycemia is also likely to cause inappropriate insulin secretion, which in return leads to the occurrence of hypoglycemia, further exacerbating fluctuations in blood glucose. Furthermore, long-term, recurrent hypoglycemia caused by

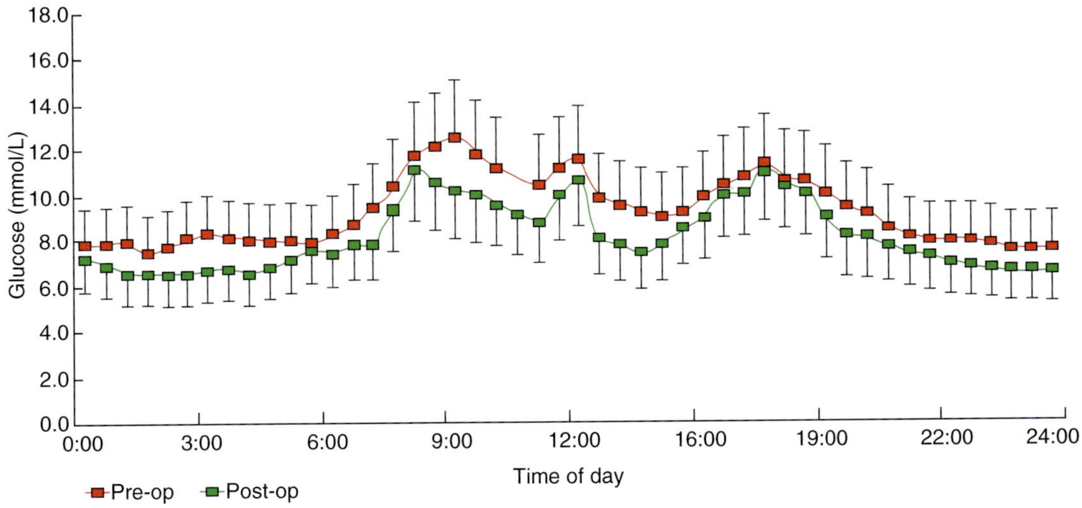

Fig. 19.1 Preoperative and 1-year postoperative CGM profiles of 27 type 2 diabetes patients who underwent RYGB surgery [21] (Reprint with permission from Surg Obes Relat Dis)

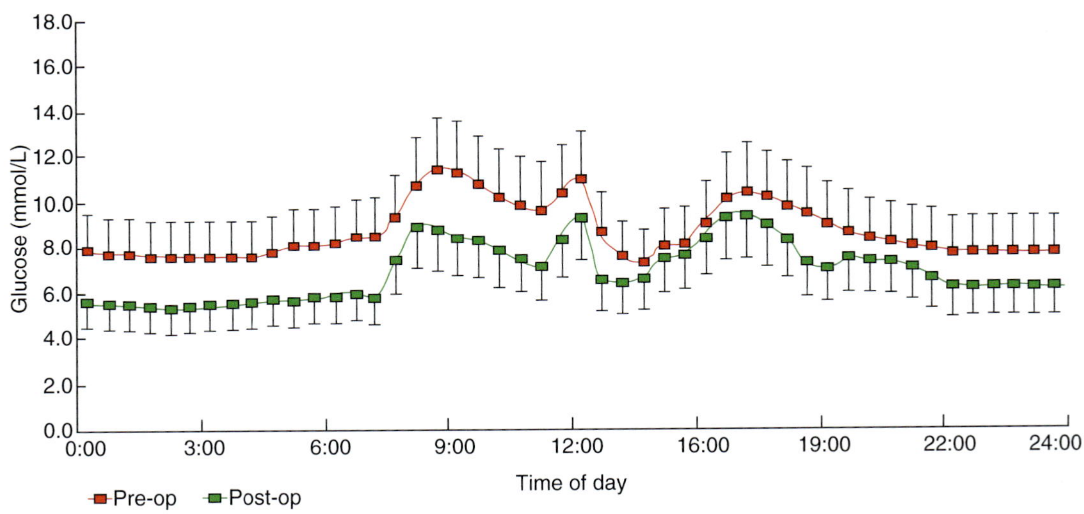

Fig. 19.2 Preoperative and 1-year postoperative CGM profiles of eight type 2 diabetes patients who achieved "dual-remission" after RYGB surgery [21] (Reprint with permission from Surg Obes Relat Dis)

increased food intake is an important factor for the recurrence of obesity and type 2 diabetes postoperatively [24].

19.3 Therapeutic Interventions for Glucose Variability After Metabolic Surgery

Postoperative interventions for glucose variability after RYGB mainly include two aspects, diet and medication. For selection of staple food, patients should consume low-carbohydrate and nutritionally balanced diets under the guidance of nutritionists. Those foods with a low glycemic index (GI), for example, cereals and grains, seem to be better options, and high-GI foods, such as white bread, fruit juice, fructose, chocolate, and glutinous rice, should be avoided. Tramunt et al. [25] found that consumption of low-GI carbohydrates for breakfast can significantly reduce the postprandial hyperglycemic peak. Moreover, the speed, amount, and frequency of meal consumption also should be noted. On the other hand, there are few studies on medication interventions for improving glucose variability after RYGB. In the study performed by Ritz et al. [26], eight RYGB-operated patients with dumping syndrome were treated with acarbose (50–100 mg TID) for 6 weeks. The dumping symptoms disappeared in seven patients. CGM showed that there was a significant reduction in the maximum glucose peak with marginal statistical difference (13.8 ± 4.4 mmol/L vs. 10.3 ± 2.2 mmol/L, $P = 0.09$) and a significant increase in the minimum glucose value (2.8 ± 0.8 mmol/L vs. 3.2 ± 0.5 mmol/L, $P = 0.04$). Also, the percentages of time (PTs) spent with glucose <3.3 mmol/L were decreased (2.5 ± 3.5% vs. 0.2 ± 0.5%, $P = 0.02$). The time to postprandial peak glucose level was significantly prolonged (52.1 ± 7.1 min vs. 98.5 ± 21.1 min, $P = 0.01$]. Thus, acarbose has a certain role in correcting postprandial hypoglycemia and improving postoperative glucose variability after RYGB. In addition, since the RYGB induced a shortened time interval to peak level, the timing of finger stick glucose monitoring should be at 0.5–1 h rather than 2 h after a meal.

We have listed two practical examples to introduce the specific application of CGM after metabolic surgery.

Case 1: A 37-year-old man was diagnosed with type 2 diabetes based on symptoms of "dry mouth, polydipsia, and weight loss for 2 months." Preoperatively, the patient was treated with gliclazide (80 mg, BID) and metformin (0.5 g, TID). On physical examination, his height was 169 cm, body weight was 90 kg, and BMI was 31.5 kg/m^2. The glycemic parameters were as follows: fasting blood glucose (FPG), 4.07 mmol/L; 2-h postprandial blood glucose, 11.88 mmol/L; fasting insulin, 8.87 μU/ml; 2-h postprandial insulin, 33.27 μU/ml; fasting C-peptide, 2.90 ng/ml; 2-h postprandial C-peptide, 6.92 ng/ml; and HbA_{1c}, 7.7% (61 mmol/mol). The preoperative CGM data are shown in Fig. 19.3. The patient underwent

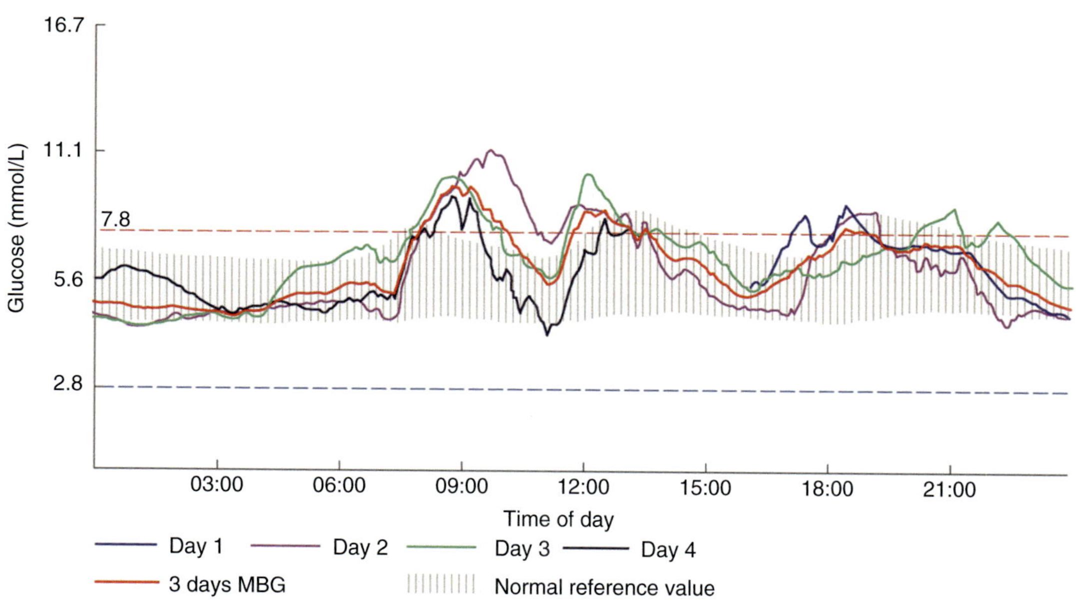

GLUCOSE EXPOSURE	GLUCOSE VARIABILITY	Dangerously Low	Low	GLUCOSE RANGES In Target Range	High	High
MBG mmol/L	SDBG mmol/L	≤ 2.8 mmol/L	≤ 3.9 mmol/L	3.9<GLUCOSE<10.0 mmol/L	≥ 10.0 mmol/L	≥ 11.1 mmol/L
6.3	**1.7**	**0%**	**2%**	**95%**	**3%**	**0%**

Fig. 19.3 Case 1: Preoperative CGM profiles of a patient with type 2 diabetes who underwent RYGB surgery. Notes: The red curve represents the mean glucose level over multiple days, and the shaded portion represents normal reference ranges for CGM parameters established in our previous study

RYGB surgery under general anesthesia, and oral hypoglycemic agents were discontinued after surgery. The changes in BMI, blood glucose, HbA_{1c}, and islet function at 6 and 12 months postoperatively are shown in Table 19.1. The postoperative CGM glucose profiles are shown in Figs. 19.4 and 19.5. Although the HbA_{1c} had gradually reduced to the normal range after RYGB surgery, glucose variability did not improve as compared with the preoperative state with occasional occurrence of postprandial hypoglycemia, which may be caused by RYGB-related dumping syndromes.

Case 2: A 59-year-old woman had a history of type 2 diabetes for 12 years. Preoperatively, the patient was treated with insulin and oral hypoglycemic agents for glycemic control. The

Table 19.1 Case 1: Changes in clinical indicators in a type 2 diabetes patient before and after RYGB surgery

	Pre-op	6 month post-op	12 month post-op
BMI (kg/m^2)	31.5	24.2	24.8
FPG (mmol/L)	4.07	4.78	5.03
2hPG (mmol/L)	11.88	5.30	5.34
FINS (μU/ml)	8.87	3.81	4.56
2hINS (μU/ml)	33.27	5.88	9.72
FCP (ng/ml)	2.90	1.67	1.77
2hCP (ng/ml)	6.92	3.17	4.53
HbA_{1c} (%)	7.7	5.3	5.2
HbA_{1c} (mmol/mol)	61	34	33

Notes: *BMI* body mass index, *FPG* fasting plasma glucose, *2hPG* 2-h postprandial glucose, *FINS* fasting insulin, *2hINS* 2-h postprandial insulin, *FCP* fasting C-peptide, *2hCP* 2-h postprandial C-peptide, *HbA_{1c}* glycated hemoglobin A_{1c}

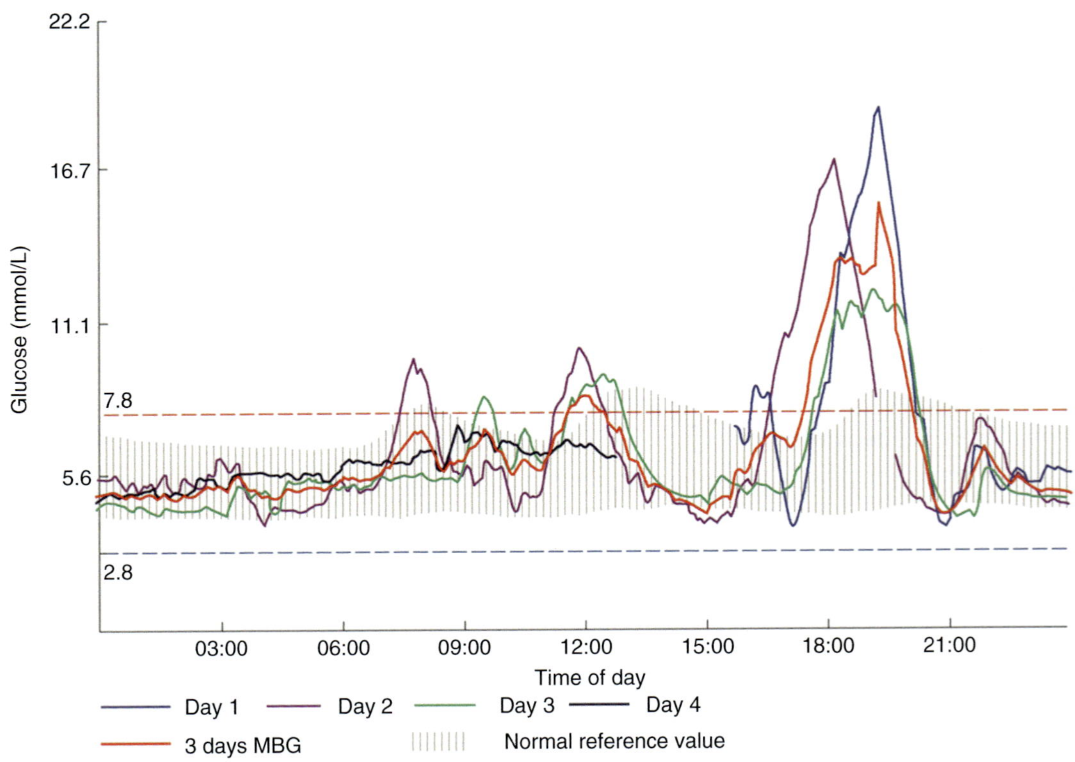

GLUCOSE EXPOSURE	GLUCOSE VARIABILITY	Dangerously Low	Low	GLUCOSE RANGES In Target Range	High	High
MBG mmol/L	SDBG mmol/L	≤ 2.8 mmol/L	≤ 3.9 mmol/L	3.9<GLUCOSE<10.0 mmol/L	≥ 10.0 mmol/L	≥ 11.1 mmol/L
6.4	**2.6**	**0%**	**1%**	**90%**	**9%**	**7%**

Fig. 19.4 Case 1: 6-month postoperative CGM profiles of a type 2 diabetes patient after RYGB surgery

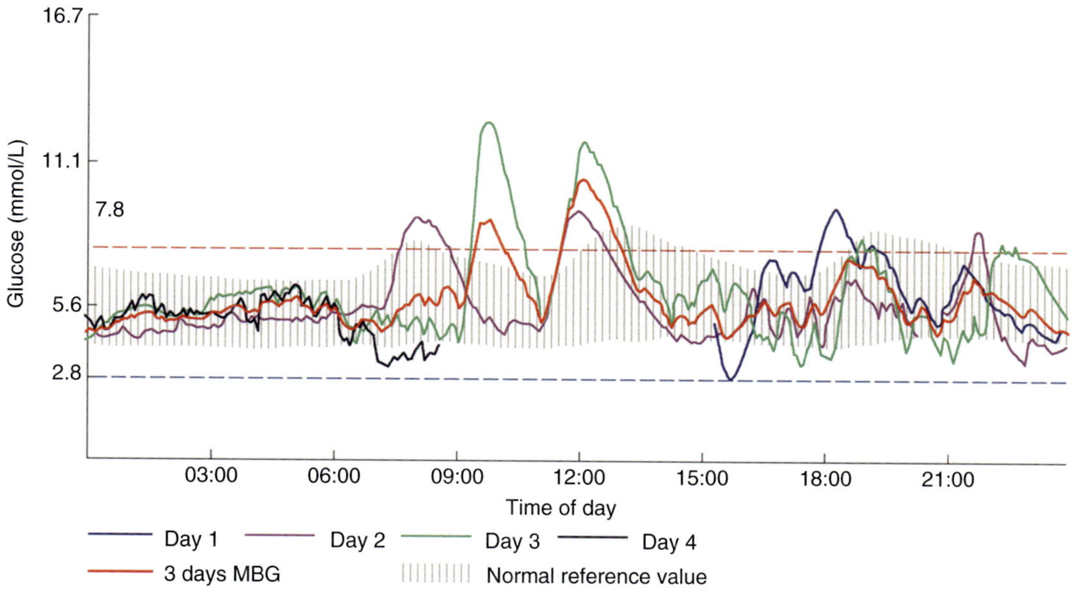

GLUCOSE EXPOSURE	GLUCOSE VARIABILITY	Dangerously Low	Low	GLUCOSE RANGES In Target Range	High	High
MBG mmol/L	SDBG mmol/L	≤ 2.8 mmol/L	≤ 3.9 mmol/L	3.9<GLUCOSE<10.0 mmol/L	≥ 10.0 mmol/L	≥ 11.1 mmol/L
5.8	**1.6**	**0%**	**5%**	**92%**	**3%**	**2%**

Fig. 19.5 Case 1: 12-month postoperative CGM profiles of a type 2 diabetes patient after RYGB surgery

Table 19.2 Case 2: Changes in clinical indicators in a type 2 diabetes patient before and after RYGB surgery

	Pre-op	6 months post-op	12 months post-op	2 years post-op
BMI (kg/m^2)	35.0	25.3	23.7	23.3
FPG (mmol/L)	10.57	4.61	4.87	5.14
2hPG (mmol/L)	20.96	7.79	6.30	7.67
FINS (μU/ml)	10.82	5.30	4.88	4.52
2hINS (μU/ml)	28.12	11.22	6.19	11.18
FCP (ng/ml)	1.91	1.27	1.68	1.76
2hCP (ng/ml)	4.33	3.48	3.09	3.78
HbA$_{1c}$ (%)	9.9	6.2	6.5	6.4
HbA$_{1c}$ (mmol/mol)	85	44	48	46

patient had comorbid hypertension and was treated with nifedipine sustained-release tablets. On physical examination, her height was 159 cm, weight was 88.5 kg, and BMI was 35.0 kg/m^2. The patient underwent an RYGB surgery, and the preoperative and postoperative data at 6 months, 12 months, and 2 years are shown in Table 19.2. The patient exhibited a significant decrease in body weight as well as HbA$_{1c}$ level, which reached the target goal within 6 months. Also, her blood pressure decreased to the normal range. Insulin and oral hypoglycemic agents were gradually discontinued. The corresponding CGM data are shown in Figs. 19.6, 19.7, 19.8, and 19.9. From the data, the patient had a high preoperative MBG and dramatic glucose variability, which were significantly decreased after RYGB surgery.

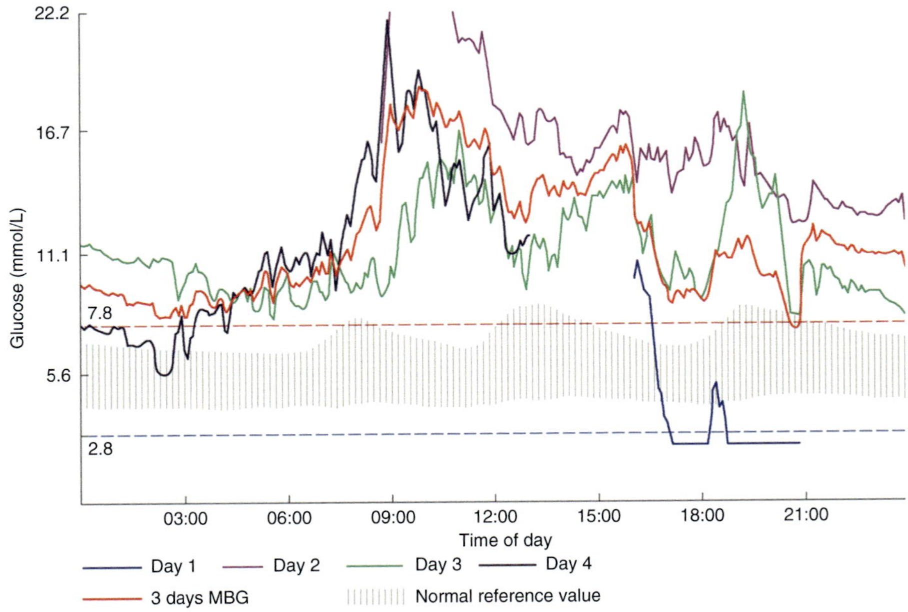

GLUCOSE EXPOSURE	GLUCOSE VARIABILITY	Dangerously Low	Low	GLUCOSE RANGES In Target Range	High	High
MBG mmol/L	SDBG mmol/L	≤ 2.8 mmol/L	≤ 3.9 mmol/L	3.9<GLUCOSE<10.0 mmol/L	≥ 10.0 mmol/L	≥ 11.1 mmol/L
11.9	**4.4**	**6%**	**6%**	**27%**	**67%**	**52%**

Fig. 19.6 Case 2: Preoperative CGM profiles of a type 2 diabetes patient who underwent RYGB surgery

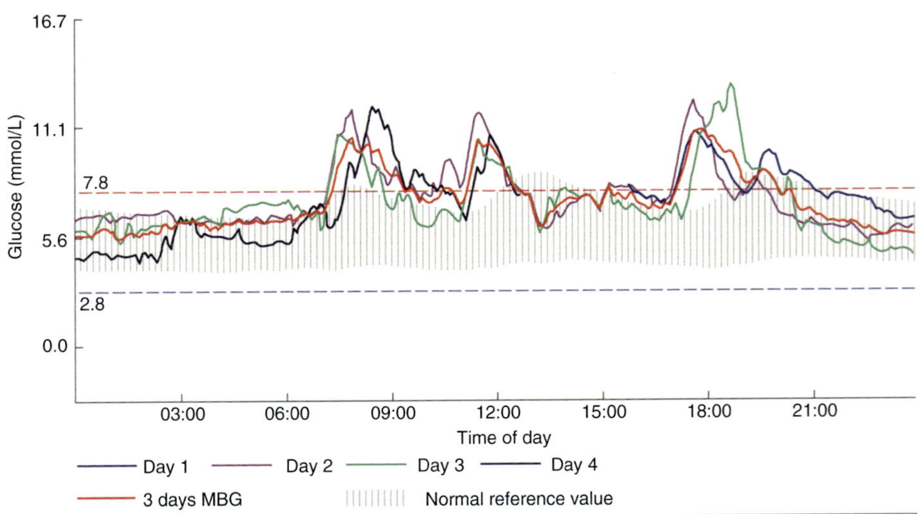

GLUCOSE EXPOSURE	GLUCOSE VARIABILITY	Dangerously Low	Low	GLUCOSE RANGES In Target Range	High	High
MBG mmol/L	SDBG mmol/L	≤ 2.8 mmol/L	≤ 3.9 mmol/L	3.9<GLUCOSE<10.0 mmol/L	≥ 10.0 mmol/L	≥ 11.1 mmol/L
7.4	**1.7**	**0%**	**0%**	**91%**	**9%**	**4%**

Fig. 19.7 Case 2: 6-month postoperative CGM profiles of a type 2 diabetes patient after RYGB surgery

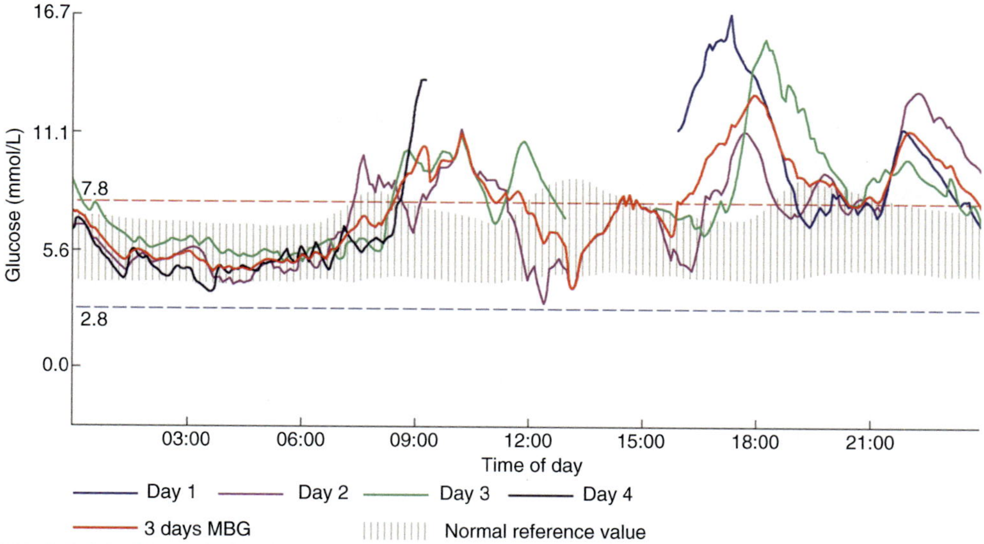

GLUCOSE EXPOSURE	GLUCOSE VARIABILITY	Dangerously Low	Low	GLUCOSE RANGES In Target Range	High	High
MBG mmol/L	SDBG mmol/L	≤ 2.8 mmol/L	≤ 3.9 mmol/L	3.9<GLUCOSE<10.0 mmol/L	≥ 10.0 mmol/L	≥ 11.1 mmol/L
7.5	**2.6**	**0%**	**1%**	**84%**	**15%**	**9%**

Fig. 19.8 Case 2: 12-month postoperative CGM profiles of a type 2 diabetes patient after RYGB surgery

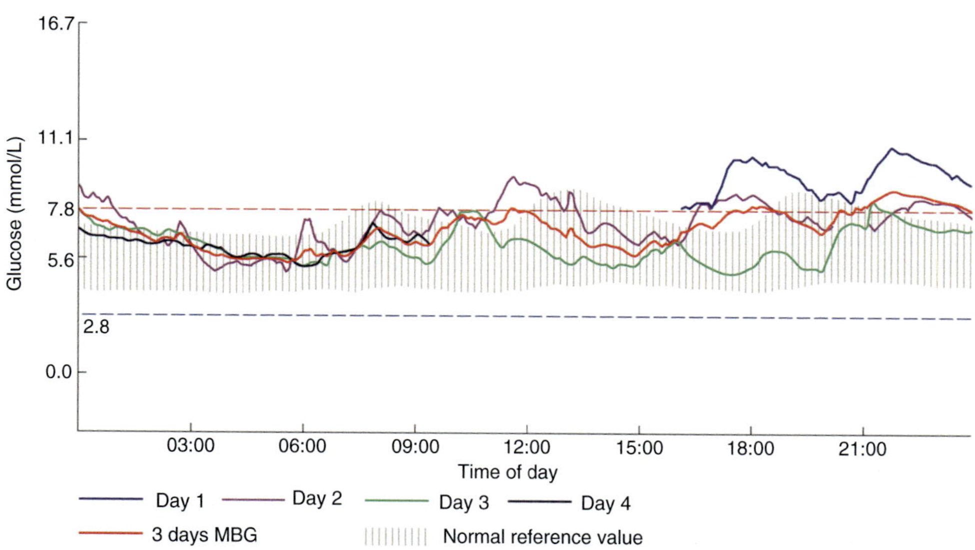

GLUCOSE EXPOSURE	GLUCOSE VARIABILITY	Dangerously Low	Low	GLUCOSE RANGES In Target Range	High	High
MBG mmol/L	SDBG mmol/L	≤ 2.8 mmol/L	≤ 3.9 mmol/L	3.9<GLUCOSE<10.0 mmol/L	≥ 10.0 mmol/L	≥ 11.1 mmol/L
6.9	**1.4**	**0%**	**0%**	**97%**	**3%**	**0%**

Fig. 19.9 Case 2: 2-year postoperative CGM profiles of a type 2 diabetes patient after RYGB surgery

Statement on Consent for Participation
All the clinical trials carried out by the authors in this book have been reported to the Ethics Committee of Shanghai Jiao Tong University Affiliated Sixth People's Hospital already and were in accordance with the Good Clinical Practice and Standards of China Association for Ethical Studies (approval number: 2007-45).

References

1. Yang W, Lu J, Weng J, Jia W, Ji L, Xiao J, Shan Z, Liu J, Tian H, Ji Q, Zhu D, Ge J, Lin L, Chen L, Guo X, Zhao Z, Li Q, Zhou Z, Shan G, He J, China National Diabetes and Metabolic Disorders Study Group. Prevalence of diabetes among men and women in China. N Engl J Med. 2010;362:1090–101. https://doi.org/10.1056/NEJMoa0908292.
2. Hou X, Lu J, Weng J, Ji L, Shan Z, Liu J, Tian H, Ji Q, Zhu D, Ge J, Lin L, Chen L, Guo X, Zhao Z, Li Q, Zhou Z, Shan G, Yang Z, Yang W, Jia W, China National Diabetes and Metabolic Disorders Study Group. Impact of waist circumference and body mass index on risk of cardiometabolic disorder and cardiovascular disease in Chinese adults: a national diabetes and metabolic disorders survey. PloS One. 2013;8:e57319. https://doi.org/10.1371/journal.pone.0057319.
3. Pories WJ, Swanson MS, MacDonald KG, Long SB, Morris PG, Brown BM, Barakat HA, deRamon RA, Israel G, Dolezal JM. Who would have thought it? An operation proves to be the most effective therapy for adult-onset diabetes mellitus. Ann Surg. 1995;222:339–52.
4. Schauer PR, Kashyap SR, Wolski K, Brethauer SA, Kirwan JP, Pothier CE, Thomas S, Abood B, Nissen SE, Bhatt DL. Bariatric surgery versus intensive medical therapy in obese patients with diabetes. N Engl J Med. 2012;366:1567–76. https://doi.org/10.1056/NEJMoa1200225.
5. Mingrone G, Panunzi S, De Gaetano A, Guidone C, Iaconelli A, Leccesi L, Nanni G, Pomp A, Castagneto M, Ghirlanda G, Rubino F. Bariatric surgery versus conventional medical therapy for type 2 diabetes. N Engl J Med. 2012;366:1577–85. https://doi.org/10.1056/NEJMoa1200111.
6. Rubino F. Is type 2 diabetes an operable intestinal disease? A provocative yet reasonable hypothesis. Diabetes Care. 2008;31(Suppl 2):290–6. https://doi.org/10.2337/dc08-s271.
7. Yu H, Zhang L, Bao Y, Zhang P, Tu Y, Di J, Han X, Han J, Jia W. Metabolic syndrome after Roux-en-Y gastric bypass surgery in Chinese obese patients with type 2 diabetes. Obes Surg. 2016;26:2190–7. https://doi.org/10.1007/s11695-016-2074-7.
8. Xu H, Zhang P, Han X, Yu H, Di J, Zou J, Wang Y, Qian Y, Tu Y, Bao Y, Yi H, Guan J, Yin S, Jia W. Sex effect on obesity indices and metabolic outcomes in patients with obese obstructive sleep apnea and type 2 diabetes after laparoscopic Roux-en-Y gastric bypass surgery: a preliminary study. Obes Surg. 2016;26:2629–39. https://doi.org/10.1007/s11695-016-2140-1.
9. Zhang H, Di J, Yu H, Han X, Li K, Zhang P. The short-term remission of diabetic nephropathy after Roux-en-Y gastric bypass in Chinese patients of T2DM with obesity. Obes Surg. 2015;25:1263–70. https://doi.org/10.1007/s11695-015-1666-y.
10. Yu H, Chen J, Lu J, Bao Y, Tu Y, Zhang L, Zhang P, Jia W. Decreased visceral fat area correlates with improved arterial stiffness after Roux-en-Y gastric bypass in Chinese obese patients with type 2 diabetes mellitus: a 12-month follow-up. Surg Obes Relat Dis. 2016;12:550–5. https://doi.org/10.1016/j.soard.2015.09.003.
11. Hoerger TJ, Zhang P, Segel JE, Kahn HS, Barker LE, Couper S. Cost-effectiveness of bariatric surgery for severely obese adults with diabetes. Diabetes Care. 2010;33:1933. https://doi.org/10.2337/dc10-0554.
12. Zimmet P, Alberti KG, Rubino F, Dixon JB. IDF's view of bariatric surgery in type 2 diabetes. Lancet. 2011;378:108–10. https://doi.org/10.1016/S0140-6736(11)61027-1.
13. Rubino F, Nathan DM, Eckel RH, Schauer PR, Alberti KG, Zimmet PZ, Del Prato S, Ji L, Sadikot SM, Herman WH, Amiel SA, Kaplan LM, Taroncher-Oldenburg G, Cummings DE, Delegates of the 2nd Diabetes Surgery Summit. Metabolic surgery in the treatment algorithm for type 2 diabetes: A Joint Statement by international diabetes organizations. Diabetes Care. 2016;39:861–77. https://doi.org/10.2337/dc16-0236.
14. Bantle JP, Ikramuddin S, Kellogg TA, Buchwald H. Hyperinsulinemic hypoglycemia developing late after gastric bypass. Obes Surg. 2007;17:592–4.
15. Hanaire H, Bertrand M, Guerci B, Anduze Y, Guillaume E, Ritz P. High glycemic variability assessed by continuous glucose monitoring after surgical treatment of obesity by gastric bypass. Diabetes Technol Ther. 2011;13:625–30. https://doi.org/10.1089/dia.2010.0203.
16. Kefurt R, Langer FB, Schindler K, Shakeri-Leidenmuhler S, Ludvik B, Prager G. Hypoglycemia after Roux-en-Y gastric bypass: detection rates of continuous glucose monitoring (CGM) versus mixed meal test. Surg Obes Relat Dis. 2015;11:564–9. https://doi.org/10.1016/j.soard.2014.11.003.
17. Abrahamsson N, Eden Engstrom B, Sundbom M, Karlsson FA. Hypoglycemia in everyday life after gastric bypass and duodenal switch. Eur J Endocrinol. 2015;173:91–100. https://doi.org/10.1530/EJE-14-0821.
18. Marfella R, Barbieri M, Ruggiero R, Rizzo MR, Grella R, Mozzillo AL, Docimo L, Paolisso G. Bariatric surgery reduces oxidative stress by blunting 24-h acute glucose fluctuations in type 2 diabetic

obese patients. Diabetes Care. 2010;33:287–9. https://doi.org/10.2337/dc09-1343.
19. Chinese Diabetes Society. Standards of care for type 2 diabetes in China (2013). Chin J Endocrinol Metab. 2014;30:893–942. https://doi.org/10.3760/cma.j.issn.1000-6699.2014.10.020.
20. Zhou J, Li H, Ran X, Yang W, Li Q, Peng Y, Li Y, Gao X, Luan X, Wang W, Jia W. Reference values for continuous glucose monitoring in Chinese subjects. Diabetes Care. 2009;32:1188–93. https://doi.org/10.2337/dc09-0076.
21. Yu H, Zhou J, Bao Y, Pin Z, Lu W, Jia W. "Dual-remission" after Roux-en-Y gastric bypass surgery: glycemic variability cannot always be improved in Chinese obese patients with type 2 diabetes. Surg Obes Relat Dis. 2016;12:1312–9. https://doi.org/10.1016/j.soard.2015.10.076.
22. Stearns AT, Balakrishnan A, Tavakkolizadeh A. Impact of Roux-en-Y gastric bypass surgery on rat intestinal glucose transport. Am J Physiol Gastrointest Liver Physiol. 2009;297:G950–7. https://doi.org/10.1152/ajpgi.00253.2009.
23. Leturque A, Brot-Laroche E, Le Gall M. GLUT2 mutations, translocation, and receptor function in diet sugar managing. Am J Physiol Endocrinol Metab. 2009;296:E985–92. https://doi.org/10.1152/ajpendo.00004.2009.
24. Roslin MS, Oren JH, Polan BN, Damani T, Brauner R, Shah PC. Abnormal glucose tolerance testing after gastric bypass. Surg Obes Relat Dis. 2013;9:26–31. https://doi.org/10.1016/j.soard.2011.11.023.
25. Tramunt B, Vaurs C, Lijeron J, Guillaume E, Ritz P, Diméglio C, Hanaire H. Impact of carbohydrate content and glycemic load on postprandial glucose after Roux-en-Y gastric bypass. Obes Surg. 2016;26:1487–92. https://doi.org/10.1007/s11695-015-1930-1.
26. Ritz P, Vaurs C, Bertrand M, Anduze Y, Guillaume E, Hanaire H. Usefulness of acarbose and dietary modifications to limit glycemic variability following Roux-en-Y gastric bypass as assessed by continuous glucose monitoring. Diabetes Technol Ther. 2012;14:736–40. https://doi.org/10.1089/dia.2011.0302.

20 Perspectives on Continuous Glucose Monitoring Technology

F. Gao and W. Jia

Blood glucose monitoring is an important part of diabetes management. Continuous glucose monitoring (CGM) can offer a panoramic view of glucose changes for both physicians and patients, providing a fully comprehensive basis for glycemic control. This technology is constantly improving, and it is expected to play an increasingly important role in diabetes management.

20.1 Real-Time CGM Technology

Compared with traditional self-monitoring of blood glucose (SMBG), CGM technology can better reflect the blood glucose levels of patients and detect asymptomatic hypoglycemia in a timely manner, thus improving the safety of hypoglycemic therapy. However, for retrospective CGM, the glycemic data cannot be downloaded instantly and clinicians can only retrospectively analyze until the end of the monitoring. Therefore, retrospective CGM is unable to give a timely alert for hyperglycemic or hypoglycemic events during the monitoring. The real-time CGM technology is designed with the aim of overcoming the shortcomings of retrospective CGM. As the name suggests, "real-time" means that patients and clinicians can easily obtain glucose readings at any time, including glucose concentration at a specific time point or the trend of glucose fluctuations. The device can be programmed to sound an alarm for readings above or below a glucose threshold. Moreover, the real-time CGM glucose data can be downloaded, retrospectively reviewed, and analyzed whenever necessary. Thus, the real-time CGM allows physicians to correct drastic glucose fluctuations as well as hyperglycemia and hypoglycemia in a timely manner and improves patients' adherence as well.

At present, the real-time CGM technology has been applied to clinical practice in China. It has been reported that the utilization of real-time CGM facilitates achievement of better glycemic control in diabetes management. Also, the decrease in glycated hemoglobin A_{1c} (HbA_{1c}) is positively correlated with the frequency of CGM usage; that is, patients who regularly use CGM devices are more likely to achieve better glycemic control. However, CGM operators are required to have good self-awareness and self-management skills of glycemic control, possessing a certain ability to utilize the real-time CGM system and interpret readings, and to manage warnings of hyperglycemia and hypoglycemia.

F. Gao · W. Jia (✉)
Department of Endocrinology and Metabolism, Shanghai Clinical Center for Diabetes, Shanghai Diabetes Institute, Shanghai Jiao Tong University Affiliated Sixth People's Hospital, Shanghai, China
e-mail: wpjia@sjtu.edu.cn

W. Jia (ed.), *Continuous Glucose Monitoring*, https://doi.org/10.1007/978-981-10-7074-7_20

20.2 Artificial Pancreas

The artificial pancreas is a system of devices that closely mimics the secretion of various hormones by human pancreas through a computer-controlled algorithm connecting the CGM and an insulin infusion pump, in order to achieve intelligent glycemic control. This intelligent control system is also known as a "closed-loop" system.

20.2.1 Low-Glucose Suspend (LGS) System

At present, the US Food and Drug Administration (FDA) has approved the use of an insulin pump system with a preliminary feedback system based on CGM data; that is, the real-time CGM system automatically suspends basal insulin delivery for up to 2 h in response to sensor-detected hypoglycemia in the absence of manual intervention [1].

The system developer has conducted a randomized, controlled, multicenter, open-label trial, namely the Automation to Simulate Pancreatic Insulin Response (ASPIRE) In-Home study. The study was conducted in 19 centers in the USA, with the primary efficacy endpoint being the area under the curve (AUC) for nocturnal hypoglycemic events, and the primary safety endpoint being the change in the HbA_{1c} [2]. The findings were published in the *New England Journal of Medicine (NEJM)* in 2013. The study included a 6-week pre-study phase (including repeated 2-week Run-In phase) to establish eligibility for the 3-month study phase. Patients were eligible for randomization if they had at least two nocturnal hypoglycemic events during the Run-In phase. A nocturnal hypoglycemic event was defined as sensor glucose measurements ≤3.6 mmol/L between 10:00 p.m. and 08:00 a.m. for more than 20 consecutive minutes in the absence of an insulin pump interaction. The study included a total of 247 eligible patients with type 1 diabetes mellitus, aged 16–70 years, randomly assigned to receive insulin-pump therapy featured with the threshold-suspend (threshold-suspend group, $n = 121$) or control group ($n = 126$). Compared with the controls, the severity and duration of hypoglycemic events were significantly reduced in the threshold-suspend group: the mean AUC for nocturnal hypoglycemic events in the threshold-suspend group was 37.5% less than that of the control group; the rate of nocturnal hypoglycemic events was reduced by 31.8%; and the percentage of nocturnal time spent with glucose <3.9 mmol/L was reduced by 40.0%. This study indicated that the use of insulin pump therapy featured with the threshold-suspend reduced hypoglycemia, without increasing HbA_{1c} values. In the same year, another randomized, controlled study was conducted to assess the efficacy of the sensor-augmented pump with automated insulin suspension with regard to the incidence of severe and moderate hypoglycemic events, and this study was published in the *Journal of the American Medical Association (JAMA)* [3]. The patients had experienced at least one moderate or severe hypoglycemic event per day, with short-time (<10 min) and long-time hypoglycemic events each accounting for a half of events. Patients also had 13% of hypoglycemic events lasting up to 2 h, and 80% occurring during the sleeping period. The results showed that there was no difference in HbA_{1c} between the low-glucose suspension group and the control group. The adjusted incidence rate per 100 patient-months was 34.2 for the control group versus 9.5 for the low-glucose suspension group. The incidence rate ratio was 3.6, indicating that sensor-augmented pump therapy with automated insulin suspension reduced the incidence rate of moderate and severe hypoglycemia in patients with type 1 diabetes.

20.2.2 Predictive Low-Glucose Suspend (PLGS) System

If the prevention of hypoglycemia by using a LGS function is like "nipping it in the bud," an analogy for the PLGS system is "no chance of budding" for hypoglycemia. Currently, the PLGS is based on real-time CGM, and is able to predict the occurrence of hypoglycemic events through a computer-controlled algorithm and will give an alarm or automatically suspend basal insulin delivery [4]. The system has the following characteristics: (1) the suspend threshold can be set between 2.8–5.0 mmol/L with a default of 5.0 mmol/L; (2) a maximum of 8 different low glycemic thresholds can be set for a 24-h period; (3) if the device predicts that hypoglycemia will occur within 30 min, it will give alarm; if the suspend threshold is set at 2.8 mmol/L, it will automatically suspend basal insulin delivery for at least 30 min, unless manually altered; if no response to the alarm is detected within 10 min, the warnings will be upgraded; (4) the insulin infusion will resume automatically after 2-h suspension or manually at any time. In addition, basal insulin will resume automatically if the glucose value is at least 1.1 mmol/L above the preset low limit and is predicted to be at least 2.2 mmol/L above the preset low limit 30 min later; and (5) The basal insulin cannot be re-suspended within 30 min after the last suspension, and the bolus function is disabled during the suspension period.

In the Predictive Low-Glucose Management in Real-time Sensing Insulin Pump Therapy (PILGRIM) Study, the investigators tested the clinical feasibility, safety, and efficacy of predictive automatic suspension of insulin delivery and its predictive capacity of exercise-induced hypoglycemia through a computer simulation test among youth patients with type 1 diabetes who were on continuous subcutaneous insulin infusion (CSII) [4]. The patients exercised until the occurrence of LGS or PLGS. The results showed that 73% of participants experienced hypoglycemic events after exercise. PLGS prevented 80% of hypoglycemic episodes, and the mean sensor glucose reading at predictive suspension was 5.1 ± 0.4 mmol/L, resulting in a post-suspension nadir of 4.3 ± 1.2 mmol/L. The suspension lasted for 90 ± 35 min, resulting in a sensor glucose level at insulin resumption of 5.4 ± 1.1 mmol/L. PLGS reduced hypoglycemic events (defined as glucose measurement <3.9 mmol/L) by 26.7% compared with no insulin suspension. LGS reduced hypoglycemic events by 5.3% compared with no insulin suspension. The duration of hypoglycemia with PLGS (58 min) was significantly less than with LGS (101 min). Real-time CGM-based predictive insulin adjustment is feasible and represents an important step in the development of an "artificial pancreas."

Moreover, there are two recent studies added to the evidence base about the effectiveness of predictive hypoglycemia management. Battelino et al. [5] found that the predictive low glucose management system with insulin suspension was associated with a significantly reduced number of hypoglycemic events. Although this was achieved at the expense of increased time in moderate hyperglycemia, there were no serious adverse effects in young patients with type 1 diabetes. Another research conducted by Biester et al. [6] came up with the conclusion that SmartGuard technology can significantly reduce the risk for hypoglycemia in pediatric type 1 diabetes patients without increasing HbA_{1c}.

20.2.3 Artificial Pancreas

Preventing hypoglycemia while achieving target glycemic control is the principal treatment goal of diabetes management pursued by both physicians and diabetes patients. The use of an "artificial pancreas" undoubtedly represents a pivotal step toward achieving this goal. In 2010, the *Lancet* published a phase II randomized crossover trial of a manual closed-loop insulin delivery system [7]. This trial included 19 type 1 diabetic children and adolescents who aged 5–18 years with duration of diabetes 6.4 years. The patients were randomly assigned to receive standard CSII or one-night closed-loop delivery in the hospital. A comparison was made in the percentage of time (PT) spent with normal glycemia (3.9–8.0 mmol/L) and the PT spent with nocturnal hypoglycemia (defined as plasma glucose ≤3.9 mmol/L, PT3.9) between the two groups. The results showed that closed-loop system could improve the glucose levels (PT4.0–8.0 was 60% vs. 40%) and reduce the risk of nocturnal hypoglycemia (PT3.9 was 2.1% vs. 4.1%). Subsequently, in 2013 *Diabetes Care* published an open-label, randomized controlled crossover study of closed-loop basal insulin delivery [8]. The study included 12 adolescents with type 1 diabetes with a mean age of 15 years old and HbA_{1c} of 7.9% (63 mmol/mol). The patients were randomly assigned to receive either closed-loop basal insulin delivery or conventional pump therapy for 36 h. The results showed that compared with standard pump therapy, closed-loop basal insulin delivery increased the PT spent with glucose in the target range (84% vs. 49%) and reduced the mean plasma glucose (MBG) levels (7.1 mmol/L vs. 9.2 mmol/L). Ten episodes of hypoglycemia occurred in patients with standard pump therapy, and 9 episodes occurred in patients with closed-loop delivery.

To confirm the findings from single-center experiences, multicenter trials were conducted by investigators. In 2013, *NEJM* published a multicenter, randomized, crossover trial, which was conducted to assess the safety and efficacy of an artificial pancreas system for control of nocturnal glucose levels [9]. The results showed that compared with control treatments, the artificial pancreas system resulted in improved glucose levels (7.0 mmol/L vs. 7.8 mmol/L) and fewer nocturnal hypoglycemia (7 episodes vs. 22 episodes). Thus, glucose levels were significantly more stable over nighttime with the artificial pancreas as compared with control treatments. Similar findings were observed in another crossover study using an overnight closed-loop insulin delivery system in 16 young subjects with type 1 diabetes, which was published in *Diabetes Care* in 2014 [10]. Recently, pivotal studies based on MiniMed 670G system also confirmed the safety and effectiveness of the hybrid closed-loop (HCL) system [11, 12].

It is worth mentioning that *NEJM* published the results of a study using an artificial pancreas for glycemic control during pregnancy in women with type 1 diabetes in August 2016 [13]. In this open-label, randomized, crossover study, 16 pregnant women with type 1 diabetes were enrolled to compare the efficacy of an artificial pancreas versus sensor-augmented pump therapy (control) in type 1 diabetes. During the first study phase, the patients were randomly assigned to receive closed-loop pump therapy (intervention) or sensor-augmented pump therapy (control) for 4 weeks. The results showed that the PT spent with overnight glucose levels within the target range (3.5–7.8 mmol/L) was higher in patients who received closed-loop therapy than in controls (74.7% vs. 59.5%), and the overnight MBG level was lower during closed-loop therapy than during control therapy (6.6 mmol/L vs. 7.4 mmol/L). There were no significant differences between closed-loop and control therapy in the PT in which glucose levels were below the target range, in insulin doses, or in the occurrence of adverse events. During the continuation study phase, 14 of the participants used the closed-loop system from antenatal hospitalization until delivery. The results showed that 68.7% of the time was spent with glucose levels within the target range, and the MBG level was 7.0 mmol/L. No episodes of severe hypoglycemia occurred during the entire study phase. Thus, the closed-loop system is able to achieve good glycemic control in pregnant women with type 1 diabetes.

20.2.4 Dual-Hormone Artificial Pancreas

Although the closed-loop artificial pancreas can significantly reduce the occurrence of hypoglycemia while achieving target glycemic control through the day, it cannot completely avoid the occurrence of hypoglycemia. Another effective measure is to inject a certain amount of glucagon in a timely manner at the onset of hypoglycemia unawareness, especially for hypoglycemia during sleep. In addition to islet β-cells that secrete insulin, the human pancreas contains another major cell type, the glucagon-secreting α cells. If an artificial pancreas is capable of simultaneously simulating the functions of both types of cells, it will reproduce a more accurate physiological state that is closely similar to the well-functioning endocrine pancreas, providing further benefits for diabetes patients.

However, practice often fails to keep pace with the theory. In 2015, the *Lancet Diabetes & Endocrinology* published an open-label, randomized, controlled, crossover trial that failed to verify the superiority of the dual-hormone artificial pancreas over the single-hormone artificial pancreas [14]. The study enrolled 56 patients with type 1 diabetes who were randomly assigned to receiving a dual-hormone artificial pancreas, a single-hormone artificial pancreas, or conventional insulin pump therapy. The primary endpoint was the PT spent with glucose in the target range (4.0–8.0 mmol/L, or 2-h postprandial glucose 4.0–10.0 mmol/L) and the occurrence of hypoglycemic events (defined as plasma glucose concentration <3.3 mmol/L with hypoglycemic symptoms or less than <3.0 mmol/L irrespective of symptoms). The results showed that the single-hormone and dual-hormone artificial pancreas systems both provided better glycemic control than conventional insulin pump therapy did. Similarly, both the single- and dual-hormone artificial pancreases could reduce the risk of hypoglycemic events. However, there was no difference in glycemic improvement as well as prevention of hypoglycemic events between the single- and dual-hormone artificial pancreas systems. A study based on pre-adolescent children (aged 6–11 years) with type 1 diabetes (diagnosed for ≥1 year) who were on insulin pump therapy found that bionic pancreas can help to improve the mean glycemia and to reduce hypoglycemia [15]. Besides, same results were found in another study on adults and adolescents [16].

The study on dual-hormone artificial pancreas systems is still in its infancy. Only few studies have been conducted on this topic, with relatively small sample size and immature equipment that needs to be further improved. More importantly, glucagon preparations used in insulin pumps must achieve certain quality traits with high stability as well as good pharmacokinetics and pharmacodynamics. However, the existing glucagon is not yet sufficient to meet this requirement. Moreover, the addition of glucagon to a dual-hormone artificial pancreas system will slightly increase production cost and may cause the following risks: increased insulin dose, masking incorrect algorithms of insulin delivery, nausea and other discomforts, consumption of hepatic glycogen, and glucagon resistance. In addition, the long-term safety with glucagon has not been established. Finally, while having a second hormone like glucagon as a "rescue" hormone would permit setting the glucose target lower than in insulin-only closed-loop systems, it may thereby introduce additional risks of severe hypoglycemia in the case of an occlusion of the glucagon infusion set. Therefore, whether the dual-hormone artificial pancreas is really superior to the single-hormone artificial pancreas is still unknown. Also, whether the addition of glucagon is "superfluous" still needs more evidence to confirm.

20.2.5 Intelligent Algorithms of the Artificial Pancreas

The artificial pancreas consists of a real-time CGM system, an insulin continuous infusion system, and an intelligent reactive control system with algorithm function. The control system acts like a brain, receiving signals from the CGM system, calculating and processing, and finally providing feedback information to the insulin continuous infusion system to control the blood glucose levels. The ideal control system should be automatic, flexible, sensitive, and capable of developing personalized insulin infusion regimens in a timely manner based on a specific situation (e.g., changes in the amount of exercise, consumption of snacks, etc.). The infusion dose of insulin is related to individual islet function, insulin sensitivity, composition and amount of food intake, food digestion and absorption, and the amount of exercise. To this end, the control system is required to have complex data processing function and precise calculation capacity. However, the current algorithms cannot meet these requirements. The traditional algorithms include the proportional integral derivative (PID) algorithm, model predictive control (MPC) algorithm, and fuzzy logic (FL) algorithm [17]. The PID algorithm estimates the required delivery of insulin based on a weighted sum of PID terms, in order to achieve the desired glucose concentration. However, this algorithm cannot meet the requirements of an artificial pancreas and easily leads to postprandial hypoglycemia [17, 18]. The MPC algorithm requires a model that can predict future glucose concentrations given known values for current glucose, insulin delivery, and food intake. Such an algorithm then calculates the appropriate insulin infusion rate by minimizing the difference between the model-predicted glucose concentration and the target glucose concentrations over a prediction time-window.

This algorithm has main shortcomings. The established model and all calculations in MPC are based on the assumption. Imperfections in the model lead to differences between the expectation and reality, and this means that each calculation step must be recalibrated. More importantly, it is unable to accurately evaluate the uncertainty of the model. In addition, conventional MPC operates on a purely dynamical systems description model, and external disruptions to the system due to, for instance, meal intake or physical activity cannot be timely captured by the model [17, 18]. Fuzzy logic algorithms should be developed with professionals since it is based on the model of a set of binary conditions instead of a clear test model of patient metabolism. Considering the algorithm cannot readily incorporate knowledge from existing biological models, there is no theoretical support and a lack of performance guarantees [17, 18].

In order to meet the complex requirements of an artificial pancreas, the "learning algorithms" seem to be a good choice [17]. Appropriate learning algorithms are able to analyze training data, recognize complex patterns, and on the basis of such patterns apply the knowledge to other data to predict their behaviors. The major difference between traditional algorithms and learning algorithms is that the latter are based on recognition of patterns instead of hypotheses, which improves the accuracy of the system. A second advantage of learning algorithms is that they consider interactions between variables instead of minimizing or maximizing them. This might result in more complex models, but justify their use for diabetes treatment. However, the learning algorithms pose the risk of developing a model that can perform perfectly on the training data but then be unable to be generalized for unseen data, which is called over-fitting. It is therefore required to correct for over-fitting by using cross-validation and regularization techniques. The first attempt applying learning algorithms into diabetes care was the use of an artificial neural network (ANN) [18]. ANN algorithms involve a calculation minimizing the errors between calculated parameters and desired parameters based on supervised training data. However, the supervised learning process needs to be performed by an expert, which is time-consuming and prone to human error. The existing evidence has shown that ANN algorithms work well in short-term prediction of blood glucose concentrations and insulin regimen recommendations. However, there is lack of reliable evidence regarding long-term prediction of blood glucose concentrations with ANN algorithms. Furthermore, glucose pattern in diabetes keeps changing. Supervised learning algorithms cannot adapt to this change, but reinforcement learning algorithms can. Such algorithms can be used on sequences of decisions along a timeline. Additionally, they can be used in decision-making progress based on current observations [17]. This is true for the artificial pancreas system, as there is a need to continuously observe glucose concentrations and determine the ideal time and amount for insulin delivery. Moreover, reinforcement learning algorithms can be applied directly using real data, or they can interact with a dynamic system represented by a mathematical model, making very modest assumptions about this system. Thus, reinforcement learning algorithms may provide a very promising approach for maintaining euglycemia as artificial pancreas system in a flexible and independent manner. Even with the most advanced algorithms, the ultimate limiting factor at this time is the current insulin pharmacodynamics and pharmacokinetics of insulin injected into the subcutaneous tissue. Either fasting-acting insulins with shorter half-lives or alternative insulin delivery sites (intra-peritoneal or intravenous) will mostly likely be necessary to achieve a fully automatic and flexible system.

20.3 Shortcomings of CGM and Prospective

Since 1999 when the US FDA approved the first CGM device, this technology has been constantly updated and improved. However, there are still shortcomings, which include the following aspects:

1. The accuracy has yet to be further improved. There is a gap between the interstitial fluid glucose level and venous glucose level, irre-

spective of the amplitude of glycemic variability [19]. Moreover, studies have shown that the accuracy and sensitivity of CGM probes decrease over time [20]. Thus, the probe should be frequently replaced with a new one during long-term use, which causes inconvenience to patients and decreased adherence. Therefore, determining how to improve the accuracy and sensitivity of CGM and to prolong the duration of probe use are common problems faced by investigators in the design of a new type of CGM in the future. What's worth looking forward to is the fact that some medical device companies are now working on a long-term CGM device, and phase II clinical trials have shown its excellent accuracy. This kind of CGM device will soon be available to patients.

2. Invasiveness. Even a tiny trauma can cause varying degrees of pain and discomfort and a possibility of infection, which appears to be a barrier to good adherence as well as promotion and popularization of a CGM device. In addition, the probe puncture site will gather a certain amount of erythrocytes, platelets, thrombin, and cell debris, which will affect the effectiveness of the probe [21, 22]. Thus, noninvasive CGM technology that is easy to wear and convenient to use is undoubtedly an emerging trend in research strategies.
3. CGM calibration. The existing CGM measurements need to be calibrated with blood glucose values, which not only brings inconvenience to the operators, but also affects the accuracy of monitoring. The finger-tip blood glucose value is first calibrated using the laboratory reference value, while the CGM glucose sensor needs calibration against the finger-tip blood glucose values, which makes CGM measurements different from the laboratory reference. Therefore, future improvement in calibration algorithms of CGM is required.
4. Physiological delay. The CGM sensor glucose physiologically lags 5–15 min behind actual changes in blood glucose [23]. Therefore, it is often necessary to re-measure the blood glucose level again before interventions for high/low glucose measurements detected by real-time CGM sensors. The future CGM technology should narrow the time lag between the change in actual glucose levels and their measurements, thereby further increasing the sensitivity of detection and improving the accuracy, flexibility, and sensitivity of the artificial pancreas as well.
5. Intelligent platform and telemedicine. Today, intelligent platforms are used everywhere. In the near future, medical personnel can interact with patients by remotely monitoring the glycemic control of patients with a CGM system and an artificial pancreas through information technology, e.g., smart phones, personal computers or other equipment, and provide timely feedback to diabetes patients. Thus, intelligent platforms bring great convenience to both physicians and patients in diabetes management.

20.4 Summary

A number of large clinical studies have shown that CGM plays an important role in glycemic control. CGM is going to become even more ideal with the introduction of new technologies. The combined use of a real-time CGM system, an insulin continuous infusion system, and an intelligent control system enables us to obtain a prototype of an artificial pancreas, which undoubtedly can benefit every diabetes patient, especially those with brittle diabetes. This technology not only facilitates the achievement of target glycemic control and delays the progression of chronic complications of diabetes, but also improves the quality of life of patients, releasing patients from the shackles of disease and allowing them to realize their dream of enjoying a better life.

References

1. Agrawal P, Welsh JB, Kannard B, Askari S, Yang Q, Kaufman FR. Usage and effectiveness of the low glucose suspend feature of the Medtronic Paradigm Veo insulin pump. J Diabetes Sci Technol. 2011;5:1137–41. https://doi.org/10.1177/193229681100500514.

2. Bergenstal RM, Klonoff DC, Garg SK, Bode BW, Meredith M, Slover RH, Ahmann AJ, Welsh JB, Lee SW, Kaufman FR, ASPIRE In-Home Study Group. Threshold-based insulin-pump interruption for reduction of hypoglycemia. N Engl J Med. 2013;369:224–32. https://doi.org/10.1056/NEJMoa1303576.
3. Ly TT, Nicholas JA, Retterath A, Lim EM, Davis EA, Jones TW. Effect of sensor-augmented insulin pump therapy and automated insulin suspension vs standard insulin pump therapy on hypoglycemia in patients with type 1 diabetes: a randomized clinical trial. JAMA. 2013;310:1240–7. https://doi.org/10.1001/jama.2013.277818.
4. Danne T, Tsioli C, Kordonouri O, Blaesig S, Remus K, Roy A, Keenan B, Lee SW, Kaufman FR. The PILGRIM study: in silico modeling of a predictive low glucose management system and feasibility in youth with type 1 diabetes during exercise. Diabetes Technol Ther. 2014;16:338–47. https://doi.org/10.1089/dia.2013.0327.
5. Battelino T, Nimri R, Dovc K, Phillip M, Bratina N. Prevention of hypoglycemia with predictive low glucose insulin suspension in children with type 1 diabetes: a randomized controlled trial. Diabetes Care. 2017;40:764–70. https://doi.org/10.2337/dc16-2584.
6. Biester T, Kordonouri O, Holder M, Remus K, Kieninger-Baum D, Wadien T, Danne T. "Let the algorithm do the work": reduction of hypoglycemia using sensor-augmented pump therapy with predictive insulin suspension (smartguard) in pediatric type 1 diabetes patients. Diabetes Technol Ther. 2017;19:173–82. https://doi.org/10.1089/dia.2016.0349.
7. Hovorka R, Allen JM, Elleri D, Chassin LJ, Harris J, Xing D, Kollman C, Hovorka T, Larsen AM, Nodale M, De Palma A, Wilinska ME, Acerini CL, Dunger DB. Manual closed-loop insulin delivery in children and adolescents with type 1 diabetes: a phase 2 randomised crossover trial. Lancet. 2010;375:743–51. https://doi.org/10.1016/S0140-6736(09)61998-X.
8. Elleri D, Allen JM, Kumareswaran K, Leelarathna L, Nodale M, Caldwell K, Cheng P, Kollman C, Haidar A, Murphy HR, Wilinska ME, Acerini CL, Dunger DB, Hovorka R. Closed-loop basal insulin delivery over 36 hours in adolescents with type 1 diabetes: randomized clinical trial. Diabetes Care. 2013;36:838–44. https://doi.org/10.2337/dc12-0816.
9. Phillip M, Battelino T, Atlas E, Kordonouri O, Bratina N, Miller S, Biester T, Stefanija MA, Muller I, Nimri R, Danne T. Nocturnal glucose control with an artificial pancreas at a diabetes camp. N Engl J Med. 2013;368:824–83. https://doi.org/10.1056/NEJMoa1206881.
10. Hovorka R, Elleri D, Thabit H, Allen JM, Leelarathna L, El-Khairi R, Kumareswaran K, Caldwell K, Calhoun P, Kollman C, Murphy HR, Acerini CL, Wilinska ME, Nodale M, Dunger DB. Overnight closed-loop insulin delivery in young people with type 1 diabetes: a free-living, randomized clinical trial. Diabetes Care. 2014;37:1204–11. https://doi.org/10.2337/dc13-2644.
11. Bergenstal RM, Garg S, Weinzimer SA, Buckingham BA, Bode BW, Tamborlane WV, Kaufman FR. Safety of a hybrid closed-loop insulin delivery system in patients with type 1 diabetes. JAMA. 2016;316:1407–8. https://doi.org/10.1001/jama.2016.11708.
12. Garg SK, Weinzimer SA, Tamborlane WV, Buckingham BA, Bode BW, Bailey TS, Brazg RL, Ilany J, Slover RH, Anderson SM, Bergenstal RM, Grosman B, Roy A, Cordero TL, Shin J, Lee SW, Kaufman FR. Glucose outcomes with the in-home use of a hybrid closed-loop insulin delivery system in adolescents and adults with type 1 diabetes. Diabetes Technol Ther. 2017;19:155–63. https://doi.org/10.1089/dia.2016.0421.
13. Stewart ZA, Wilinska ME, Hartnell S, Temple RC, Rayman G, Stanley KP, Simmons D, Law GR, Scott EM, Hovorka R, Murphy HR. Closed-loop insulin delivery during pregnancy in women with type 1 diabetes. N Engl J Med. 2016;375:644–54. https://doi.org/10.1056/NEJMoa1602494.
14. Haidar A, Legault L, Messier V, Mitre TM, Leroux C, Rabasa-Lhoret R. Comparison of dual-hormone artificial pancreas, single-hormone artificial pancreas, and conventional insulin pump therapy for glycaemic control in patients with type 1 diabetes: an open-label randomised controlled crossover trial. Lancet Diabetes Endocrinol. 2015;3:17–26. https://doi.org/10.1016/S2213-8587(14)70226-8.
15. Russell SJ, Hillard MA, Balliro C, Magyar KL, Selagamsetty R, Sinha M, Grennan K, Mondesir D, Ehklaspour L, Zheng H, Damiano ER, El-Khatib FH. Day and night glycaemic control with a bionic pancreas versus conventional insulin pump therapy in preadolescent children with type 1 diabetes: a randomised crossover trial. Lancet Diabetes Endocrinol. 2016;4:233–43. https://doi.org/10.1016/S2213-8587(15)00489-1.
16. Russell SJ, El-Khatib FH, Sinha M, Magyar KL, McKeon K, Goergen LG, Balliro C, Hillard MA, Nathan DM, Damiano ER. Outpatient glycemic control with a bionic pancreas in type 1 diabetes. N Engl J Med. 2014;371:313–25. https://doi.org/10.1056/NEJMoa1314474.
17. Bothe MK, Dickens L, Reichel K, Tellmann A, Ellger B, Westphal M, Faisal AA. The use of reinforcement learning algorithms to meet the challenges of an artificial pancreas. Expert Rev Med Devices. 2013;10:661–73. https://doi.org/10.1586/17434440.2013.827515.
18. Bequette BW. A critical assessment of algorithms and challenges in the development of a closed-loop artificial pancreas. Diabetes Technol Ther. 2005;7:28–47. https://doi.org/10.1089/dia.2005.7.28.
19. Ginsberg BH. The FDA panel advises approval of the first continuous glucose sensor. Diabetes Technol Ther. 1999;1:203–4. https://doi.org/10.1089/152091599317431.
20. Baek YH, Jin HY, Lee KA, Kang SM, Kim WJ, Kim MG, Park JH, Chae SW, Baek HS, Park TS. The correlation and accuracy of glucose levels between inter-

stitial fluid and venous plasma by continuous glucose monitoring system. Korean Diabetes J. 2010;34:350–8. https://doi.org/10.4093/kdj.2010.34.6.350.
21. Klueh U, Liu Z, Feldman B, Henning TP, Cho B, Ouyang T, Kreutzer D. Metabolic biofouling of glucose sensors in vivo: role of tissue microhemorrhages. J Diabetes Sci Technol. 2011;5:583–95. https://doi.org/10.1177/193229681100500313.
22. Kenneth Ward W. A review of the foreign-body response to subcutaneously-implanted devices: the role of macrophages and cytokines in biofouling and fibrosis. J Diabetes Sci Technol. 2008;2:768–77. https://doi.org/10.1177/193229680800200504.
23. Wentholt IM, Vollebregt MA, Hart AA, Hoekstra JB, DeVries JH. Comparison of a needle-type and a microdialysis continuous glucose monitor in type 1 diabetic patients. Diabetes Care. 2005;28:2871–6.

MIX
Papier aus verantwortungsvollen Quellen
Paper from responsible sources
FSC® C105338

If you have any concerns about our products,
you can contact us on
ProductSafety@springernature.com

In case Publisher is established outside the EU,
the EU authorized representative is:
Springer Nature Customer Service Center GmbH
Europaplatz 3, 69115 Heidelberg, Germany

Printed by Libri Plureos GmbH
in Hamburg, Germany